# DRUG DEVELOPMENT
# AND MARKETING

# DRUG DEVELOPMENT AND MARKETING

A conference sponsored by the
Center for Health Policy Research of
the American Enterprise Institute

*Edited by Robert B. Helms*

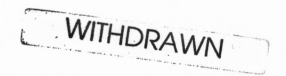
The American Enterprise Institute for Public Policy Research
Washington, D. C.

381.4561
~~D~~

ISBN 0-8447-2062-3 (Paper)
ISBN 0-8447-2063-1 (Cloth)

Library of Congress Catalog Card Number L.C. 75-4389

*Printed in the United States of America*

To

Robert D. Dripps, M.D.

who contributed so richly to the study of the impact of public policy on the discovery, development, and application of drugs and who encouraged the type of discussion among physicians, businessmen, policy makers, and economists that is exhibited in these proceedings.

Irvine H. Page, M.D

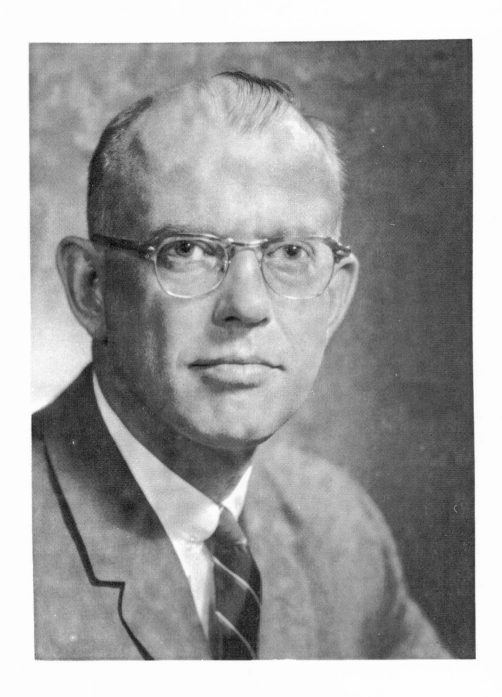

Robert D. Dripps, M.D.

# CONTRIBUTORS

*Robert Ayanian*
Instructor of Business Economics, University of Southern California

*Martin J. Bailey*
Professor of Economics, University of Maryland

*Mitchell B. Balter*
Chief, Special Studies Section,
Psychopharmacological Research Branch, National Institute of Mental Health

*Yale Brozen*
Professor of Business Economics,
Graduate School of Business, University of Chicago

*John P. Bunker*
Visiting Professor of Preventive and Social Medicine,
Harvard Medical School

*Rita Ricardo Campbell*
Senior Fellow,
The Hoover Institution on War, Revolution and Peace

*Harold A. Clymer*
Vice President for Planning and Business Development,
SmithKline Corporation

*Douglas L. Cocks*
Associate Economist, Eli Lilly and Company

*J. Richard Crout*
Director, Bureau of Drugs,
Food and Drug Administration

*J. F. Dunne*
Senior Medical Officer
Secretariat of Committee on Safety of Medicines, United Kingdom

*Aaron J. Gellman*
President, Gellman Research Associates

*Leon I. Goldberg*
Chairman, Committee on Clinical Pharmacology, Department of Pharmacological
and Physiological Sciences, University of Chicago

*Bernard A. Kemp*
Professorial Lecturer, Department of Clinical Engineering,
George Washington University Medical Center

*Edmund W. Kitch*
Professor of Law, University of Chicago Law School

*Louis Lasagna*
Professor of Pharmacology and Toxicology,
School of Medicine and Dentistry, University of Rochester

*Stanley Lebergott*
Chester D. Hubbard Professor of Economics, Wesleyan University

*Alex R. Maurizi*
Economist, Federal Energy Administration

*Kenneth L. Melmon*
Professor of Medicine and Pharmacology,
San Francisco Medical Center, University of California

*John A. Oates*
Professor of Medicine and Pharmacology,
School of Medicine, Vanderbilt University

*Irvine H. Page*
Editor, *Modern Medicine,* and Chairman, Advisory
Committee, Center for Health Policy Research

*Sam Peltzman*
Professor of Business Economics,
Graduate School of Business, University of Chicago

*Barr Rosenberg*
Assistant Professor of Business Economics,
School of Business Administration, University of California, Berkeley

*Frederic M. Scherer*
Director, Bureau of Economics, Federal Trade Commission

*David Schwartzman*
Professor of Economics, New School for Social Research

*Lewis B. Sheiner*
Assistant Professor of Medicine, Clinical Pathology, and Laboratory Medicine,
San Francisco Medical Center, University of California

*Thomas F. Stauffer*
Lecturer in Economics and Research Associate
Center for Middle Eastern Studies, Harvard University

*Robert B. Stobaugh*
Professor of Business Administration, Harvard Business School

*Lester G. Telser*
Professor of Economics, University of Chicago

*William M. Wardell*
Assistant Professor of Pharmacology and Toxicology, and of Medicine,
School of Medicine and Dentistry, University of Rochester

*Murray L. Weidenbaum*
Director, Center for the Study of American Business
Washington University

# CONTENTS

## PART THREE
### External Determinants of
### Drug Innovation

## PART FOUR
## Factors Affecting Drug
## Industry Structure and Costs

# PREFACE

In early 1974 the American Enterprise Institute established the Center for Health Policy Research to study some of this country's policy issues relating to health care and drugs. The first major activity of the center was a two-day conference on drug development and marketing held in Washington, D. C., in July 1974. This volume presents the papers and proceedings of that conference.

A common theme of several previous conferences on drugs has been that there is insufficient data upon which to base hard analysis of issues relating to the benefits and risks of drug therapy and the performance of the drug industry. The purpose of this conference was to present for public debate a number of pieces of research containing new data that might contribute to a better understanding of some of the major policy issues. Experts from a wide range of disciplines and backgrounds were assembled to present papers and provide critical commentary. Also attending were approximately seventy-five public officials, scholars, and businessmen who had a particular interest in the availability and development of drugs.

The conference was in a way my own introduction to the drug industry and the controversy surrounding it. As one who believes that economics can contribute to the analysis of public policy issues, I was not surprised to find that the conference offered some interesting lessons in economics that should prove useful to both the policy analyst and the student of economics interested in applications of economic theory. It is hoped that a few brief remarks about some of these economic applications will introduce the reader to the subject matter of the proceedings.

A common criticism of drug companies is that advertising and promotional activity is in general wasteful and results in higher drug prices because it supposedly pushes up costs and enhances the monopoly power of the companies. Several of the conference papers dealing with various aspects of drug promotion tell a quite different story. We do not have to look to the monopoly motive to explain drug advertising.

While Sam Peltzman's paper does not consider the form of drug promotion, the evidence he presents that the immediate therapeutic benefits of rapid diffusion of information about new drugs helps explain the market demand for advertising services and hence the existence of this market activity. In addition to the obvious benefits of reduced illness and longer life, advertising can be said to build up "brand-name capital," the economists' term for the consumer's knowledge of the existence, uses, and quality of a manufacturer's product.

The development and use of drugs require the knowledge of complex and continually changing technical information. Information on the quality and efficacy of drugs is, therefore, a valuable complement to the actual drug product. Telser's finding that the promotion of drugs is positively associated with market entry reinforces this interpretation of drug advertising: advertising provides information demanded by drug prescribers and users rather than acting as a means to restrict entry and monopolize the industry. In fact, relatively high advertising expenditures are associated with high rates of innovation. It follows from this analysis that government policies tending to reduce the complementary information provided by advertising and brand names will also reduce the value and usefulness of drugs for treatment.

A second area of interest was the process of competition in the drug industry. Again, a commonly voiced complaint about the industry is that much of its research is unproductive—that it is carried out in order to circumvent a competitor's patent rather than to discover new drugs. The implication is that government-sponsored research would be more productive.

The usual counterargument to this complaint is that competitive research does two things. (1) It produces products that are more effective because of improved composition, assimilation, convenience, or taste. (2) The research often proves to be productive in unforeseen ways: usage sometimes shows that a drug is effective for a medical problem different from the one for which it was originally intended.

The papers by Telser, Cocks, and Kemp defend drug industry research, also, by showing that research is the basis of the competitive process in the drug industry and that the outcome of competition through innovation is new entry into therapeutic drug markets, unstable market shares, and declining drug prices. While patents obviously give some protection to new drugs, several sets of data indicate that patent protection may not provide effective, long-term protection. The main policy implication of these findings is that the industry behaves competitively. The relatively large size of research-intensive drug firms can probably be explained by economics of scale in drug research, manufacturing, or promotion. It is likely, therefore, that government policies (such as requirements for increased proof of efficacy and higher safety standards) raising the cost of research will impair the competition that has traditionally operated within the drug industry. Less competition through research will result in fewer new drugs and higher drug prices.

However, as Dr. Crout of the Food and Drug Administration noted in one of the discussions, the FDA congressional mandate has been to promote more safety and not worry about economic efficiency. Doctors Wardell and Lasagna, drawing upon their experiences with drug treatment, have called for a redefinition of this mandate to put more emphasis on the medical benefits of drugs. The economic evidence about the competitive process in the drug industry reinforces concern about the impact of drug safety legislation. If research costs could be reduced, the effect would be to lower drug prices and encourage the development of new drugs.

In short, it is my view that the proceedings of this conference provide good lessons about how markets work. Much of the criticism of economics derives from the fact that we economists have not effectively demonstrated the uses of economic theory for the analysis of real-world problems. Perhaps this volume will contribute to public awareness and understanding by presenting empirical evidence of the practical applicability of economic theory.

The highlights of the floor discussions contain both criticism of and support for the above interpretation of the conference papers. I have tried to organize and paraphrase the commentary to emphasize what seemed to be the essential points rather than to provide a verbatim account.

I would like to express my gratitude to the various authors and discussants for their cooperation in preparing their contributions for publication.

ROBERT B. HELMS

*Director, Center for Health*
*Policy Research of the*
*American Enterprise Institute*

# PART ONE

## THE CONSUMER'S INTEREST IN PHARMACEUTICALS

# CHAIRMAN'S COMMENT

*Irvine H. Page*

This is an interesting time to discuss drug development and marketing because of the very active role government has come to play in the area.

As I have watched the medical scene for the past half-century, many changes have occurred, not only in the drugs used but also in those who use them. I recall that when I was on the staff of the Rockefeller Hospital in New York, I heard Leonard Colebrook give his first paper in the United States on sulfanilamide. And it was when I was living in Germany, long before there was any hint of penicillin, that I had the privilege of getting to know Howard Florey quite well. At this early time, the physician's drug list was short, and there were few drugs effective against infection. No thought was being given to what were called "chronic degenerative diseases," that is, atherosclerosis and hypertension. Indeed, even though as a student I had Harold Pardee as my teacher of electrocardiography, I learned nothing of myocardial infarction. Heart attacks seemed scarcely to exist in 1924.

Another aspect of that day, in contrast to the present, was the dominance of the clinician. When I began medical research in 1922, laboratory studies were considered largely a waste of time. Not much money was "wasted" on research chiefly because there was little money to waste. There was little thought of government support for drug research, and if government had proposed to enter any domain of medicine except public health, physicians would have been scandalized.

But this atmosphere was not to last. In the course of the next forty years research became dominant. This was the era of the discovery and exploitation of large numbers of valuable drugs—an era in which industry played a critical role, since the majority of the new drugs were discovered not in academia but in industrial laboratories. To a large extent, clinical medicine was placed in limbo and professorships in medicine came to be granted on the basis of research contributions, no matter how trivial!

This emphasis upon research opened the gates to extensive government participation—which, as you are well aware, has steadily grown in importance. Indeed, government has become the major force in medicine and in the rules and regulations of the pharmaceutical industry. It is this concern for the hegemony of government that will lie at the heart of much of the discussion in this symposium.

The trend toward increasing government influence has been accompanied by the appearance of a large number of people who call themselves "health professionals." It is impossible to describe a uniform educational background for them, but generally they are identified with the academic world. From this very articulate, often verbose, group has come a plethora of suggestions, demands, and criticism regarding pharmaceutical development. They have often been joined by interested and activist laymen, such as Benno Schmidt and Mary Lasker.

Now problem solving, whether dealing with the manufacture and sale of drugs, their use by physicians, or their abuse by the public, is very complex. To make headway is not easy, especially when recommendations are being offered by so many obscure sources. It is little wonder that the majority of practicing physicians are thoroughly confused. They have neither the time nor the patience to follow the complexities of drug development and marketing.

This does not alter the fact that decisions made by the practicing physician will determine the success or failure of a drug. Government may make all the rules it likes, but if those rules receive only grudging acceptance by physicians, they are not likely to be helpful or permanent. A recent example is furnished by the unlamented regional medical programs.

Thus, strong winds are blowing, the barometer is falling, and there is every reason to conduct ourselves with both caution and imagination. We are not yet in a crisis in medicine, and crisis psychology should not be used to force premature guidelines and prohibitions on either physicians or manufacturers.

Although it may be difficult, I hope during these discussions that we all aim at trying to help the physician provide better care. None of us has the exclusive answer, and a touch of humility always makes for a better dialogue.

# MEDICAL BENEFITS
# AND RISKS ASSOCIATED
# WITH PRESCRIPTION DRUGS:
# FACTS AND FANCY

*Kenneth L. Melmon, Lewis B. Sheiner, and Barr Rosenberg*

## Introduction

Physicians and patients continue to use and demand prescription drugs in ever-increasing numbers despite precious little documentation of the benefits and risks associated with drug therapy. In 1971 we became interested in reviewing the data on the risks involved in using prescription drugs. Some data were available on the subject, but they were scientifically inadequate and incomplete. Most data had been collected in university hospital settings and had been taken from the results of surveys on internal medicine wards. Obviously, considerable bias was introduced into these studies. Nevertheless, the extrapolated results might be summarized as follows: (1) between 150,000 and 450,000 patients per year enter hospital wards in the speciality of internal medicine either with or solely because of a drug reaction; (2) those being treated for a drug reaction have a 30 percent chance of developing another while being treated for the first (perhaps a measure of our therapeutic sophistication); (3) the consequences that correlate with, and perhaps are caused by, the reactions include doubling of the hospital stay of the affected patients.[1]

Whether these figures represent the tip of an iceberg or the base of a pyramid no one can say. With our current information we do not know if the incidence of drug reactions is a "mere" 150,000 patients per year [2] or 1.5 million; whether treating such reactions costs 1.5 million patient-days per year or 50 million; whether it accounts for only a few or as many as 140,000 avoidable deaths per year. Each figure has been quoted but, in each case, it has been based on what is probably unwarranted extrapolation of perfectly good, but limited, information. Furthermore, we have no estimate of the costs of the adversity to the patient, to the doctor, or to society.

This work was supported in part by USPHS grants GM-16496, GM-00001, HL-15851, and GM-01791.

[1] K. L. Melmon, "Preventable Drug Reactions—Causes and Cures," *New England Journal of Medicine,* vol. 284 (1971), p. 1361.

[2] H. Wiener, "Letter to Editor," *Science,* vol. 181 (1973), p. 110.

One fact is certain: There is no longer any room for complacency about the safety of drugs, including those prescribed to patients in every doctor's office. In Osler's time it was thought that most drugs did no good but, by and large, did little harm either. Then came the era of seeing drugs as "magic bullets." In a few cases, but by no means all, the "magic" was justified, but now we are concerned that whether or not drugs are magic, they certainly can be "bullets." Clearly, drugs can be both useful and dangerous, but the extraordinary fact is that we are woefully ignorant of the real incidence and consequences of either the efficacy or toxicity of our drugs.

A first priority of those concerned with the economy of drug use is to encourage epidemiologic study of drug use and adverse reactions to drugs and to secure solid facts and figures. A few investigators have already obtained useful information, and the project is likely to be feasible. Paul Stolley of Johns Hopkins University, for example, has found that in one small county virtually all of the inappropriate prescriptions of chloramphenicol, a potentially toxic antibiotic, were written by a tiny minority of physicians and that "good" prescription writing correlated well with the educational level of physicians.[3] This study and analogous data encourage academicians and allow us to support education of physicians. Physicians surely intend to do the best they can for their patients; however, they may not always know what is best. Hershel Jick and his collaborators have discovered new and unsuspected adverse effects of drugs by careful epidemiologic study of hospitalized patients.[4] Thus, even small-scale epidemiologic studies have been able to define problems in therapeutics and to suggest solutions.

Epidemiologic work is needed on a large scale to elucidate the character of efficacy, or the reaction to an administered drug. This country has no way of retrieving information concerning the incidence, degree, and consequence of either efficacy or adverse reactions once the drugs are released onto the market. We simply do not know whether the adverse reaction data that we have mentioned can be extrapolated either to areas outside the hospital or to medical experience inside the hospital in specialities other than internal medicine. It is hard for us to believe that reports from the Johns Hopkins and Massachusetts General Hospitals represent the poorest examples of the national experience with prescription drugs or that internists in academia do poorer jobs in using drugs than do internists in practice, or surgeons, pediatricians, or obstetricians wherever their base of practice. Nevertheless, we do not know the answers to these relatively straightforward

---

[3] P. D. Stolley et al., "Drug Prescribing and Use in an American Community," Annals of Internal Medicine, vol. 76 (1972), p. 537. P. D. Stolley et al., "The Relationship between Physician Characteristics and Prescribing Appropriateness," Medical Care, vol. 10, no. 1 (1972), p. 17. P. D. Stolley and L. Lasagna, "Prescribing Patterns of Physicians," Journal of Chronic Diseases, vol. 22 (1969), p. 395.

[4] D. J. Greenblatt and J. Koch-Weser, "Adverse Reactions to Spironolactone: A Report from the Boston Collaborative Drug Surveillance Program," Journal of the American Medical Association, vol. 225, no. 1 (1973), p. 40.

questions, and we have no way at present to begin to determine the balance of benefit versus risk.

Moreover, learning the answers will not be a simple task. We probably need a central clearinghouse for reports both of efficacy and adverse drug reactions, but before such an effort would be effective we must train people to obtain useful information. Data acquisition requires the efforts of as yet untrained epidemiologists (both health-oriented and economics-oriented) working with highly qualified statisticians and with individuals who can separate the complex chemical environment we have created for man from the drug environment. Without answers, we cannot plot important long-range corrective measures.

However, even if we were to provide for training of these investigators and funding for their research, the costs of *present-day* prescribing patterns must still be dealt with. Although we have indicated to you some of our ignorance about these costs, we are now going to try to define them in more detail. We must stress that what follows is based largely on judgment and experience, and only partially on demonstrable fact.

### Costs of Prescribing Patterns

In the United States these are roughly of three types, one having to do with dollars, one with sickness and death induced by drugs (which might also be crudely related to dollars), and the third related to prolongation of illness or delay in diagnosis resulting from the choice of an inappropriate drug or drug regimen. We also may say that this misuse of prescription drugs results in lack of benefit in at least three sets of circumstances. One is when no treatment, or the wrong treatment, is given for a disease that is treatable. A second is when patients do not comply with a proper therapeutic regimen. The third is when drugs are given for inappropriate reasons but do produce an effect.

**Costs.** It appears that in some cases patients are paying excessive sums for some drugs that produce the same benefit as other, less expensive ones. Steps are being taken at a federal level to decrease this phenomenon. If a drug producer markets a brand name drug that he says is both chemically and clinically equivalent to the same drug marketed by other producers, he should have evidence that this is so. So far, that evidence is lacking. If the original producer of the drug claims superiority for his product—that is, nonequivalence—this should be demonstrated also. Such proof undoubtedly will raise the developmental costs of generics. However, even in the absence of such validation, it is not clear to us that the prices of drugs truly reflect their cost plus a reasonable profit. In fact, the data gathered by Lee and Silverman seem to suggest otherwise.[5]

---

[5] M. Silverman, and P. R. Lee, *Pills, Profits, and Politics* (Berkeley: University of California Press, 1974).

The second category of costs associated with prescribing patterns is drug toxicity to patients. Some drug toxicity appears to be unavoidable, as with rare and unpredictable "idiosyncratic" reactions and some hypersensitivity reactions. However, what evidence we have suggests that the great majority of drug toxicities are predictable and may be avoidable.

There appear to be at least three causes of such avoidable reactions: One occurs when appropriate drugs are given in inappropriate doses. Eighty percent of the adverse drug reactions seen in a number of studies were due to the known pharmacologic effects of drugs that were selected correctly but given in the wrong doses (improper quantitative therapeutic decisions). Examples include unnecessary production of hypokalemia while using diuretics for the treatment of hypertension, production of digitalis-induced arrhythmias in the course of treating a patient for congestive heart failure, or bleeding caused by an inappropriate dose of, or an unanticipated drug interaction with, an anticoagulant. Most distressing is the possibility that 60 percent or more of the adverse effects in some studies could have been avoided without compromise of the therapeutic benefits of the drug had it been given with the understanding of dosage that we presently possess. We emphasize that about 80 percent of the adverse reactions that occurred on those medical wards could, in theory, have been avoided and did not necessarily represent inherent and unavoidable risks of therapy. A second cause of avoidable reactions is the fact that drugs are given inappropriately, that is, drugs that can produce toxic reactions are given when they should not be. Perhaps the best-known example of this is the use of antibiotics for irrational and ineffective prophylaxis.[6] This practice literally has produced new types of infectious diseases (although not as dramatically or as avoidably as Jack Anderson might want us to believe). The third cause of avoidable reactions is that drugs in general are probably prescribed far too often;[7] a particularly striking example is the use of potent antibiotics for the common cold.

The third category of the costs of the misuse of drugs relates to the unnecessary prolongation of a treatable illness. These costs are the consequences of unwise qualitative therapeutic decisions. Thus, there may be a delay in discovery of a curable disease because inappropriate symptomatic therapy is given. For example, if a physician gave vitamin $B_{12}$ to correct an anemia actually caused by folic acid deficiency, such a cost would result. A variant of this is the prolongation of a disease. For example, if a physician gave the wrong antibiotic for the treatment of a curable pneumonia, unnecessary extended morbidity could result.

---

[6] C. M. Kunin, T. Tupasi, and W. A. Craig, "Use of Antibiotics: A Brief Exposition of the Problem and Some Tentative Solutions," *Annals of Internal Medicine*, vol. 79 (1973), p. 555.

[7] U.S., Department of Health, Education and Welfare, Task Force on Prescription Drugs, *Current American and Foreign Programs* (Washington, D. C.: Government Printing Office, December 1968).

**Lack of Therapeutic Benefit.** In some settings inappropriate drug administration can result in an unnecessary lack of benefit of drug therapy to the patient. Perhaps the most costly example of this lack-of-benefit category occurs when inadequate therapy is offered to the patient with a treatable disease. For example, more than 25 million people in this country are suffering from an easily diagnosed, potentially lethal, but substantially reversible disease—hypertension. Despite the availability of adequate, if not ideal, drugs to prevent the crippling or death caused by complications of the disease, less than one-eighth of the patients who are at high risk of untimely and unnecessary death are being given adequate drug therapy; only one-fourth are receiving drugs at all. Of the more than 25 million people in our population with this easily diagnosed disease only 3 million are being effectively treated, even though more than 90 percent of hypertensives *can* be effectively treated. Treatment experience in hypertension has also produced another example of therapeutics with a lack of benefit. Apparently we do not know enough about factors that positively influence the compliance of patients with suggested therapeutic regimens. In the case of hypertension, in one group of patients more than 50 percent would not follow a relatively simple and efficacious drug program. Not only are we unable to judge who is and who is not going to adhere to a regimen, but we also often find it difficult to ferret out those who are complying from those who do not take the drug but do not wish this fact discovered.

Finally, benefit of therapy is absent if a physician gives a drug that produces the effect he desires, but that effect has no positive bearing on the outcome of the fundamental disease. For example, selected drugs used to lower fats, cholesterol, or fatty acids in the blood (estrogen-like hormones and derivatives of thyroid hormone) are commonly administered to patients with lipid abnormalities with the hope that coronary artery diseases will be reduced. These drugs are still commonly used, despite information that they increase the rate of mortality in patients taking the drugs. An analogous example is the common use of oral hypoglycemic agents in the "treatment" of asymptomatic hyperglycemia (early diabetes). These drugs are very commonly administered, despite extraordinarily convincing information that they do not alter the course of diabetes and that they may expose the diabetic patient to an increased mortality rate. What prompts a physician to allow drug administration that offers no hope of efficacy, but does carry a possible risk of toxicity?

## The Current Problem

Why are drugs prescribed inappropriately and excessively? Here, again, we must note that we are not speaking *ex cathedra,* but rather that lack of data obliges us to express our judgment on a question that needs much more careful investigation.

One reason for excessive prescribing is obvious: drug companies need sales to make money. This must account, in large part, for drug advertisements in medical journals and the large investments made by the pharmaceutical industry in attempts to sell doctors on their products. But why are these advertisements, which are so often misleading, so effective in selling the product?

Chauncey Starr (former dean of the School of Engineering and Applied Science at the University of California, Los Angeles) may provide part of the answer. He states that the time necessary to develop the technology from a scientific discovery (in our case, develop a pill from a drug) has remained relatively constant throughout the last several decades; however, the rate of widespread use of a technological development recently has accelerated. Thus, he points out that wide use of a technological development occurs with ease before its social impact can be properly assessed.[8] Drug use in our society seems to be an almost involuntary activity. Although the consumer knows nearly nothing about this product, he demands it and blithely accepts the risk, of which he is usually ignorant. Any knowledge of risk appears to come primarily from advertisements of non-prescription drugs and from his doctor. In other words, his psychological acceptance of risk stems from an apparent acceptance of the influence of authorities or dogma. One might go so far as to venture a guess that the doctor too is greatly influenced in his therapeutic decisions by authorities (the drug salesman) and dogma (the drug advertisement). Starr tells us that even if the public knew and was concerned about the risks associated with drug therapy, advertising the benefits of drug consumption would probably increase public acceptance of even higher levels of risk.[9] All too many examples are available to prove his points in health related matters—witness the unabated use of ethanol and tobacco despite well-known risks that are essentially nullified, in the public's mind, by misleading advertising.

There have been no studies of the effects that advertising of over-the-counter drugs has on the public demand for non-advertised prescription drugs. Industry has clearly profited from the sale of both proprietary and prescription drugs despite regulatory measures begun in 1938.[10] Most regulatory procedures have been directed toward stopping unethical procedures, bad business practices, violation of interstate commerce laws, or unethical advertising. In many instances, in the past at least, such advertising promoted the sales of drugs irrespective of the health consequences of such sales. Indeed, little, if anything, has been done to determine what health consequences the availability of drugs has on the population as a whole.

Some of the consequences of poor data related to drug therapy have been mentioned in the introduction. We are now entering a period when general academic concern about therapeutics is noticeable, some would say for the first

---

[8] C. Starr, "Social Benefit versus Technological Risk: What Is Society Willing to Pay for Safety?" *Science*, vol. 165 (1969), p. 1232.

[9] Ibid.

[10] Silverman and Lee, *Pills, Profits, and Politics*, pp. 27–31, 212–14.

time in medical history, and clinical pharmacology is being fostered in some medical schools. Attention to the area of therapeutics also appears politically attractive and has resulted in recent proposals of bills that are likely to have substantive effects on therapeutics, for example, bills S.3441 and S.966 and the recent actions of the Office of Technology Assessment (OTA).[11] Similarly, consumer advocates such as Sydney Wolfe and Ralph Nader are turning their attention toward problems of drug therapy. Among other approaches, the psychology of both the physician and the patient in relation to drug use is being examined.

Although the physician tends to over-prescribe for subjective and frequently irrational reasons (his wish to be or to appear to be effective, decisive and helpful), the patient may also irrationally demand prescriptions. We are a society that believes in the magic of technology: surely "miracle drugs" exist even for life's inevitable woes. Physicians have described to us the bewilderment and indignation of their patients when prescriptions were not offered. Furthermore, it has been pointed out that a prescription represents an effective termination strategy for the doctor-patient encounter: [12] it is a symbol of the physician's concern; it terminates the current encounter, yet promises a future one; and it is something that serves to symbolize and render concrete the act of healing. But surely drugs are likely to be too efficacious and dangerous to be used as simple symbolic tokens.

## Approaching the Problem of Data Collection in Drug Economics

In our opinion it is entirely appropriate and timely for a group like the American Enterprise Institute to begin examining the economic impact of drugs on society. We hope that it will be possible to weave in some suggestions for the standards that the public probably will want. These must be based on acceptable estimates of risks and benefits in any category of drug treatment.

Although we profess no expertise in the special areas of concern that this conference is examining, we would like to suggest that certain questions might best be answered by the people with special talents assembled for this conference.

A cost-benefit analysis on drug use in this country probably has eluded us because we have not medically defined a utility function for the state of health. Only minor efforts have been made to put a value on health or to establish what fraction of disability is amenable to drug therapy and what the overall utility of such therapy is. Although it may be relatively easy to estimate the cost to society of a disease that requires hospitalization or results in loss of life, limb function.

---

[11] Office of Technology Assessment, *Drug Bioequivalence* (Washington, D. C.: Government Printing Office, 15 July 1974).

[12] C. Muller, "The Overmedicated Society: Forces in the Marketplace for Medical Care," *Science,* vol. 176 (1972), p. 488.

limb, or eyesight,[13] what are the costs of mild anxiety, acne, acute upper respiratory illness or mild asthma?

Besides lack of useful estimates of the utility of health, we have almost no data related to the probabilities of attaining adequate health in a spectrum of diseases with or without medical or surgical therapy. We know that withholding therapy for hypertension leads to a poorer prognosis than if the patient were treated, but hypertension is the exception. It is by no means obvious that the course of many of the life-threatening diseases we face are positively affected by drug treatment. The therapy for hypercholesterolemia may be efficacious, but it may not reduce the incidence of coronary artery disease; the treatment of hyper-glucosemia may be possible, but it may not reduce the morbid events associated with diabetes; the antineoplastic agents may reduce signs of cancer, but they may not prolong useful life; diuretics may cosmetically alter a patient's appearance, but they may not provide better function to his heart or lungs or alter the course of his renal disease; artificial sweeteners may allow low calorie substitutes for food, but they do not appear to reduce obesity; sweeteners may increase use of tooth-paste, but there is some question of the efficacy of toothpaste. Although, since the 1962 Kefauver amendments to the Food and Drug Act, we test widely for the potential efficacy and safety of new drugs, we know almost nothing about the utility of these drugs when they are used by the general public. Obviously we must begin to audit the effects of all drugs used in therapeutics, regardless of when or how these drugs appeared on the marketplace, if we are to develop estimates of the probability of various states of health resulting from their use. Such audits undoubtedly would initially increase the costs of care to society, but they might substantially alter treatment habits presently based on dogma and tradition.

If an audit were to be accomplished, additional factors of economic interest might appear. We might begin to learn of the true probability of risk to patients created by errors in the physician's therapeutic judgments. The audit must be designed so that it can detect the separate types of consequences of inappropriate uses of drugs listed in the introduction.

If we learned how to establish a utility function for various states of health, and if we could define the probability of reaching these various states with and without drugs and then could establish the probability of risk to a patient by inappropriate physician judgment and patient behavior, we could then progress to a comparison of the expected utility of treatment of a patient with the cost of using the drug. In approaching this category of data gathering, we would consider the cost of developing a drug or drug product (if indeed such information could actually be gleaned from industry). In addition, we would be able to estimate the costs of developing drugs for the treatment of rare diseases and alternative (inter-changeable) drug products that may be required by a few patients with a disease

---

[13] Silverman and Lee, *Pills, Profits, and Politics;* P. C. Reynell and M. C. Reynell, "The Cost-Benefit Analysis of a Coronary Care Unit," *British Heart Journal,* vol. 34 (1972), p. 897.

that is already treatable by available drug products. Furthermore, we would be in a position to determine who would or should be responsible for developing drug products necessary for the treatment of rare diseases when there would be relatively little, if any, economic incentive for a drug manufacturer to do so. Information on this topic would make possible much more reasonable decisions on compendium standards and government reimbursement for available therapeutic agents than those made at this time.

If all the above topics could be discussed from a base of useful data, then the economics of a more complicated matter could be anticipated and acted upon. As drugs continue to proliferate and become more specific in their effects, fundamental decisions as to the costs of alternatives in education of the drug prescribers can be approached. Today, education of the physician in therapeutics is not systematically or thoroughly taught by academic medical centers. Instead, suboptimal education is being given the physician by the *Physician's Desk Reference* (PDR) and drug industry representatives (detail men) at no small cost. A burning question in our minds is whether a convincing rally can be started to switch primary education in therapeutics from the shoulders of industry to those of academia. If so, what will the cost be and who will bear it? What will the results be in terms of the cost of therapy per patient treated? Clearly, it is not only the cost of developing and distributing a drug that must be considered in the economy of drug use; the cost of educating the physician in optimal drug use is an additional concern that must be considered in order to arrive at our fixed costs or overhead.

If and when we are truly able to use real figures for overhead, patient risk, the utility function of the state of health, the probabilities of reaching a state of health by using therapy, and the probability of success of alternative modes of patient management without drugs (perhaps requiring comparisons of disease management between countries), we will then be able to separate facts from fancy about the medical benefits and risks associated with prescription drugs. The task is formidable but imperative. It is difficult to conceive how rational medical and nonmedical decisions about drugs can be made without real data.

# THE DIFFUSION OF
# PHARMACEUTICAL INNOVATION

*Sam Peltzman*

This paper discusses the benefits, but not the costs, of different rates of diffusion for pharmaceutical innovation. It also discusses the role of promotion in attaining these benefits without evaluating the relative efficiency of promotion and other methods of altering diffusion rates. These caveats are meant to show by implication what further research is required for an evaluation of the present methods by which an innovation is delivered from the laboratory to the patient. The major point I wish to make is that some market forces create a bias toward too little promotion of innovation. The particular manifestation of this bias that I focus on concerns the speed with which innovation is spread. An innovation will remain a laboratory curiosity until a physician is made aware of its properties, so that the time it takes for the innovation to get to the patient can be reduced by expenditures on the informing of physicians. If the bias that I shall describe is important, then too little promotion implies too slow a diffusion of innovation, in the sense that more promotion and faster diffusion would provide benefits greater than their costs. I then examine the diffusion rates of some major past innovations to show the potential order of magnitude of the benefits of accelerated diffusion of such innovations. Depending on the frequency of such innovations, this magnitude can be substantial enough to pay for rather extensive promotion activities that might enable realization of the benefits.

## Incentives to Promotion of Innovation

I wish to argue, in nontechnical language that inevitably ignores some complications, that the benefits derived from a speedier diffusion of innovation than occurs in a typical market may exceed the costs of acceleration. Implicit here is the notion that diffusion rates are not immutably fixed but can be altered by activities, such as information dissemination, that entail expenditures. This means that one can characterize an efficient rate of diffusion as one in which the benefit from increasing the rate just pays the costs required to do so. For example, there would surely be more benefits realized than is usually the case if every sufferer from a disease were discovered, informed, and transported to the factory door the moment a drug that could cure the disease went into production. The costs

15

of so drastic an acceleration of diffusion might strike us as extravagant, which is simply to say that they would exceed the relevant benefits; whatever we claim, we do not act as if health were infinitely precious. On the other hand, regaining health today rather than tomorrow is worth something, so it might be equally extravagant if the discoverer of the drug were to rely entirely on cocktail party acquaintances to spread word of the drug. Typically, there will be some pace between the most forced and most leisurely at which benefits from accelerating diffusion will no longer pay the costs. My point is simply that there are forces at work making the actual pace more leisurely than this optimum. The relevant inhibitions arise from competition among innovators and constraints on their ability to charge discriminatory prices.

I can best illustrate the way these inhibitions work by using stereotype examples. To elaborate the role of competition among innovators, imagine a drug worth $10 to any potential user, because it saves one the need for another treatment that costs $10. If the drug can be produced and sold for less than $10, the user would obviously wish to buy it. Suppose that all the costs connected with developing, producing, and distributing the drug—apart from informing physicians currently ignorant about the drug—in fact amount to $1 per application. Now, suppose further that among these ignorant physicians are some with patients who could benefit tomorrow from the drug. But, of course, these physicians will not know of the drug tomorrow unless someone tells them, and this is costly. If the cost of doing just this sort of informing is under $9, there would be at least the potential for net benefits to be shared among patient, doctor, and drug producer. In terms of the conditions for an efficient diffusion rate, the benefits from the drug's use tomorrow rather than later (that is, $10, and I am assuming, only to avoid a complication that is not essential to the argument, that postponement of the drug's use is not a relevant alternative for this patient) exceed the costs of securing this use ($1 plus some amount less than $9). Indeed, if the cost of a quick trip by the detail man were, say, $5, there would appear to be room for a profitable deal all around—at a retail price of $8, a net gain of $4 could be split evenly between producer and doctor-patient. However, the deal will not be struck and these benefits will be forgone if the drug producer faces competition sufficient to drive the drugstore price down to less than $6. A competitor may not be able to duplicate the drug, or to do so for $1 per application, but few innovators can expect to be in a position in which they can hope to realize all of the benefits of their innovation.

The history of drug innovation shows very few exceptions to this generalization: Major innovation is frequently followed by competition from related products. This competition does produce benefits; it keeps prices down and expands the market. But in the matter at issue, some benefits will be lost. If the competitor's higher cost required him to price an equivalent drug (or dose) at say, $5.50, the innovator's product could not sell for more than that. Neither he nor his competitor will pay the $5.00 that it takes to inform the ignorant physician in our example, and a benefit will be lost. In this case, the innovator will pay no more than $4.50 to bring about an application of the drug that might not otherwise occur, and the diffusion rate of the innovation will be slower than it would be without the competition.[1]

To elaborate the role of constraints on price discrimination in retarding the diffusion of information, it is useful to introduce the possibility that drug benefits differ among patients. For example, some patients might have to undergo twice as much, or $20 worth, of the more expensive therapy as others to cure the same malady that our hypothetical drug cures. They could share with the drug seller and their physicians a net benefit from immediate use of the drug as long as the cost of providing immediate information to doctors is under $19, but if the cost of providing such information is this high, it will be provided only if the producer of the drug can recoup the cost in an atypically high price. This may prove difficult, even if there is no explicit competition from other producers. For example, if the majority of users get no more than $10 benefit from the drug, that figure will set an upper limit to what the producer can charge these customers. Should the producer seek much more than this from a minority of customers, he faces the problem of preventing this minority from discovering and purchasing at the lower price. Given the current organization of drug prescribing and distribution, this would have to be accomplished by somehow ensuring that the wholesale price of the drug prescribed by some physicians exceeds that of the same drug prescribed by others. Even where this feat can be brought off—perhaps by selling to hospitals at wholesale prices different from those paid by pharmacies—the market segmentation that is feasible may not correspond to the one desired by the producer; the high-benefit patients, for example, may be scattered among both hospital outpatients and general-practice patients. More generally, the producer will have to expend resources in an attempt to achieve the desired segmentation. For example, he may engage in the much-maligned practice of developing "artificially differentiated" alternative brands of the same general drug formula that are sold at different wholesale prices. However well the practice may work in some cases, there will be others in which either the costs of developing the high-priced brand or the incentives for doctors and patients to seek and use the low-priced alternative after they are informed about the high-priced counterpart are too great to make price discrimination practicable. In these cases, some potential

---

[1] This assumes that promotion expenditures are to be recouped in a uniform retail price, or at least one that does not differ systematically among customers. I treat the alternative of systematic price differences—say $5.50 to everyone else but $8.00 to our ignorant doctor's patient—below. Another alternative would be for innovators to charge for information and drugs separately. This rarely happens, in part because as information-seller the innovator would have to contemplate the prospect of competition from his first customers, and in part because it is difficult for the potential customer to guess whether the information is worth the asking price. Few producers find it worthwhile to ask their customers to become, in effect, gamblers about the value of information.

17

patient benefits will simply be lost until doctors have acquired information through some more leisurely information dissemination process.

## Benefits of Rapid Diffusion of Innovation

If market forces retard the spread of some benefits, one would like to know whether the retardation is substantial or trivial. To shed light on this issue, I examine the diffusion of benefits from three major postwar drug innovations: antituberculosis drugs, major tranquilizers, and Salk polio vaccine. Most of the data I use here are derived from other research on drug innovation, to which the reader is referred for greater detail.[2] The reader should also keep in mind that innovations of similar importance occur rarely and that technological factors can affect the diffusion process importantly. For example, unlike the tranquilizers, TB and polio drugs treat communicable diseases, so the successful treatment or prevention of one case spreads benefits to other potential victims.

These three innovations do have a particular advantage for the purpose of getting at the interaction of information and the diffusion of benefits. The drugs differed greatly in the speed with which information about them was spread. In marked contrast to the other drugs, Salk vaccine received the benefit of immediate nationwide publicity in the aftermath of an extensive field trial of the drug. Nearly 500,000 children participated in the trial, and the ubiquitous interest in the results among patients as well as doctors led to quick adoption of the drug. Something like three-fourths of the entire population under twenty had received at least one dose of the drug within two years of the end of the trial.[3] Neither of the other drugs received such immediate widespread publicity or acceptance. In fact, the acceptability of the tranquilizers appears to have been retarded by professional skepticism, which took as long as a decade to dispel, regarding their value.[4]

In light of this experience, I shall treat the diffusion of benefits from Salk vaccine as the prototype for drugs that receive widespread publicity, and then compare the diffusion rate of these benefits with those of the other two drugs. Such a comparison should, of course, be treated with caution. It ignores the costs of different levels of publicity, the important technological differences among the innovations, and the differences in market receptivity to similar promotion efforts for different types of drugs. The main purpose of the comparison is simply to establish the order of magnitude of benefits from diffusion of innovation at rates that are greater than historical averages but still within the realm of experience.

---

[2] See Sam Peltzman, *Regulation of Pharmaceutical Innovation* (Washington, D. C.: American Enterprise Institute, 1974), and "The Benefits and Costs of New Drug Regulation," in R. Landau, ed., *Regulating New Drugs* (Chicago: University of Chicago Center for Policy Study, 1973).

[3] American Medical Association, *Report of the Commission on the Cost of Medical Care*, vol. 3 (Chicago: American Medical Association, 1964), p. 31.

[4] See L. Goodman and A. Gilman, *The Pharmacological Basis of Therapeutics* (New York: Macmillan, 1965), pp. 163, 177.

For this limited purpose, the Salk vaccine experience is at least a benchmark for the kind of experience that we might practically hope to duplicate.

I will present here only the skimpiest outline of the nature of the benefits from the three drugs in question.[5] The drugs that acted directly against the TB bacteria (streptomycin, PAS, and isoniazid) were the first chronologically. Other modes of TB therapy and prophylaxis—patient confinement, public health measures, x-ray detection, and so forth—had been successful in reducing the death rate from TB by something like 4 or 5 percent annually over most of this century. The major benefit of the new drugs, first introduced in the late 1940s, appears to have been a marked acceleration of this decline—to something like triple the historical rate in the years immediately following introduction. There were also important benefits resulting from improved TB morbidity experience, but I will focus only on mortality effects here.

The major tranquilizer, chlorpromazine, was introduced in 1954. The drug family of which it was part (phenothiazines) proved useful in the management of psychoses that had previously entailed lengthy confinement in mental hospitals. The drugs do not prevent psychoses, so that growth in hospital admission rates has not slowed. They do, however, permit some patients to function outside of a hospital sooner than previous treatment proved capable of doing. Thus, their major benefit has been a reduction in the average length of confinement for mental hospital admittees.

The Salk vaccine and subsequent variants immunize most recipients to poliomyelitis, a disease whose incidence had previously remained resistant to medical advance. The disease has by now been virtually eradicated.

Among the many problems of measuring the diffusion of benefits from these or any similar innovations, I want to focus on those connected with the time-span over which the diffusion takes place. Even if one innovation preempts the market for any other, we cannot assume that the relevant benefits continue perpetually. For, in the absence of the first innovation, a market for another would have existed and might have permitted development of the alternative. In that case, one would wish to attribute to a specific innovation only those benefits produced prior to the introduction of the hypothetical alternative in addition to any subsequent benefits in excess of those attainable from the alternative. Given the effects of an initial innovation on the market for alternatives, we are inevitably left to guess how long it would have taken for an alternative to appear. My procedure here will be to assume arbitrarily that the benefits from an innovation reach a peak a decade after introduction and that any benefits from more rapid diffusion can be achieved only within this decade.

The assumption that benefits peak within a decade is perhaps plausible for something like polio vaccine. In fact, because of its rapid acceptance, polio was

---

[5] For further details, see Peltzman, *Regulation of Pharmaceutical Innovation,* and references therein.

virtually eradicated only five years or so after the vaccine was introduced. However, the assumption may be overly stringent for TB drugs and tranquilizers. In the case of the former, the decline of TB death rates has moderated, but it is even now about double the pre-drug decline. Similarly, the decline in per patient confinement at mental hospitals does not yet appear to have run its course, and part of the reason may be the slowness of the medical profession's acceptance of tranquilizers. This means that the benefits from more rapid diffusion of innovation may be much greater than is implied by estimates confined to a decade of experience.

Table 1 indicates something of the magnitude of the benefits that might be attained from faster diffusion of an innovation within a decade of its introduction.

## Table 1
### DIFFUSION OF BENEFITS FOR
### THREE MAJOR DRUG INNOVATIONS

| | (1) Actual Loss from Disease as Percent of Loss Expected without Drug | | | (2) Saving from Drug as Percent of Tenth Year Saving | | |
|---|---|---|---|---|---|---|
| | (a) | (b) | (c) | (a) | (b) | (c) |
| Years after Introduction of Drug | Polio (paralytic cases) [a] | TB (deaths) [b] | Mental hospital stay (patient-days) [c] | Polio | TB | Mental hospital |
| 1 | 59 | 93 | 98 | 41 | 11 | 5 |
| 2 | 31 | 86 | 94 | 69 | 22 | 15 |
| 3 | 10 | 77 | 86 | 90 | 36 | 35 |
| 4 | 14 | 72 | 76 | 86 | 44 | 60 |
| 5 | 22 | 59 | 79 | 78 | 64 | 53 |
| 6 | 9 | 48 | 81 | 91 | 81 | 48 |
| 7 | 3 | 41 | 75 | 97 | 92 | 63 |
| 8 | 2 | 39 | 67 | 98 | 95 | 83 |
| 9 | 1 | 37 | 67 | 99 | 99 | 83 |
| 10 | nil | 36 | 61 | 100 | 100 | 100 |

[a] Actual number of new paralytic cases of polio reported in each year, 1955–64, divided by number of cases expected if Salk vaccine had not been introduced. Expected cases for 1955–61 estimated in American Medical Association, *Report of the Commission on the Cost of Medical Care,* vol. 3, 1964; the 1961 estimate is used for 1962–64.

[b] Actual death rate from tuberculosis in each year, 1948–57, divided by 1947 rate × exp − .045 × number of years from 1947. This exponent is the average annual decline of the TB death rate from 1920 to 1947, which, it is presumed, would have continued in the absence of any drug innovation.

[c] Patient-days in mental hospitals per new admittee in each year, 1955–64, divided by 800, which approximates the level prevailing in the decade prior to introduction of chlorpromazine.

Each entry in column 2 is derived from its counterpart in column 1 as follows: the column 1 value is subtracted from 100 and divided by the resulting number for the tenth year after introduction. Column 1 of the table expresses the observed toll from a disease as a percent of what could have been expected without the drug in each of the ten years following a drug's introduction. For example, the entry for year 8 in column 1(b) means that the TB death rate was only 39 percent as large as (that is, 61 percent below) the level that could have been expected if TB deaths had declined only as rapidly as they had in the pre-drug era. In column 2, the implied saving in each year is expressed as a percent of the tenth year saving, which is the presumed maximum. Thus, to continue the example, the maximum saving for TB drugs is assumed to be a 64 percent reduction of the death rate from its expected level (that is, the actual rate in year 10 is 36 percent of expected). The entry for year 8, column 2(b), indicates that 95 percent (61/64) of this reduction was achieved by year 8.

The pattern emerging from this exercise is not surprising, given the previous discussion. The benefits of polio vaccine were diffused much more quickly than those of the other innovations: for most years the "saving index" in column 2 of Table 1 is substantially higher for polio vaccine than for either of the others. Of the two laggards, the tranquilizer benefits are fairly consistently the slowest to accrue. To put the potential saving from more rapid diffusion into some sort of context, I estimate the additional savings that might have been realized had the laggards been diffused as rapidly as polio vaccine. These estimates are in Table 2. To illustrate the derivation of these estimates, consider first the entries for year 2 in Table 1 for both TB and polio. The TB death rate is 14 percent below the expected level, and this represents a saving that is 22 percent of maximum (a 64 percent reduction). But suppose the saving were the 69 percent of maximum characteristic of polio. This would mean a 44 percent (.69 $\times$ 64) rather than a 14 percent reduction of the TB death rate that year. The expected death rate in the relevant year was in fact 307 per million population; the 14 percent saving produced an actual rate of 263. A 44 percent saving would have produced a rate of 172 or an additional saving of ninety-one lives per million population. This would translate into 19,200 lives on the current population base, which is the figure shown in Table 2 for TB drugs.

Quite clearly if even a fraction of the saving that this rough calculation produces had been attained, the gross benefits would be prodigious. To provide some common denominator for the relevant magnitudes, one can convert the savings into dollars, although this has its own formidable problems. Nevertheless, if one considers only the added earnings of potential TB victims who might be saved, a present value of $50,000 per life would be quite conservative—much less than conventional calculations of this sort that have emerged from accident-liability court causes and recent economic research. Using this figure and a

## Table 2
### POTENTIAL GAIN FROM MORE RAPID DIFFUSION, TB DRUGS AND TRANQUILIZERS

| Years after Introduction of Drug | TB Drugs (lives saved, in thousands) a | Tranquilizers (patient-days saved, in millions) b |
|---|---|---|
| 1 | 13.1 | 78 |
| 2 | 19.2 | 119 |
| 3 | 21.5 | 117 |
| 4 | 15.8 | 58 |
| 5 | 4.9 | 50 |
| 6 | 3.2 | 90 |
| 7 | 1.9 | 70 |
| 8 | 0.8 | 29 |
| 9 | 0.2 | 34 |
| Total | 80.6 | 645 |

a A hypothetical TB death rate series is computed by assuming a diffusion pattern for savings equal to that for polio vaccine in column 2 (a), Table 1. The difference between the observed series and the hypothetical series is multiplied by 211 million, the 1973 U.S. population, to get the potential saving in lives on the current population base. See text for example of computation.

b A hypothetical series of average length of stay per new mental hospital admittee is derived by assuming a diffuson pattern for reduction of this figure equal to that for polio vaccine. The difference between the observed series (365 × average daily census in mental hospitals in year/new admissions that year) and the hypothetical series is multiplied by 700,000, the approximate number of 1973 mental hospital admissions, to get the potential saving in patient-days on a current basis.

10 percent discount rate, the present value at the year of innovation of increased rapidity of diffusion of something like TB drugs works out to roughly $3 billion. In the case of tranquilizers, one can ignore completely any added productivity due to shorter patient confinement, and, in terms only of the saving of hospital costs (about $20 per patient-day currently), come up with a potential saving of almost $9 billion in present value. Again, the point of these calculations is not that exactly $12 billion in extra benefits could in fact have been realized for smaller costs, but only that the potential benefits of more rapid diffusion of major innovations are hardly trifling. By way of comparison, gains of this order once per decade could easily pay for a doubling of current drug promotion expenses, if that is what it takes to realize them.

In the light of the previous analysis, it is worth looking more closely at some of the data to see why these potential benefits may have been missed. The average length of stay at mental hospitals declined from about six hundred days to five hundred from 1961 to 1964. While the communicable aspect of polio may make application of its diffusion rate to tranquilizers unrealistic for early years, the differences in receptivity to the drugs loom correspondingly larger in the later years. If this is so, our estimates imply that had the medical profession been as receptive to tranquilizer therapy as to polio vaccine, the 1964 average patient stay would have been attained by 1961. Given then prevailing mental hospital expenditures of about $5 per day this would have meant a saving of $500 in hospital costs alone for the average 1961 admittee. For the admittee in whom we are particularly interested, the one who would not have used drugs in 1961, the drug therapy promised a hospital cost saving on the order of $1,500 or more. (The pre-drug average stay was eight hundred days, or three hundred more than the 1964 average, which itself does not reflect full exploitation of tranquilizer benefits.) The principal and interest from such sums could have paid for a great deal of drug therapy: specifically, the 1966 cost for maintenance users of Thorazine (the trade name for chlorpromazine) was 37 cents per day of therapy.[6] At this price, and discounting by the long-term average rate of return on equities (10 percent per year) the $500 saving represents the present value of about five years of continuous daily drug therapy, and $1,500 would more than pay for a lifetime of such therapy. In short, there must have been some patients in 1961 who would have gained more than the cost of drugs, but who did not use them. In part, this may be attributable to insufficient incentive on the part of drug sellers to spend what was required to overcome the skepticism of some doctors. This sounds peculiar, since Thorazine was among the more profitable of postwar innovations. However, examine these incentives in the "best" (from the seller's view) circumstance, that of a prospective lifetime daily user. The present value of sales at 1966 prices to such a user was about $1,300. Given the prevailing wholesale-retail margin for drugs, the manufacturer could expect to realize about half of this in sales, and of course less still in pretax profits. Thus, something under $650 represents the maximum additional promotion effort the seller would be willing to undertake to secure this particular drug use. But this still overstates the incentive to secure a use in 1961 instead of a few years later. For the type of user who will benefit from long-term maintenance, the drug producer may well view the relevant alternative as one in which the maintenance will begin a few years later if no additional promotional effort is made today. In that case, the maximum promotional expenditure would be considerably under $650—in fact, under $175 to secure the maintenance three years earlier than otherwise. Given the extreme length of confinement for some of the disorders treated by the drugs, it is not unreasonable to expect that several hundred extra days of institutional confinement would be the probable cost for a patient who delays drug therapy for three years, and that consequently there would be a considerable net savings for commencing drug treatment earlier. (Each one hundred days of confinement costs $500, while three years of drug use cost around $350 at retail.) However, we have

---

[6] U.S., Department of Health, Education and Welfare, Task Force on Prescription Drugs, *The Drug Users* (Washington, D. C.: Government Printing Office, 1968), p. 125.

just seen that those net benefits would not be realized if the promotion required to secure them cost over $175, even though the size of benefits could well pay for a greater effort. The constraints imposed by competition among tranquilizer producers and the difficulty of collecting abnormal selling expenses by price discrimination would militate against the extra effort.

## Implications

It would be simplistic to jump to a conclusion that less competition and more price discrimination would yield net benefits to patients. Price discrimination may not, as I have indicated, be a practicable alternative, and reduced competition would benefit some patients only at a cost to others. Even if the benefit exceeded the cost, a more specific mechanism for hastening the diffusion of innovations might widen this excess.

Unfortunately, one can only speculate about the nature of such a mechanism. I have suggested that there is a link between seller promotion and the rate of diffusion. However, finding the empirical magnitudes involved in the link remains a major research task yet to be done. Some very crude data I have examined indicate that the research could prove fruitful. From data on sales of new chemical entities introduced from 1961 to 1967 and promotion expenses for them,[7] I compiled measures of diffusion and promotion intensity for successful new products, by which I mean entities that had at least $1 million in sales in some year and whose 1967 sales were within 20 percent of peak annual sales in the 1961–67 period. The measures are, respectively, the ratio of sales in the early years of the period (1961–64 for drugs introduced in 1961 and 1963–65 for those introduced in 1963; only two 1962 drugs met the criteria) to sales in the later years, and the ratio of promotion expenses to sales for the entire period. The former ratio will be higher the more quickly sales build up from date of introduction, and the latter ratio is a measure of promotional effort relative to the drug's market size. For the 1961 entities the coefficient of rank correlation between these ratios is +.43, while for 1963 entities the rank correlation is +.30. Since there are only six and five drugs respectively in these samples, the results should be greeted cautiously. The rank correlations could have been improved by the inclusion of conspicuous failures—drugs whose sales peak early but then decline sharply. However, it would be unclear in these cases whether the relatively high promotion for these drugs is responsible for quick discovery of their characteristics or merely reflects the inherent risk of the large initial promotional expenses typical of new drugs. What the data do at least hint at is that drugs that have durable applications tend to be accepted more quickly the greater the promotional effort on their behalf. If further research indicates that the promotion-diffusion relationship is

---

[7] The data are from D. Schwartzman and R. Druckman, "Size of Firm, Research, and Promotion in the Drug Industry," mimeographed (New School for Social Research, 1972).

indeed persistent and important, we ought then to examine the productivity of alternatives to promotion. At this point we lack a comparison of the effects of seller promotion and other forms of information dissemination, such as more formal training of physicians, publicity aimed at patients (as in the case of polio vaccine), and so forth. In addition, we would like to know to what extent other market forces counter those that lead to underproduction of information. For example, if drug sellers produce too little information, doctors will have an incentive to pool information. This incentive may help explain the growth of institutions such as group practice that facilitate pooling of information. The one generalization that can, I think, be made at this point is that the benefits from accelerating the diffusion of innovation can rival in magnitude the benefits from having the innovation in the first place. This is, at least, the case for the innovations I have examined here.[8] Under those circumstances we should at least be wary of overemphasizing the costs attributable to activities that assist the diffusion process. As just one example, the current ability of firms to treat promotion expenditures affecting sales over a long period as a current expense for tax purposes might appear to be an uneconomic subsidy of this particular form of investment. However, if it indeed turns out that the other forces keeping the private returns to promotion below the social returns are sufficiently important, this tax subsidy could on balance improve the allocation of resources. In that case, it would be policies that retard rather than subsidize the dissemination of information that would be uneconomic.

Promotion and other forms of direct dissemination of information are not the only means of hastening the diffusion process to which the points I have made are applicable. For example, constraints similar to those operating on promotion can retard investment in improvement of a basic innovation and thus retard the rate at which benefits from the basic innovation are spread. In the light of the payoff to increasing the rate of diffusion of innovation, even apparently minor improvements can be highly productive. A case in point appears to be the TB drugs. Here it turned out that one of the pioneer drugs, PAS, was unpleasant to take and required large doses. In consequence, until more palatable forms were developed, some patients tended to discontinue use of the drug before they were cured.[9] Given the magnitude of losses from TB, we might have reason to regret the lag of approximately a decade between the discovery of the basic drug and development of the more palatable forms. Similarly, we have all the more reason to regret more recent public policies that appear to have increased drug development time and reduced the extent of product improvement.

---

[8] While my estimates of the benefits from more rapid diffusion of TB drugs and tranquilizers may be sanguine, it is worth noting that they are on the order of half the *total* benefits I was able to attribute to these innovations. For details of the latter estimate, see Peltzman, *Regulation of Pharmaceutical Innovation*, pp. 58–66.

[9] See American Medical Association, *Report of the Commission on the Cost of Medical Care*, p. 70.

# COPING WITH ILLNESS: CHOICES, ALTERNATIVES, AND CONSEQUENCES

*Mitchell B. Balter*

## Thesis

This paper finds current frameworks for examining the costs, benefits, and risks of drug development and treatment inadequate. It suggests that a careful analysis of coping behavior and factors affecting the flow of persons into treatment can provide some valuable insights and help us develop the framework we seek. It sees us in the midst of a consumer overreaction that could stifle therapeutic progress, and it recognizes a pressing need to enlighten the public on the subject of costs, benefits, and risks in drug development, treatment, and research.*

## An Overview

Let me begin with the notion that, at any given time, there is a large but finite number of persons in the community suffering from somatic and/or psychic disruptions, dysfunctions, or perturbations ranging from moderate to very severe that might reasonably be termed illnesses or regarded as abnormal states of health. Many of those illnesses lack classical form, are vague or complex in origin, and are very difficult to either label or diagnose. But nonetheless, they constitute a serious problem—an intolerable state or a crisis situation and perhaps a risk—for the individuals experiencing them. Furthermore, only a certain proportion of the individuals thus afflicted or incapacitated are officially identified, assume the status of patient, and become candidates for therapy. Many others similarly situated never become patients and never appear for treatment in an institutional setting.

In general, the more acutely life-threatening or the more socially disruptive the illness or trauma, the greater the likelihood that the person will surface somewhere in the extended health care system. However, the fact remains that among the many persons with disabling illnesses, some seek treatment and some do not; and in several instances, such as hypertension and depression, the untreated cases may be in the majority. The pathways to treatment are diverse, and who is seen

* The ideas and opinions expressed in this paper are the views of the author and are not necessarily those of The National Institute of Mental Health or any other component of the Department of Health, Education, and Welfare.

and what eventually gets treated in the health care system is the outcome of a highly selective process in which non-illness factors such as sex, age, income, and ethnicity play important roles.

The mass of persons who finally get diagnosed or treated by the medical system constitutes what is commonly known as "treated prevalence." And it is on various portions of this very large but highly selected group of individuals that our thinking about therapeutic utility—drug utility—is characteristically based. Little is known about the fate of persons who are ill but do not appear for treatment.

Our base of information on illness and medication—our national drug experience, if you will—may also be limited and unrepresentative on matters other than drug utility. It may be somewhat misleading on the subject of adverse reactions, for example.

Reports of serious drug adversities from which national extrapolations are currently being made are frequently a reflection of drug experiences with hospitalized patients who are severely ill, undergoing multiple drug therapy, or receiving types or doses of drugs that would be infrequently administered outside of the hospital. In other cases, the conditions of illness are such that the therapeutic options of both doctor and patient are markedly reduced, as in the treatment of geriatric patients with multiple illnesses and complications. Yet the bulk of medication—approximately 65 percent—is dispensed on the basis of prescriptions issued by physicians in private practice to outpatients who differ from hospitalized patients in many important respects. Outpatients are in better general health, their illnesses are less severe, and they are generally younger. In addition, daily doses of drugs are significantly lower, and the route of administration is much more frequently oral. All of these factors tend to reduce the probability of serious adverse reactions.

The only segment of the hospital data on adverse reactions directly applicable to patients being treated in the community is that portion dealing with persons admitted to the hospital for such reactions. The proper base for interpreting figures on hospitalizations for adverse reactions is not all hospital admissions, but rather, all persons in the community who have been treated with the drugs concerned. For completeness, data on hospitalizations for adverse reactions should be supplemented with data on the occurrence of lesser drug reactions among drug-treated patients living at home. If these procedures are followed, a much more balanced and conservative picture of adverse reactions will no doubt emerge.

The issue is important because the threat of adverse reactions is likely to be a source of great apprehension for consumers who require drug treatment, and the subject of adverse reactions is frequently misunderstood by the general public—partly because the concept of risk is difficult to convey in probabilistic terms. Public confusion on the subject of adverse reactions, if uncorrected, could have serious negative consequences for all drug treatment and all clinical research.

Maintaining a balanced national perspective on adverse reactions is clearly in the best interest of everyone.

In this context, it is interesting to note that in a 1971 probability-based national household survey concerned with the acquisition and use of psychotherapeutic drugs,[1] my colleagues and I encountered very few reports of serious adverse reactions among the users of prescription drugs. All respondents who had taken a medically prescribed psychotropic drug during the past year (in most instances a minor tranquilizer or a sedative), but had not taken it for the three months preceding the interview, were asked why they had stopped; the question was repeated for each drug taken. In 53 percent of the instances, the reason given for stopping minor tranquilizers and sedatives was that the respondents felt better and no longer needed the drug. These drugs were seldom discontinued because of serious side effects. However in 11 out of 114 instances, 9 percent of the cases, minor tranquilizers and sedatives were stopped for lesser reasons such as drowsiness, headaches, stomach upsets, and drug hangover.

Our experience in that study leads me to believe that systematic household interviewing of community-based samples of persons being treated with various drugs may be a feasible technique for establishing base rates for certain kinds of drug adversities (those involving events that can be directly observed or subjectively experienced). In several respects, the community survey approach may be superior to a system of spontaneous but unsystematic reporting of drug adversities by physicians in private practice. In a well-designed community study, interviews would be repeated at intervals within large samples of persons reflecting both acute and chronic experience with the drugs in question. Similar interviews would be conducted with control groups of persons who were not being treated with drugs.

Household interviewing techniques for the detection of drug adversities might be employed in a sequential approach to the marketing of new drugs, wherein all early recipients of the drug would be clearly identified and carefully followed in the community. Additional clinical and laboratory observations would of course be required. The design could incorporate some of the best features of test marketing and applied clinical research. It may be worth a trial and some further examination.

## A Coping Paradigm

Since most illnesses are neither immediately life-threatening nor of the type where there is but one therapeutic recourse, coping with illness can be generally viewed as a process of choosing among available therapeutic alternatives or socially defined

---

[1] H. J. Parry et al., "National Patterns of Psychotherapeutic Drug Use," *Archives of General Psychiatry*, vol. 130 (1973), pp. 769–83.

pathways. The process of choice need not be explicit nor strictly rational nor the actor consciously aware of the set of forces affecting his decision. The individual may seek conventional treatment of some type within the health care system or he may decide to treat himself outside that system—with or without drugs.

**Coping outside the System.** If the individual decides to treat his illness outside the health care system he may self-medicate with products purchased in a drug-store or liquor store, employ home remedies, or follow folk practices. He may seek faith healers, purchase esoteric potions, or he may, if his problem is essentially psychic, hie himself off to a local encounter group or become a devotee of transcendental meditation. He may struggle for control at Weight Watchers or Alcoholics Anonymous. He may use illicit drugs (such as marijuana, LSD, or heroin) or prescription drugs obtained illicitly, in quasi-therapeutic fashion, with the attendant risks, costs, and benefits. He may do nothing about his illness, but exact a high cost from his family or co-workers, or he may simply stay at home and experience a significant loss of earnings. If he chooses to ignore his illness, he may suffer a great deal or possibly put himself and others in jeopardy.

It is important that we recognize that there are both physical risks and possible therapeutic benefits, as well as extended cost-benefit consequences of a more external and social nature, associated with all of these choices. It is also essential that the costs, benefits, and risks of these extramedical alternatives be taken into account in our debates about the relative utility of conventional therapies. It would seem that, all other things being equal, conventional therapies have merit to the extent that they have greater utility—are more advantageous to the individual and society—than these extramedical alternatives.

**Coping inside the System.** A view of coping as a semidiscretionary process implies that, in most instances, when a person elects to visit a physician he has already made some personal decisions about his illness and chosen among alternatives. To illustrate this point, let me once again draw upon the national survey data which indicate that during the preceding year approximately 9 percent of American adults had used an over-the-counter (OTC) tranquilizer or sleeping pill, 22 percent had used a psychotherapeutic drug prescribed by a physician, and 14 percent were likely to increase alcohol consumption as a means of coping with psychic distress.[2] Yet the use of alcohol or the OTC drugs or both as a means of coping with psychic distress seldom overlapped the use of the medically prescribed drugs. These medical and nonmedical pathways tended to be mutually exclusive. Further, the use of medically prescribed psychotherapeutic drugs was much more frequently associated with a high level of psychic distress than was increased use of alcohol

---

[2] H. J. Parry *et al.*, "Increasing Alcohol Intake as a Coping Mechanism for Psychic Distress," in R. Cooperstock, ed., *Social Aspects of Medical Use of Psychotropic Drugs* (Addiction Research Foundation of Ontario, 1974).

or the use of OTC drugs when employed with the same therapeutic intent. However, it is also true that in general persons with high levels of distress were more likely to have sought relief in more than one way.

I do not yet have analogous data on medical versus nonmedical strategies for coping with somatic illnesses or infectious diseases, but I suspect that there are major similarities in coping related to severity of illness as well as important differences associated with the availability of more potent OTC drugs. There are also coping choices to be made within the health care system, although these are less obvious and the patient's contribution is often of lesser importance than the treatment recommendations of the doctor or some other health professional. The nature of these choices becomes clearer once a decision to seek professional help has been made.

If he is free and able to do so, the typical patient will proceed to choose a practitioner or select a treatment facility with some foreknowledge or expectations, however limited, about the type of therapy he is likely to receive. After checking around, one patient may choose to see a chiropractor about his persistent wry neck rather than visit an orthopedic specialist or neurologist, or he might do the opposite. Another may decide to take his blue mood, low energy, and loss of appetite to the medical clinic, or he may opt for the psychiatric clinic. A third may take his extreme nervousness to an internist or a general practitioner with expectations of short-term drug treatment, or he may try to make arrangements for psychotherapy.

The typical patient is in no position to make truly sophisticated cost-benefit-risk choices among therapeutic alternatives. However, he may approximate that process to some extent, albeit in much more emotional and far more personal terms, in his original choice of a health practitioner or treatment facility. Money, time, family obligations, embarrassment, travel distance, as well as some primitive fears, may enter his personal equation. There are some patients who in truth have almost no medical options because of such things as advanced age, very low income, ignorance, geographic area of residence, or the limited character of available treatment resources. These are the people who often try to maintain themselves outside the health care system and, when they finally enter it, are more frequently found to be severely ill.

If the typical patient who enters therapy has some problem with the treatment that has been provided—and let us assume that it is a medication prescribed by his physician—he is very likely to complain about it. If the problem persists, the doctor is likely to stop the drug and try another or try something else. If the doctor is either unwilling or unable to provide a treatment that eliminates the problem or meets the patient's needs, the patient is likely to drop out of treatment or change physicians. If the condition is resistant to treatment, another round of failures of this type is likely to lead to a search for relief outside the conventional treatment system. Thus, *both* the patient and the doctor have choices within the medical system.

31

An interactive process of this type operating over a period of time would tend to enhance the popularity of some drugs and reduce the popularity of others within the same therapeutic class. It would also tend to isolate the distinguishing features of drugs with similar indications for use. Inadequacies in the treatment system might also be attested to indirectly by the relative popularity of certain self-help organizations like Weight Watchers and Alcoholics Anonymous.

Despite the fact that it is the physician who is doing the prescribing and recommending, there is a powerful element of consumer satisfaction in all of this that must be afforded an important place in our thinking about drug utility and in our attempts to explain the relative popularity of particular drugs. How often physicians prescribe drugs in a particular therapeutic class, and to whom, is another question.

**Consequences of Treatment.** A systematic analysis of consequences, similar to the one proposed for coping choices and alternatives outside the health care system, should be carried out for the more traditional therapeutic alternatives. Questions about relative costs, benefits, and risks can be legitimately applied to a variety of clinical choice situations: the use of drugs versus the use of one or more nondrug therapies, the use of one type or class of prescription drug versus the use of another, the use of drugs versus surgical intervention, the use of drugs in an otherwise hopeless or ultimately hopeless situation—any situation where, in effect, drug therapy stands in opposition to some other therapeutic maneuver or to no treatment at all. However, very encompassing cross-modality treatment comparisons are seldom undertaken, whether in the form of logical analyses of costs, benefits, and risks or in the form of controlled clinical evaluations.

If we speak about relative efficacy, we should also speak relatively about other aspects of the costs, benefits, and risks of treatment. In the terms of a currently fashionable joke, the sour philosophical observation, "Life is unbearable," is met with the highly practical retort, "Compared to what?" The same question should be posed in any serious examination of the virtues and drawbacks of current treatment practices—and hopefully in the same practical spirit.

### What Influences Coping Behavior and Treated Prevalence?

To gain a better understanding of the consumer's use of pharmaceuticals, it is helpful to identify some of the factors that may influence coping decisions and treated prevalence—factors that affect the flow of persons into treatment in the health care system. I think we can agree, at least logically, that severity of illness is probably the primary determinant of coping behavior and treated prevalence. Coping begins with illness, and it is severe illness that propels people to the doctor. However, as I have previously indicated, that still leaves a great deal of variance to be explained.

Among the more basic considerations affecting that flow of persons into the treatment system are personal and cultural criteria of illness, the kind of critical thresholds that are exemplified in the following questions: At what point does a person admit to illness? How does he label his illness? To what does he attribute it? How much discomfort or incapacity is he willing to tolerate? When does he admit to defeat or helplessness? At what point does he decide to seek help from the physician and adopt the sick role? What is being explored in these questions is the outline of a deep-seated characterological orientation akin to the puritan ethic. In a contemporary drug context this orientation has been termed "pharmacological Calvinism." [3]

Demographic factors, such as sex and age, and specific attitudes and beliefs about drugs and illness are also likely sources of explanation for observed variations in coping behavior; in conjunction with more potent disease factors, they may play a significant role in establishing treated prevalence—that is, in determining both the type and proportion of persons from our hypothetical pool of illness who seek treatment at any given time. However, the number of persons in treatment is probably much less expandable than is commonly believed, because illness is not a simple matter of consumer preference. Much more basic biological, social, and economic forces are involved—ones that are not so readily influenced by sophisticated marketing and promotional activity. In the case of prescription pharmaceuticals, marketing and promotional activities are directed exclusively to the physician, a fact that is often overlooked in current dialogues about medication practices.

Logic notwithstanding, the more popular view is that we are in a period of treatment excesses, and many people are quick to accept annual increases in the volume of prescriptions as rather direct evidence that there are questionable forces at work to create illnesses where they did not exist before. There is, for example, a widespread belief that the antianxiety agents and many other kinds of drugs are being needlessly and inappropriately prescribed on a large scale, to the detriment of the patients and of society at large. The fault is variously attributed: Deficiencies in the physician's attitudes, training, or knowledge, and the built-in shortcomings of the current systems of medical practice may be blamed, or the broad-ranging, well-financed promotional and marketing activities of the drug industry may be held responsible. Or, in what is probably the most popular view, the putative overuse may be attributed to a general decline in public standards and a decay of traditional values, evidenced by a general unwillingness to persist or endure in the face of adversity and, in matters of health, to cope with illness by nondrug means.

In the light of these contentions, it is interesting that our survey findings on antianxiety drugs indicate that over two-thirds of the persons for whom these drugs had recently been prescribed evidenced high levels of psychic distress or life

---

[3] G. L. Klerman, "Drugs and Social Values," *International Journal of the Addictions*, vol. 5 (1970), pp. 312–19.

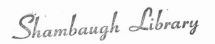

crisis or both, equivalent in degree and kind to those observed in a carefully defined population of psychiatric outpatients receiving drug treatment for anxiety neuroses.[4] Approximately three-quarters of the respondents who had taken the antianxiety agents regularly for two months or more met the severity criterion for psychiatric outpatients; another 22 percent of these regular users scored moderately high on either psychic distress or life crisis; and only 3 percent of these regular users were low on both indices.[5]

If we look at another side of the question, the side concerned with untreated prevalence, and ask what proportion of persons evidencing both a high degree of psychic distress and life crisis did *not* take medically prescribed antianxiety drugs in the year preceding interview, the answer is a surprising 65 percent for women between the ages of 18 and 74 and 79 percent for men in the same age range.

These findings do not fit conventional stereotypes; contrary to expectations the data argue that Americans are not prone to rush into treatment for minor ills and with minor provocation, at least where the antianxiety agents are concerned. The data also argue that the body of illness in the community is greater by a substantial margin than that observed in the health care system. But whether it is possible or even desirable to treat all these people in the health care system, with drugs or anything else, is a very difficult question with important economic, pharmacologic, social, and political implications.

In the case of hypertension the official position is that drug treatment is both possible and desirable.[6] This position implies that we know the morbidity and mortality of the disease, that we have effective drugs that can reduce both morbidity and mortality, and that we both know and are willing to accept the consequences of long-term use of these drugs. In the case of psychic disturbances and the antianxiety agents, the sentiment is to allow the untreated cases to remain untreated and to reduce the number of persons in treatment, on the assumption that most of those seeking treatment do not merit it. Whether these contrasting positions on hypertension and psychic disturbance can be justified on the basis of lifetime morbidity and mortality is open to question. Over the past ten years, evidence has been accumulating that life crisis and stress may be etiological factors in a wide variety of illnesses, but the effects of intervention with psychotropic drugs have yet to be determined.

---

[4] M. B. Balter, "An Analysis of Psychotherapeutic Drug Consumption in the United States," *Proceedings of the Anglo-American Conference on Drug Abuse, 16–18 April 1973* (London: Royal Society of Medicine, 1973).

[5] G. D. Mellinger *et al.*, "Psychic Distress, Life Crisis and Drug Use: National Drug Survey Data" (Paper presented at the Conference on Prescribing and Use of Anti-Anxiety Agents in Outpatients: Clinical, Pharmacologic, and Social Considerations, Bethesda, Maryland, 2–3 May 1974).

[6] U.S., Congress, Senate, Committee on Labor and Public Welfare, Statement by Charles C. Edwards, M.D., Assistant Secretary for Health, Department of Health, Education, and Welfare, 25 February 1974.

The crucial point of all of this is that, both as a society and as professionals, we often speak glibly about the overuse of pharmaceuticals without ever having established the true prevalence of the diseases for which the drugs are intended. If by overuse we mean that drugs are being prescribed for the wrong people or for the wrong reasons or that their potential for harm is worrisome, we should say so and then separate these more refined judgments from vague negative generalizations about sheer increases in the volume of prescribing. It is important to remember that better treatment of many diseases and better health care for previously neglected subgroups in the population are quite likely to produce what most people would regard as laudable increases in the overall volume of drug consumption.

In recent years there has developed a highly generalized tendency to equate drug treatment with "the bad" and getting along without drugs with "the good." Yet the consequences of no treatment, in terms of personal costs to the individual, remain essentially unstudied in a whole range of self-limited illnesses of both short and long duration and in chronic conditions of lesser severity. If the sheer ability to survive or weather a storm of illness without drugs is the test of appropriate prescribing or responsible patient behavior, then there is obviously little need for most pharmaceuticals.

Before we get further enmeshed in struggles over the costs of quality health care under one or another form of health insurance, it would be wise to remember that shifts in prescribing behavior under economic or regulatory pressures, although conceivably substantial, may tell us precious little about the estate of patients or the wisdom and rectitude of policy decisions, unless these changes are accompanied by enlightened analysis of the attendant costs, benefits, and risks.

Earlier, it was suggested that attitudes and beliefs about drugs and illness might influence coping decisions and thus affect the size and nature of treated prevalence. Data on the distribution of various public attitudes and beliefs about tranquilizing drugs and the relationship of these attitudes and beliefs to use of psychotherapeutic drugs prescribed by a physician are available from our community surveys in the United States [7] and western Europe.[8] In several studies in the United States, we have found attitudes toward tranquilizers to be essentially conservative. Almost three-quarters of American adults feel that minor tranquilizers are effective calming agents, but this judgment about effectiveness is relatively independent of other notions about tranquilizing drugs. One can entertain the idea that the drugs work very well and yet hold negative attitudes toward them, as most Americans do.

---

[7] D. I. Manheimer et al., "Popular Attitudes and Beliefs about Tranquilizers," *American Journal of Psychiatry*, vol. 130 (1973), pp. 1246–53.
[8] M. B. Balter, J. Levine, and D. I. Manheimer, "Cross-national Study of the Extent of Anti-Anxiety/Sedative Drug Use," *New England Journal of Medicine*, vol. 290 (1974), pp. 769–74.

As we have stated elsewhere,[9] doubts about the virtues of using tranquilizers encompass immediate and long-term physical effects as well as such potential moral and behavioral consequences as loss of control over one's actions or a reduced sense of responsibility. In addition, many people feel that the use of drugs that simply alter a mood or emotional state may mask symptoms or reduce motivation to change, thus interfering with the solution of underlying problems. Others feel that such drug use is evidence of moral or characterological weakness.

We also find consistent differences in attitude between users and nonusers of minor tranquilizers, that is, between people who have been treated with them by a physician and those who have not. These differences are clear-cut and highly reliable. They hold in the United States [10] and every country that we have studied in western Europe [11] or elsewhere, with users everywhere being much more positively disposed toward the drugs. However, because the data on attitudes and use were collected simultaneously, we cannot be certain that the attitudes preceded the use.

In the United States, interestingly enough, the significant differences in attitudes toward tranquilizing drugs between users and nonusers are obtained on the issues of morality, negative behavioral consequences, and efficacy, rather than on issues of safety, side effects, and long-term physical consequences. It is also worth mentioning that, differences notwithstanding, a large percentage of users hold unfavorable attitudes toward tranquilizers—a further indication of the conservative orientation of the American public and of the potential conflict situations in which they may find themselves.

A more refined analysis of the data for the United States indicates that, at all levels of psychic distress, persons with positive attitudes toward tranquilizers are more likely to have used such drugs than persons with negative attitudes. These data also suggest that strong negative attitudes and beliefs about tranquilizing drugs are a relatively greater deterrent to their use among persons with high levels of psychic distress than among persons with low levels of distress.[12]

When attitudes are measured by asking people whether they would condone the use of drugs in highly practical situations reflecting different degrees of interference with social functioning (in what is essentially a cost-benefit-risk framework), a majority of persons will sanction the use of psychotropic drugs if the individual is so distressed that he cannot meet his everyday work or family obligations.[13] This approach to attitude measurement may have virtue for what

[9] Manheimer et al., "Popular Attitudes and Beliefs about Tranquilizers."

[10] Ibid.

[11] Balter, Levine, and Manheimer, "Cross-national Study."

[12] I. H. Cisin, D. I. Manheimer, and S. T. Davidson, "The Mediating Effect of Attitudes and Beliefs on Psychotherapeutic Drug Use" (Paper presented at the Conference on Prescribing and Use of Anti-Anxiety Agents in Outpatients: Clinical, Pharmacologic, and Social Considerations, Bethesda, Maryland, 2–3 May 1974).

[13] Manheimer et al., "Popular Attitudes and Beliefs about Tranquilizers."

I am going to propose later—namely, that we obtain some input from the general population on what are currently considered to be esoteric cost-benefit-risk questions in the domain of drug development, research, treatment, and regulation.

## A Question about Drug Consumption

What do increases in the annual volume of prescriptions mean? It is important that we find out, because a clearer understanding of the phenomenon could alter some of our current assumptions about illness, coping, and health care.

Data on the annual volume of prescriptions for various classes of psycho-therapeutic drugs filled in U.S. drugstores for the years 1964 through 1973 are presented in Table 1 and displayed graphically in Figure 1. In 1973 there were 223.2 million prescriptions for all psychotherapeutic drugs filled in U.S. drug-stores, of which 104.5 million or 47 percent were for antianxiety agents (minor tranquilizers).[14] In that same year, drugstores filled 1.5 billion prescriptions for all drugs.

Over the past ten years, percentage increases in the annual volume of prescriptions for the antidepressants and antianxiety agents have been substantial, with antidepressants leading the way. However, because of sheer magnitude, the absolute increase in the number of prescriptions for antianxiety agents has captured much more attention. In Table 1 it can be seen that between 1964 and 1973 the number of prescriptions for antianxiety agents filled annually rose from 45.1 million to 104.5 million, a difference of nearly 60 million. During the same period, the yearly total of prescriptions for the sedatives, mainly phenobarbital and butisol, declined by approximately 4 million.

Trends in the annual volume of prescriptions for each of the principal drugs in the antianxiety-sedative category can be followed in Table 2. Three of the drugs selected, diazepam (Valium), chlordiazepoxide (Librium) and meprobamate (Equanil, Miltown) account for approximately 90 percent of the prescriptions in the antianxiety class.

What is important but not completely evident from the data presented is that since the mid-1950s drugs in the antianxiety-sedative category have been rapidly overtaking each other in a process that might be termed drug cannibalism. By the late 1950s phenobarbital had been exceeded and its market partially can-nibalized by meprobamate. This process continued, and in the early 1960s meprobamate was in turn superseded by chlordiazepoxide. Figure 2 indicates that

---

14 In this paper the term "antianxiety agents" refers to drugs with primary indications for the treatment of anxiety-tension states, for example, diazepam (Valium), chlordiazepoxide (Librium, Libritabs), meprobamate (Equanil, Miltown, and so on). Also known as minor tranquilizers, they can be distinguished from the sedatives—drugs such as phenobarbital and butabarbital—which produce more drowsiness and have some different indications for use. The antianxiety and sedative classes of drugs are sometimes treated as a single category because their indications partially overlap.

## Table 1

## PSYCHOTHERAPEUTIC DRUGS: PRESCRIPTIONS FILLED IN U.S. DRUGSTORES, 1964–73

**Prescriptions**
(millions)

| Drug Class | 1964 | 1965 | 1966 | 1967 | 1968 | 1969 | 1970 | 1971 | 1972 | 1973 |
|---|---|---|---|---|---|---|---|---|---|---|
| Antipsychotics | 14.3 | 14.8 | 16.9 | 16.5 | 17.8 | 20.2 | 21.9 | 22.2 | 23.2 | 23.8 |
| Antianxiety agents | 45.1 | 51.7 | 58.8 | 59.7 | 67.8 | 77.4 | 83.2 | 89.1 | 95.1 | 104.5 |
| Antidepressants | 9.5 | 9.8 | 12.6 | 14.8 | 16.3 | 19.1 | 19.8 | 23.1 | 25.0 | 28.5 |
| Stimulants | 26.7 | 28.0 | 26.1 | 26.8 | 27.2 | 26.9 | 28.2 | 21.3 | 11.6 | 8.6 |
| Sedatives | 24.1 | 25.0 | 23.8 | 22.4 | 22.1 | 22.2 | 23.8 | 22.5 | 20.7 | 20.3 |
| Hypnotics | 29.4 | 31.8 | 35.7 | 33.4 | 33.8 | 35.9 | 37.5 | 39.6 | 38.7 | 37.5 |
| Total [a] | 149.2 | 161.0 | 173.9 | 173.6 | 185.1 | 202.1 | 214.4 | 217.8 | 214.5 | 223.2 |

[a] Columns may not add because of rounding.

**Source:** *National Prescription Audit*, IMS America Ltd. Drugs have been reclassified and original data reorganized by Balter and associates, Psychopharmacology Research Branch, National Institute of Mental Health.

**Figure 1**
PSYCHOTHERAPEUTIC DRUGS: PRESCRIPTIONS FILLED
IN U.S. DRUGSTORES, 1964–73

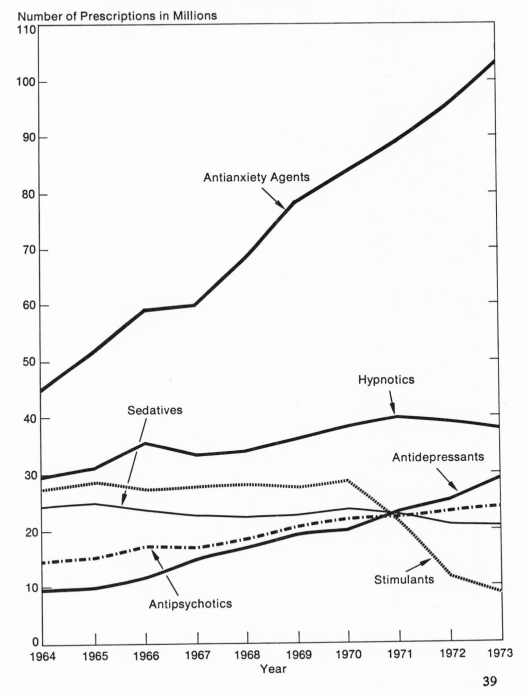

Number of Prescriptions in Millions

Antianxiety Agents

Hypnotics

Sedatives

Antidepressants

Antipsychotics

Stimulants

Year

## Table 2

## SELECTED ANTIANXIETY AGENTS AND SEDATIVES:
## PRESCRIPTIONS FILLED IN U.S. DRUGSTORES, 1964–73

**New and Refill Prescriptions**
(millions)

| Drug | 1964 | 1965 | 1966 | 1967 | 1968 | 1969 | 1970 | 1971 | 1972 | 1973 |
|---|---|---|---|---|---|---|---|---|---|---|
| Chlordiazepoxide | 20.6 | 21.1 | 24.8 | 24.1 | 25.6 | 27.2 | 26.9 | 25.2 | 23.2 | 22.7 |
| Diazepam | 4.6 | 8.2 | 10.2 | 12.8 | 18.7 | 24.9 | 31.8 | 40.7 | 50.3 | 58.4 |
| Meprobamate | 17.2 | 18.6 | 18.6 | 17.3 | 18.2 | 18.9 | 16.8 | 15.9 | 13.9 | 13.5 |
| Phenobarbital | 10.3 | 10.7 | 9.9 | 10.2 | 10.5 | 10.3 | 10.8 | 11.2 | 11.1 | 10.8 |
| All sedatives a (barbiturates) | 23.9 | 24.7 | 23.4 | 22.1 | 21.7 | 21.7 | 23.2 | 22.4 | 20.5 | 20.2 |

a Hypnotics are not included.

**Source:** *National Prescription Audit,* IMS America Ltd.

diazepam, which began its startling rise in 1964, passed phenobarbital in 1966, meprobamate in 1966, and by 1970 had gone ahead of chlordiazepoxide. In 1973, the 58.4 million prescriptions for diazepam alone exceeded the combined total of 56.4 million for chlordiazepoxide, meprobamate, phenobarbital and all other barbiturate sedatives.

Beginning in 1969, there has been a small but steady decline in the annual number of drugstore prescriptions for chlordiazepoxide and meprobamate. By 1973 these annual totals were down by 28.5 percent for meprobamate and 16.5 percent for chlordiazepoxide. Prior to 1969, increases in drugstore prescriptions for diazepam were accompanied by increases for chlordiazepoxide and by a general leveling off of prescriptions for meprobamate and phenobarbital. Since 1969, only phenobarbital has held its own, but it no longer has the same basic spectrum of use as the other drugs.

It is of interest that, between 1964 and 1973, annual increases in prescriptions for antianxiety agents *as a class* have fluctuated in nonsystematic fashion between 5.9 and 9.6 million per year, irrespective of what has occurred for particular drugs

**Figure 2**

SELECTED ANTIANXIETY AGENTS AND SEDATIVES: NEW AND REFILL
PRESCRIPTIONS FILLED IN U.S. DRUGSTORES, 1964–73

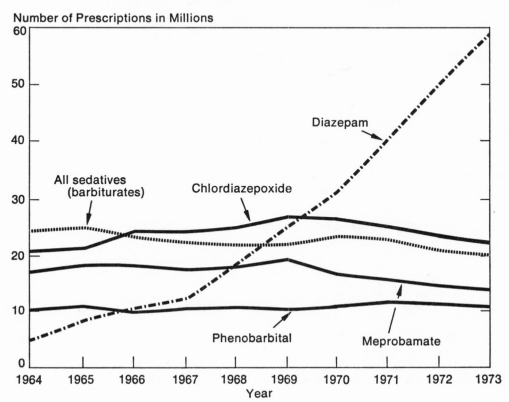

41

within the class or the size of the annual base.[15] It also appears that over the past ten years there has been very little change in the distribution of prescribing by diagnosis in instances of new therapy for the antianxiety agents as a class.[16] No matter what drug was in the ascendancy, be it meprobamate, chlordiazepoxide or diazepam, and despite promotional activities that tend to emphasize the differences between the drugs, the overall pattern of use by diagnosis for the class as a whole has remained fairly constant. What emerges is the strong impression that there is a definite place in the general practice of medicine for a safe and effective all-purpose sedative with muscle relaxant properties, and the drug that best meets those requirements at a particular time is the one that comes to be prescribed most frequently.

The rapid rise in popularity of diazepam is difficult to explain, at least for me, without some resort to a joint prescriber-consumer satisfaction model of the type discussed earlier, in which both doctor and patient have made an independent contribution. It may be that diazepam is effective in a wider range of conditions or that doctors favor it because it is less lethal or there is simply something more satisfactory about its overall clinical performance and effects on the patient. Another possibility is that the various drugs in the antianxiety class do not really differ from one another in any important respect and the dramatic rise of diazepam is simply the end product of a very ambitious promotional campaign. My best guess is that the startling success of diazepam in the outpatient market is the result of a potent interaction between a moderate to high level of prescriber-consumer satisfaction and a highly effective promotional effort.

A proper explanation of the rapid rise in the volume of prescriptions for the whole class of antianxiety agents is also elusive. For example, it is estimated that between 1964 and 1973 the annual number of physician visits (office, home, and telephone contacts) increased by 187 million, from 844.4 million to 1.031 billion.[17] In that same period, the annual volume of drugstore prescriptions for the combined category of antianxiety-sedative drugs increased by 55.6 million, from 69.2 million to 124.8 million. On the basis of these figures it would appear that an antianxiety or sedative drug was prescribed on 8 percent of all patient visits in 1964 and on 12 percent in 1973.

However, it remains unclear whether the increase in the annual volume of prescriptions is a reflection of more persons in treatment, of more chronic use, or of a higher rate of prescribing for the persons who come. It also remains unclear

---

[15] The period 1966–67 is an obvious exception. There was atypical growth for most classes of psychotherapeutic drugs between 1966 and 1967 because of uncertainties about the interpretation of the drug abuse control amendments that were enacted at that time.

[16] In this context, an instance of new therapy means the first use of a drug for a particular diagnosis in a particular patient. These instances are then summed across patients. Data on new therapy are collected routinely by the National Disease and Therapeutic Index (NDTI) of IMS America, Ltd.

[17] Unpublished data, U.S. Department of Health, Education, and Welfare, Health Interview Survey, National Center for Health Statistics.

whether the increases in patient visits have occurred in particular demographic or illness groups in which antianxiety-sedative drugs have been characteristically prescribed, or whether the increases have been more general. Also unknown is whether a higher proportion of the patients are chronic. These are difficult questions and in many instances cannot be answered because the required data are not available.

It is difficult to develop any fixed opinions about the factors responsible for the increases in the annual volume of prescriptions for the antianxiety agents. What has yet to be determined is the relative importance of promotional activities aimed at the physician, of increases in the volume of patients and patient visits, of changes in the age and illness characteristics of the patient population, and of shifts in the criteria of illness or in the popularity of various coping styles.

## A Call for More Enlightened Consumerism

While the consumer is busy coping with illness, others are making decisions about what is treatable, what therapeutic alternatives can and should be made available, how these may be obtained, and how they may be employed. This seems right and proper when the issues are basically scientific, technical, or medical, but they often are not.

Until now, most parties who have had a major voice in the varied processes of drug development, marketing, treatment, regulation, and control—and I include here government, industry, the scientific community, practicing physicians, and consumer protectionists—have subscribed to the general thesis that the public is basically uninformed and untrustworthy. People are seen as mainly childish, incapable of managing their own affairs in matters of illness and medication, and in need of protection from themselves, as are little children who lack critical judgment. Protecting the public often consists of preventing people from making any important decisions about their personal use of potent medications and excluding them from any meaningful participation in the development of major public policy in the area of drug safety, regulation, and control.

In the process of developing standards or policies for the protection of human subjects in research, or in similar standard-setting activities in the domains of drug development, treatment, and marketing, it would seem almost mandatory that the public be consulted or, if possible, enter the process in some more active way.

If past experience is an indication, advance publication of proposed policy guidelines, regulations, or action plans, although necessary and desirable, is not sufficient. Advance announcements will mainly elicit responses from individuals, groups, or institutions with a professional interest in the support and conduct of research or from organized lobbies with a specific point of view or an economic or political axe to grind. Such reaction is likely to be parochial and, to some extent, self-serving.

I propose a major research effort to determine what public attitudes are and to use the public as an active resource in the development of standards and basic principles just as certain professional organizations have used their membership to develop codes of ethics for research and treatment—by asking people to project themselves into hypothetical situations where they must make painful choices among alternatives or suggest acceptable courses of action. In this manner, it is possible to pose classical dilemmas and to gauge public sentiment on some crucial issues of cost, benefit, and risk.

Technical and scientific questions about the potential risks and probable benefits of certain types of clinical research or particular treatment procedures, or disagreements about legal rights, obligations, and consequences, are obviously not matters to be decided by public sentiment. They require special education, special experience, and a high level of professional competence. However, a great deal of what presently needs clarification or adjudication in the fields of science and medicine are questions about ethics and values or the setting of priorities in human affairs—issues that can properly be submitted to the public for decision. If we can require a jury, after clarification and instruction, to render decisions about life and death or settle complex questions of liability, then we can certainly ask the public, after proper orientation, to make difficult decisions about costs, benefits, and risks that affect their personal health and welfare.

Many people appear to speak directly for the public on the subjects of research ethics, drug safety, and the like, particularly the leading consumer advocates in the field of health. But, in actuality, policy positions are being taken by all concerned in the absence of any reliable knowledge about what informed public preferences or thinking might be.

Can complex value questions about what constitutes tolerable levels of risk in drug development, research, and treatment be conveyed to the general public in an intelligible fashion? Are people willing and able to enter judgments on such matters and suggest courses of action? Can they make difficult choices among hypothetical alternatives in the types of critical situations that would help us define a practical ethic or provide us with a set of general principles for weighing and balancing the benefits and risks in matters concerning drugs? As long as we insist on a principle of informed consent, as we no doubt should, we must presume that the answer to these questions is "yes." We should then proceed to probe public views through an active program of research. A well-designed study on the subject of costs, benefits, and risks that was aimed at the general public could also help us define the limits of informed consent.

Given what I consider to be a growing need for public input on sensitive policy issues and the growing emphasis that is being placed upon ethical standards, individual rights, and safety in both treatment and research, it seems imperative that we launch a massive and continuing program of public information and education concerned with the subtleties and complexities of cost-benefit-risk thinking.

The public must also be made aware of the probable long-term consequences of the various health policies and actions that are currently being proposed.

In my opinion we are in a difficult period of overreaction on matters of safety and ethics in drug treatment and research; and much of current consumer thinking and advocacy in this realm is based upon standards and expectations so high that they may be self-defeating in the long run. This stringent form of consumer advocacy, although welcome and admirable in many respects, is often unenlightened and may, in conjunction with other contradictory social forces, actually be impeding our movement toward safe and effective therapies. What is needed is more, not less, consumer involvement—but of a different type.

## Some Final Comments

There are inherent dangers to the public in the processes of drug development and research, in the aggregate therapeutic acts of the physicians who treat millions of people with marketed drugs, and in our system of opportunities for self-medication with over-the-counter drugs. The inevitability of these dangers must be acknowledged and dealt with in responsible community fashion by government, industry, consumers, physicians, and scientists alike, for it is pointless to simply deny or decry the existence of such risks or to demand that they be completely eliminated.

Once the inevitabilities of the situation are generally accepted, the major problem becomes one of defining a tolerable level of risk for the society at large. What is required for that task and presently unavailable is a very broad but highly discriminated framework for evaluating our national experience with pharmaceuticals—one that can accommodate economic, medical, pharmacologic, social, psychological, and ethical considerations. If we do not develop such a framework, it will be extremely difficult to achieve or maintain a happy balance between therapeutic and societal benefits and risks.

What I am suggesting is that we approach our national drug experience from the vantage point of the consumer who is coping with illness rather than that of the practicing physician, the regulatory agencies, the research community, or the drug industry. The individual who must cope with illness seeks relief in any way he can. At least in theory, all the choices and alternatives are available to him, both within and outside the health care system. He is also the most representative locus for the analysis of consequences. Almost any other orientation that might be entertained is more limited in scope and less appropriate to the task of attaining a balanced societal appraisal.

The problem of getting the public to think about drug development, treatment, and research in a realistic framework of costs, benefits, and risks is probably paramount. I am afraid that little else can be accomplished without some significant movement in that direction.

# COMMENTARIES

*John P. Bunker*

My comments on these papers will be from the vantage point of a quarter-century in the operating room, and I will attempt to draw lessons from studies of costs, risks, and benefits of surgical care that may be useful in this conference's scrutiny of the costs, risks, and benefits of drugs.

Dr. Melmon has called attention to the risks of drug therapy and has pointed out how little we know about the benefits, and, therefore, how little we can say about the relative value of costs (including risks) compared with benefits. This is certainly true of surgery as well.

I particularly like his point as to how little we know about the costs, risks and benefits of medicine as practiced throughout the country and how different these may be from the results of the few limited studies that find their way into the literature. I espouse his plea that we begin to develop data on what he calls a utility function by which we might try to quantify the quality of life, whatever this may be. For unless we begin to understand and develop such data on the quality of life, it is going to be very hard to draw any conclusions about what the effects of treatment may be on this quality.

Professor Peltzman calls attention to a somewhat different set of problems or needs: the potential benefits of more rapid introduction of drugs. In a sense, he is calling attention to large unmet medical needs. I am intrigued by his calculations and cannot really argue with them, but I would like to ask that in developing this interesting approach he consider the costs of the unnecessary use of drugs, or their overuse, or their use in situations where, perhaps, the patient might be better off without.

As an example, he has focused attention on the unnecessary days of hospitalization that result from failure to use tranquilizing drugs. I suggest that he ask, in addition, what is the loss in productivity and the possible loss in the quality of life of people who are taking tranquilizers. Might they be better off without them? This is clearly the kind of problem Dr. Balter has in mind in his discussion of how people cope with life.

I really do not know whether one patient or another is better off coping unassisted, assisted with drugs, assisted by group therapy, or what-have-you. But

I do think that Dr. Balter has put his finger on an essential—perhaps the most important—element in the decision process, the role of the consumer or patient. His ideas on how to enhance consumer involvement are fascinating, and I should like to come back to these in a moment.

What are the similarities of drug therapy to surgery? There are some dissimilarities, of course. Surgery is under much less restraint or regulation than the drug industry. The introduction of a new operation faces virtually no impediments or obstacles, as opposed to the very formidable ones which are of concern to Professor Peltzman.

Thomas C. Chalmers and David H. Spodick, in recent editorials, have specifically alluded to this double standard, but even with the lack of restrictions on surgery, many believe that there are large unmet surgical needs in the population. Others cite the observation of substantial geographic variations in operation rates as evidence of unnecessary surgery. But, as has been mentioned already this morning concerning drugs, we really do not have the data to allow us to make reliable cost-benefit decisions.

Without knowledge of the benefits of surgery or drugs, how can one say whether we are over-utilizing or under-utilizing—or whether both are occurring simultaneously? Indeed, I think it quite possible that we are under-utilizing our potential in some areas while over-utilizing it in others. We ordinarily blame practicing physicians for over-utilization of medical care, but the patient himself must assume some of the responsibility. The patient comes to the doctor because he wants something done, and his demands for treatment often exceed potential benefits. If the physician declines to provide the expected medicines or operation, the patient may simply look for another physician who will accede.

At this point it might be appropriate to make a comment about risks. Americans are risk takers, as Chauncey Starr points out, and we are willing to take large risks in the pursuit of things that we perceive to be desirable. In surgery, I think it is reasonable for a patient to accept a large risk of death in the pursuit of relief from disability, disfigurement, or discomfort. It is perfectly reasonable to accept, say, a mortality of 2 percent for a reconstructive hip operation, if you are in constant pain and are not able to walk in an acceptable fashion or do your job.

Unfortunately, we lack the information on which to base such a decision. We have no comprehensive data on benefits, and even our risk information is fragmentary. Worse yet, we do not really use, or are unaware of, existing data. I have come to the gloomy conclusion that when the risk of something as dramatic as death is below 1 percent in surgery, it sinks below the level of consciousness of physicians and surgeons and perhaps even anesthesiologists, although we are, perhaps, a little more risk conscious than surgeons.

There are a lot of other factors that provide incentives for medical and surgical intervention. Dr. Melmon has talked about the natural desire of the physician to be effective, decisive, and helpful. Eliot Friedson has called this the "bias toward illness." Then there is the very strong bias to be active and the strong motivation to avoid missing some potentially serious disturbance.

All of these biases provide strong motivation toward an active intervention that I believe must extend beyond any positive benefit-to-risk ratio. I would take as an example the appendectomy, where the risk of taking out an appendix that may turn out to be normal is one with which we do not very much concern ourselves. On the other hand, the risk of overlooking appendicitis is one with which physicians are very concerned indeed. There is some evidence, with which you may be familiar, that we are performing appendectomies well beyond the point of a positive benefit-to-risk ratio. When we do appendectomies at higher and higher rates for smaller and smaller indication, we eventually must come to the point where the risk of dying from the operation today, tomorrow, or next week is greater than the risk of dying from appendicitis sometime in the future.

I would like to join with Dr. Balter in making as strong a plea as I can for consumer involvement and for consumer education to prepare the public to assume responsibility for decisions concerning its own health care. When the femoral artery is cut and the patient is bleeding to death, you do not need to ask his permission to try to save his life. But when the quality of the patient's life is at issue, he or she must make the decision. Most patients today are not sufficiently well informed to assume this responsibility, of course, and the problem of education will be a formidable one. We may have to start back in high school and educate the public at that level, but one way or another I would like to see the public much more in control of its own medical fate. (Indeed, is that not what our children are complaining about today—their failure to be allowed to determine their fate politically, medically, and in every other way?)

I should like to see the establishment of a new cadre of para-professionals to carry out the systematic interviewing of patients, including the objective assessment of drug reactions, as suggested by Dr. Balter. Let the physician make the diagnosis and choose the treatment, but do not expect him to monitor the results. He is both biased and bored with such work and, as a result, he does a very bad job of it. In the clinical research laboratory, we assign a nurse to assess the effects of drugs, using double-blind techniques whenever possible. Why should not the monitoring, the surveyance of drugs, follow a similar pattern in practice? Ultimate responsibility for monitoring must, of course, remain with the physician. The report of a possible adverse reaction would be returned to the physician who then would make the decision to correct the dose, alter treatment, or take other action as appropriate.

Finally, I would like to comment on an approach we have taken to try to bridge the information gap on costs (including risks) and benefits. In a free enterprise economy, informed consumers ultimately must judge for themselves between costs and benefits. However, as we have seen and as the economists point out, in the medical care industry the consumer is not informed. There is, of course, at least one group of patients who must qualify as informed consumers, the physicians themselves, when they are ill and become patients. Therefore, we have looked at the numbers of operations that physicians and their families in California undergo; my prediction was that physicians, cognizant of risks as well as benefits, would have fewer operations, but I was quite wrong. It turns out, for example, that of wives of physicians in Santa Clara County, California, a very wealthy area, 50 percent will have had a hysterectomy by the age of 65.- This is a higher rate than for any of the other professional groups we studied, and 50 percent higher than for the country as a whole. It can be assumed that many were performed for sterilization or convenience rather than for conventional medical indication. It can be assumed that many would be deemed unnecessary by criteria that have been used by others. Yet, to the extent that hysterectomy was demanded by a knowledgeable consumer, one might reasonably argue that the operation did represent a perceived need. We did not collect data on how many drugs physicians take, and so I can only speculate about whether they are as casual in prescribing drugs for themselves and their families as they are enthusiastic about potential benefits of surgery. Based on our surgical data, I predict that the physician as informed consumer will be found to utilize drug therapy in excess of conventional medical indication. It will be an interesting study to carry out.

## Alex R. Maurizi

My remarks will be largely confined to the first two papers.

Dr. Melmon's paper is an extremely useful investigation of what constitutes the costs to the patient of the use of prescription drugs. These costs entail not only the purchase price of the drug but also the risk of toxic reaction to the prescribed drug. These costs can amount to considerably more than they ought to. In connection with the purchase price, although Dr. Melmon does not elaborate, I would think the high money price may be due to reduced competition among physicians, to the lack of incentive the physician has to minimize his patient's drug expenses, and to the inability of the patient to do so by shopping around since prescription is frequently by brand name rather than generic name. Dr. Melmon's suggested remedy is to make physicians less dependent on what is referred to as the "authority" and "dogma" of the drug salesman and drug advertisement and consumers less dependent on the authority of the physician. Regarding toxic reaction, Dr. Melmon informs us that these high costs are due to the physician's prescribing an inappropriate dosage of an appropriate drug or prescribing an inappropriate drug. The patient may also suffer, of course, if the physician fails to prescribe a drug when one is appropriate. The suggested remedy in this instance is further education of the physician in the administration of drugs. It would be helpful in this connection, he suggests, to collect reliable data indicating how a given drug would affect the state of the patient's health.

While it is desirable to have more reliable data and more educated physicians, I believe the key suggestion is that the patient's reliance on the authority of the physician should be reduced. The best way, of course, to grant the patient independence is to make available to him the information he needs to make the decision concerning treatment. The data to be collected on the risks involved in using drugs should ultimately be available to patients and in a form intelligible to *them*, not just to physicians. The patient has been forced to rely on the authority of the physician because physicians have effectively reduced the quantity and quality of information that patients have about the care they are getting and about alternatives to that care. It is not surprising, for example, that physicians have focused so much on treatment and have provided the patient with relatively little information about the prevention of illness and disease. In fact, it might be inferred from available evidence that the most important contributor to a person's lifetime state of health might be his mother, who provides most preventive treatment and instruction.[1]

Current government policy involves providing consumers with some information about drugs by assuring not only that only "safe" drugs are on the market, but that only "safe and effective" drugs are on the market. As Professor Peltzman has indicated in a recently published study,[2] however, efforts in this direction do entail a cost in the form of a reduction in the activity of developing new drugs. These costs are shown to be far greater than the benefits to patients that result from preventing wasted expenditures on safe but ineffective drugs. Policy should instead be directed, I think, toward ensuring that patients are properly informed about the properties of the drugs the physician suggests they use. The patient, after all, is the one who should make the final decision on whether to take the risk.

Professor Peltzman's current paper attempts to demonstrate that competitive market forces can reduce drug diffusion activity. His model assumes that new drugs reach the patient by being produced and then advertised or promoted to physicians. Competition from producers of related products (close substitutes), he claims, will tend to reduce retail prices and, hence, given the fixed costs of production and promotion, reduce the profits to the innovating firms and, therefore, the production of the new drug. The difficulties the producer faces in separating some kinds of customers from others prevent him from continuing production of a new drug at the same rate by selling it at a higher price to those willing to pay more than the majority, that is, by price discrimination.

---

[1] Charles Stewart and Corazon Siddayao, *Increasing the Supply of Medical Personnel* (Washington, D. C.: American Enterprise Institute, 1973), p. 65.

[2] Sam Peltzman, *Regulation of Pharmaceutical Innovation* (Washington, D. C.: American Enterprise Institute, 1974), pp. 54, 56, 72–73, 81.

He presents us with an enlightening illustration of the benefits of more rapid diffusion of the use of several drugs; the benefits can indeed be very substantial. The impediment to the distribution of these benefits is supposed to be the physicians who would not prescribe the drugs immediately because they were not convinced of their efficacy.

I have several comments to make concerning Professor Peltzman's discussion. First, it is based on assuming fixed production and promotion costs. As retail prices fall, profits must fall, and less of the new product will be produced. But competition at the wholesale level can be expected to drive production costs down, just as competition at the retail level will drive retail prices down. Added producers of a new commodity will ordinarily tend to operate at a lower average production cost since the demonstration of a proven market and profits will enable the later entrants to plan for a slower rate of production and a larger volume or longer run than the first firm. Suppose, for example, that production costs fall from $1.00 to $.25 in Peltzman's example. Given a $5.00 promotion cost, a profit of $.25 would be made even if retail prices did fall to $5.50. Which price falls more rapidly from competition (retail or wholesale), and hence which direction profits go (down or up), cannot really be determined from the theory. Moreover, it is also possible that increased competition will also reduce the costs of promotion.

Second, the evidence presented on the gains from more rapid diffusion does not constitute a true test of the model. An implication of the model is that less retail competition (hence, higher retail prices) will produce a more rapid diffusion, yet there is no evidence presented that there was less retail competition for polio vaccine than for TB drugs and tranquilizers.

Finally, the model ignores the possible benefits from increased production activity directed toward creating a well-informed patient. Those informed patients could search out physicians who were willing to prescribe the new drugs immediately. Indeed, if all the needed information about drugs could be made available to the patient, it is not at all clear that the physician should have final authority over whether the patient should consume the drug. As I understand it (from the data Dr. Balter reported concerning the rate of drug use in France and Italy of drugs that are available in the U.S. by prescription only) the often expressed fears that making prescription drugs available without a prescription will result in enormous increases in the use of these drugs seem to be unfounded. The reference to a study which concluded that consumers choose over-the-counter drugs rather wisely tends to support the reasonableness of removing the final authority the physician now has over certain drugs.

Let me return for a few comments relating to Dr. Melmon's framework, namely, the reasons for the high cost of drug use. It should not be forgotten that even if we know all that can be known about the various effects of drugs, a substantial cost of using drugs, their high monetary price, will remain. This is undoubtedly due in part to the extensive regulation of the retail end of the pharmaceutical industry.

It is difficult for me to understand how the public interest is served by requiring pharmacists to spend five or more years in training when in 1970 over 98 percent of all prescriptions were compounded by the manufacturers, not by the pharmacist at the retail pharmacy.[3] The retail pharmacist does little more than transfer pills from one bottle to another, and he sometimes does not need to do even that. Nor do I understand how the public interest is served by regulations like the following:

(1) Prohibition of advertising of drug prices or of the fact that drugs are sold at discount prices [4] (when chain prices are 12 to 14 percent lower on the average than independent prices).[5]

(2) The requirement that pharmacy floor space be a minimum of 10 to 15 percent of the store's total floor space (when chain pharmacies typically are less than 5 percent and independent pharmacies between 10 and 15 percent of total floor space).[6]

(3) The requirement that pharmacies be owned or managed only by a pharmacist.[7]

(4) The requirement that a pharmacy be fully stocked and ready to open for business before granting it a license to operate.[8]

(5) The requirement that members of state boards of pharmacy be approved by or be members of the state pharmaceutical association (when most state associations are dominated by independent pharmacists).[9]

The effect of these regulations at the retail level has been to reduce the competition facing independent or self-employed pharmacists from more efficient chain pharmacies, which typically dispense 60 percent more prescriptions annually using about 6 percent more space, operating about 20 percent longer hours, and using about 30 percent more pharmacist man-hours than the typical independent.[10] Historically, competition from the chains in all the products sold in drugstores

---

3 Horst Brand, "Productivity in the Pharmaceutical Industry," *Monthly Labor Review,* March 1974, p. 13.

4 F. Marion Fletcher, *Market Restraints in the Retail Drug Industry* (Philadelphia: University of Pennsylvania Press, 1967), pp. 224–39.

5 George F. Slavin, ed., *The Lilly Digest: A Survey of Community Pharmacies* (Eli Lilly and Company, 1973), pp. 7, 18–19; William J. Turenne, ed., *The N.A.C.D.S.-Lilly Digest: A Survey of Chain Pharmacies* (Eli Lilly and Company, 1973), pp. 5, 12–13.

6 Slavin, *Lilly Digest,* pp. 7, 18–19; Turenne, *N.A.C.D.S.-Lilly Digest,* pp. 5, 12–13; Fletcher, *Market Restraints,* pp. 214–16.

7 Fletcher, *Market Restraints,* pp. 137–60, 242–55.

8 Ibid., p. 297.

9 Ibid., pp. 40–53.

10 Slavin, *Survey of Community Pharmacies,* pp. 7, 18–19; Turenne, *Survey of Chain Pharmacies,* pp. 5, 12–13.

was stifled by fair trade laws.[11] More recently, as these laws have been felled by the courts, chain competition for the prescription drug business has been stifled in some states by the kinds of regulations just mentioned. The preliminary results from a study currently under way by a colleague, Fred Siskind, and myself indicate that, using 1970 census data on individuals, the earnings of self-employed pharmacists are significantly higher per hour in states with many such regulations than in states without such regulations, after controlling for the experience of the pharmacist, the per capita income of the state, and the ratio of pharmacists in community pharmacies per 100,000 population of the state in which he practices. Moreover, the earnings of employee pharmacists are also significantly increased in the more restricted states. This latter result is probably due to the fact that regulations reducing entry by new chain stores reduce competition among the chains and hence tend to increase the earnings of their employees, including pharmacists.

The results also suggest that pharmacist earnings are about as much influenced by changes in the number of pharmacists per capita as they are by the presence of regulations. The two variables having to do with price advertising had an effect either opposite to their expected one or no effect at all on earnings, incidentally. We understand from conversation with Dr. F. Marion Fletcher, however, who gathered all the data on state restrictions, that the price-advertising restrictions data is not reliable. There evidently is little or no price advertising even in states where it is allowed, and Dr. Fletcher suggests that there are other ways for independent pharmacists to prevent price advertising. Data on one variable, the pharmacist-manager requirement (to be carefully distinguished from the pharmacist-owner requirement, which recent court action has indicated does not constitute a denial of due process, thus reversing a long-standing decision and setting the stage for further state restriction), indicate that pharmacist earnings are *less* in states with this requirement, an unexpected result. Could it be that pharmacists sometimes do not understand what is really in their best interest?

Matters such as these, in addition to those touched on by the panel members, will need careful attention if the public interest is to be served.

---

[11] Fletcher, *Market Restraints*, pp. 54–68.

# HIGHLIGHTS OF
# THE DISCUSSION

The floor discussion dealt with one central topic—the lack of precision in current attempts to measure the costs and benefits of prescription drugs. Dr. Louis Lasagna pointed out that we do not have the hard data needed to say anything definite about how much of a problem there actually is with bioavailability of drugs or how many adverse reactions result from drug therapy. He said, "The only thing we know for sure is that drugs capable of producing good effects and bad effects can be around for a long time and can be widely used without people being aware of a serious bioavailability problem. . . ." Dr. Melmon essentially agreed with Dr. Lasagna on this point, adding that he had tried to note this lack of information in the Office of Technology Assessment (OTA) report. Melmon stated, "The rather passive way that we investigate bioavailability as it relates either to efficacy or to drug toxicity is something that really cannot be condoned. . . . Considerably more study should be made."

Two possible procedures for testing drug costs and benefits were proposed. Dr. Rita Campbell suggested a comparison of the number of days worked by patients before drug therapy with the number worked after drug therapy to determine if and when drugs have a significant positive benefit. This test would be particularly important for evaluating treatment of ambulatory patients, since studies of hospital drug use are biased against drug benefits. This is because adverse drug reaction cases are more concentrated in hospitals than in the general population. We have no idea of the benefits the population receives from drugs since those people who experience no problems with drugs are not in the hospital when the studies are made.

Dr. John Bunker suggested that studies of how doctors prescribe for themselves (and their immediate families) would give us information about how they judge the relative benefits of drugs in treating illness. This test would be similar to the procedure for the study of surgical practices among doctors, on which Dr. Bunker reported in his comments. In terms of the overall topic of cost-benefit analysis, Dr. Melmon concluded, "It would certainly help if this whole subject were treated as a more scientific venture. It is a bad thing when people think fancy is fact."

Commenting on Peltzman's study of the benefits of more rapid diffusion of drug information, Dr. Edward Burger of the National Science Foundation made the point that when we know a great deal about a disease such as polio and the effect of a drug on this disease, it is relatively easy to associate the use of the drug with the measured benefit. But when we have very little scientific information, as in the case of tranquilizers, about how drugs affect the various conditions they are used to treat, it is quite difficult to associate the use of a drug with some measure of benefit. As Dr. Burger concluded, "One really does not know whether or not the utility of tranquilizers in the conditions [Peltzman] has alluded to really make the differences that he talked about."

In reply, Peltzman said that his conclusions about the benefits of tranquilizers in reducing the length of hospital stay of mental patients was based on what he "read from the data." He summarized his findings as follows: "Before those drugs were introduced, the average stay in a mental hospital was eight hundred days. It is now on the order of four hundred days." He added that if doctors had been less reluctant to adopt tranquilizers, there could have been large benefits to counter whatever risks the doctors thought they were taking. Peltzman concluded that "given the kind of experience we have had with pharmaceutical agents, I am suggesting it is a good risk to try something that promises some reduction in [hospital stays] earlier than we might otherwise have."

# PART TWO

## FACTORS AFFECTING DRUG COMPANIES' INCENTIVES AND PERFORMANCE

# CHAIRMAN'S COMMENT

*Murray L. Weidenbaum*

The three papers to follow are variations on a common theme: the reported profitability (rate of return on investment) in the drug industry differs from the true rate of return because of accounting conventions, notably the treatment of research and development (R&D) and advertising as current expenses rather than as capital outlays.

Professor David Schwartzman of the New School for Social Research attempts to estimate the expected rate of return on investment in the pharmaceutical industry. He also offers some interesting empirical data, such as the estimate that it takes about ten years to discover and develop a new chemical entity and that the average R&D cost per entity comes to $24.4 million. Dr. Schwartzman concludes that, assuming the average life of a new drug to be fifteen years, pharmaceutical companies can expect to earn 3.3 percent on their investment in R&D; an alternative estimate based on an assumed twenty-year life yields an expected rate of return of 7.5 percent. He terms both rates "quite low," and states that the expected rate of return in 1960 was much higher than it is now, because the number of new drugs that were coming out was much larger and the research period much shorter.

Professor Robert Ayanian of the University of Southern California presents a model that incorporates advertising and R&D as well as the more traditional types of investment. He points out that these additional items should be treated as investments because of the long time-lag between the expenditure in advertising and R&D and the revenue that results from the outlay. As is the practice with conventional capital investment, he charges off against current income the annual depreciation of what he calls ARD capital (advertising and R&D). He also treats the interest forgone on the funds devoted to ARD capital as a cost of earning the resultant revenues. For a sample of six pharmaceutical firms, Ayanian estimates that their average return on investment, with his modifications, was about 14 percent in 1973. This compares with the reported return of 17.7 percent.

Professor Thomas Stauffer of Harvard University applies to the drug industry a model that he developed originally to measure the rate of return in the oil and gas industry. He points out the considerable number of difficulties that exist in estimating the true rate of return for a company because the problem of the time-lags in the R&D process persists throughout the accounting process. He states that, under certain—but not all—conditions, capitalizing R&D yields an improved measure of the profitability of a company. And he warns us that we cannot use standard accounting techniques to measure profitability whenever there are time-lags involved, particularly as prices change. In general, the greater the R&D intensity of a firm, the greater will be the overstatement of profits. The overstatement decreases as the company's growth rate increases.

According to Professor Stauffer, the real rate of return is also sensitive to the length of the period required for developing a new product. Companies with high ratios of working capital to fixed assets exhibit smaller errors in the rate of return than do companies with lower ratios. Stauffer's data for a number of drug companies show that, in most cases, capitalizing R&D and advertising yields a lower rate of profitability than that actually reported. In a few cases, however, the adjustment results in higher rates of return.

In his discussion of the papers, Dr. Frederic Scherer of the Federal Trade Commission states that it is not altogether surprising to find in an industry with advertising, high research costs, and also rapid growth that the current practice of treating R&D and advertising costs as expenses tends to lead to an overstatement of accounting profit rates. He raises the question of whether the bias is more serious in the drug industry than it is in other industries. He offers a series of technical criticisms of the formal models presented in the three papers.

In terms of public policy implications, Dr. Scherer pursues the consequences that may arise from a cutback in drug research due to the low return on investment in R&D. He questions whether the cutbacks would center on drugs of entirely new therapeutic value or on those that are just slightly better than the existing chemical entities.

The second discussant, Professor Edmund Kitch, of the University of Chicago Law School, focuses on the criticisms that have claimed that the high reported rates of return in the drug industry indicate a lack of competition. He states that sustained high profits by a firm may be consistent with a competitive industry structure; they may be explained by such hypotheses as that a growing industry needs a superior rate of return to attract capital from other investment sectors or that high returns are a reward for superior management.

Professor Kitch maintains that if we expect private firms subject to competition to continue to be important providers of information about their products, the incentives provided by the patent and trademark laws are required. He also points out problems that would arise from current proposals that drugs be procured or prescribed only on a generic basis and not by trade or brand name. He notes the incentive that the approach would provide for drug producers to meet, but not to exceed, the standards set by government.

The third discussant, Professor Martin Bailey of the University of Maryland, analyzes the models underlying each of the papers. He points out that the accounting rate of return is higher than the true rate of return when both are greater than the rate of growth of capital. The accounting rate of return is less than the true rate of return if both are less than the growth rate of capital. If the rate of growth of the firm's capital is the same as its true profit rate, then there is no error in the accounting. He emphasizes Professor Stauffer's point that accounting practices increase the dispersion of reported rates of profit compared to the dispersion of true profit rates.

Professor Bailey also raises the question as to whether the drug industry is going through a transient phase as it adjusts to a new set of ground rules by the Food and Drug Administration (FDA) and whether ultimately its financial position will look like that of other industries. With the tougher rules, according to Bailey, it will not be profitable to develop as many new drugs, and the R&D pattern will change. He wonders, as does Dr. Scherer, whether the reduction in the rate of innovation of new drugs will affect mainly "mediocre" ones.

In the discussion period, some attention was given to the term "mediocre." It was pointed out that the term may be misleading if the drugs that are produced are those offering a high economic promise of return, that is, if they treat conditions experienced by large numbers of people. In this sense, the "mediocre" drugs not developed may be those that would have treated conditions experienced by a relatively small number, but that would have been excellent in a medical sense.

The discussion also brought forth a number of other issues, such as the need to take account of the valuation of inventories and other assets, the methods of depreciation, and similar factors that can distort profitability comparisons, particularly in an environment of inflation.

# PHARMACEUTICAL R&D EXPENDITURES AND RATES OF RETURN

*David Schwartzman*

## Introduction

Investment in drug R&D will be maintained only if the expected rate of return at least equals that expected from alternative investments. Accordingly, I will estimate the expected rate of return from drug industry investment in R&D, and I will discuss it in relation to what appear to be reasonable estimates for other industries.

The estimate will refer only to the return from investment in R&D. The income on which this return is computed is adjusted for a group of costs associated with the production of the newly developed drugs, including the costs of financing plant and equipment and providing working capital. The estimate thus will not refer to the return from total investment in the drug industry.

We must also distinguish this expected rate of return from the accounting rate of return on investment. The expected rate at any moment is estimated on the basis of an expected stream of future investment and income. The estimate of the investment is based on projected costs of the required services, goods, equipment, and so forth. The estimate of the income is based on expected prices and associated costs. By contrast, the accounting rate of return for any year is calculated on the basis of the book value of investment and the income of that year. The expected rate of return is forward looking, as the name suggests, and thus is the relevant criterion for investment decisions, while the accounting rate is a measure of the success of past investments. The accounting rate frequently is used as a measure of the expected rate, and the distinction is not always made. In the drug industry the resulting error is likely to be large because of the long R&D period for a new drug and the consequent long lag of income behind investment. Thus, one reason the current accounting rate of return on total investment, measured by the rate of profit on stockholders' equity, is relatively high in the drug industry compared to what it is in other industries is the continued large sales of some major drugs introduced in the late 1950s and early 1960s. In recent years innovations have not been as numerous, so the expected rate of return on investment is not likely to be as high as the accounting rate.

The estimate of the expected rate of return will be for the industry as a whole. The average, it should be noted, is weighted, with the large firms given a greater weight than the smaller ones. Thus to obtain the average expected rate of return, we compute the average cost of R&D per new single chemical entity (NCE) using industry aggregates. Since large firms contribute most of the total R&D expenditures and discover most of the NCEs, the average reflects their experience more heavily than that of small firms.

Since the investment in the R&D for a new drug spans several years, our equation represents it as a stream of discounted expenditures. These expenditures are offset by the resulting stream of discounted income. The equation determines the rate of return yielded by the projected stream of investment and income. If this expected rate of return is high compared to that available for other investments, then the investment is attractive. The formula is as follows:

$$\frac{c_1}{(1+i)} + \frac{c_2}{(1+i)^2} + \cdots + \frac{c_n}{(1+i)^n} + \frac{y_{n+1}}{(1+i)^{n+1}}$$
$$+ \frac{y_{n+2}}{(1+i)^{n+2}} + \cdots + \frac{y_{n+m}}{(1+i)^{n+m}} = 0,$$

where $c$ = cost of research, $y$ = net income after associated costs, $i$ = discount rate, and the subscripts refer to years. The $c$s have negative signs. The problem is to solve for $i$, given estimates of the $c$s and the $y$s.

## The Expected Rate of Return on R&D Performed in 1973

**Estimating Costs.** If the goal of public policy is to encourage *significant* therapeutic discoveries, then we must estimate the current (1973) expected rate of return on investment directed only to such discoveries.

The list of significant discoveries used in this study is based on Paul de Haen's list of new single chemical entities (NCEs), which excludes new combination drugs and new dosage forms. Since a close inspection of de Haen's NCEs reveals derivatives of other more basic agents and other minor additions, my own list is even more restrictive.[1]

---

[1] Paul de Haen, Inc., *de Haen Nonproprietary Name Index*, vol. 8 (New York: Paul de Haen, Inc., 1971). I removed from de Haen's list of NCEs the following items: diagnostic aids, hospital solutions, nonabsorbed high molecular weight compounds, impure extracts of natural origin, new uses and formulations of previously marketed drugs, new single components included in previously marketed mixtures, new salts and esters of previously marketed drugs, and drugs which were later withdrawn.

The list excludes those drugs discovered and developed by foreign companies that were not members of the Pharmaceutical Manufacturers Association (PMA) in the period on which the estimate of the cost of R&D was based. These drugs are excluded because the estimate of the cost of R&D is based on PMA's estimate of R&D expenditures, which includes only members' expenditures. PMA's estimate includes world expenditures of U.S.-based companies but only U.S. expenditures of foreign-based member companies. Thus NCEs introduced by foreign-based members are included in the list of discoveries, but only part of their R&D expenditures are included. Hence the average R&D investment per discovery will be understated, and the expected rate of return will be overstated.

The estimation of the expected rate of return from R&D investment requires certain assumptions. Specifically, I assume here that the discovery and development of a new drug will require as much effort in the future as was required for the drugs introduced in the period 1966–72, and that the R&D period is ten years. This estimate of the required period is based on previous estimates by Dr. Lewis Sarett and Harold Clymer. According to Dr. Sarett, the time required to develop a product after completion of the discovery stage is five and one-half to eight years, exclusive of the average two-year period that he estimates is required for a company to obtain FDA approval. The total development period thus is seven and one-half to ten years. Dr. Sarett does not estimate the length of the discovery period, nor has anyone else in the industry done so explicitly, probably because the beginning date of research on a particular compound is difficult to identify. The exploratory research in a disease area that eventually leads to a drug may have begun many years before identification of the compound that leads directly to the final drug, and over the years many compounds that turned out to be false leads may have been synthesized.[2]

Harold Clymer estimated the development period inclusive of FDA approval to be five to seven years. Clymer's estimate of the entire R&D period is ten years, which implies a discovery research period of three to five years.[3] Adding this estimate to Sarett's more recent estimate of the development research period of seven and one-half to ten years yields a total of five and one-half to fifteen years. Thus my estimate of ten years for the entire R&D period is less than the lower limit of the range derived from the Sarett and Clymer estimates and is therefore conservative.

To obtain the expected rate of return we will estimate the R&D cost per NCE of drugs introduced in the 1966–72 period. The research period for those drugs appearing in 1966 was 1956 through 1966, of which 1961 is the middle year. Similar reasoning for each of the other years of the 1966–72 period results in the selection of the years 1961 to 1967 as the period on which we base the estimate of R&D cost. The average annual expenditure of the industry during these years, according to the Pharmaceutical Manufacturers Association (PMA), was $281.4 million.

To obtain the current cost of R&D, we must adjust this figure for the increase in prices since 1961–67. For this purpose I use 1964, the middle year of this period, as the point of reference, and I estimate that the rise in the cost of R&D

[2] L. H. Sarett, "Impact of FDA on Industrial Research and Development" (Paper presented at the University of Chicago Conference on Drug Regulation, 18 October 1973).

[3] H. Clymer, "The Changing Costs and Risks of Pharmaceutical Innovation," in J. D. Cooper, ed., *The Economics of Drug Innovation* (Washington, D. C.: American University, 1970), pp. 115–16, and "The Economics of Drug Innovation" in M. Pernarowski and M. Darrach, eds., *The Development and Control of New Drug Products* (Vancouver, B. C.: Evergreen Press, Ltd., 1972), pp. 110–29.

due to price changes between 1964 and 1973 was 48 percent.[4] Since no further correction is made for the increase in cost due to the greater demands of the Food and Drug Administration (FDA) for evidence of efficacy and safety in a new drug application (NDA), the total current cost of industry research that would result in the same number of NCEs, new combinations, and new dosage forms would equal 148 percent of $281.4 million, or $416.5 million.

We must now estimate the part of this R&D total that is allocable only to NCEs. Since the industry's discovery, as opposed to developmental, effort is devoted wholly to the search for NCEs, its cost must be allocated entirely to these drugs. My estimate of discovery research's share of total R&D cost is 50 percent,[5] yielding an estimated annual cost of a contemporary discovery research program of the same size as that which resulted in the NCEs discovered in 1966–72 to be equal to 50 percent of $416.5 million, or $208.2 million. Since the average number of NCEs produced each year by the industry was 12.3, the average discovery cost per NCE would be $16.9 million.

Developmental costs of R&D must be distributed between NCEs and other new products, including combination and dosage forms.[6] The resulting estimate

---

[4] Prices of goods and personnel services used in academic research increased by 36.4 percent between 1964 and 1971. Between 1968 and 1971, the rate of increase of prices was about 6 percent per year and accelerating (see National Science Foundation, *A Price Index for the Deflation of Academic R&D Expenditures*, NSF 72–310 (Washington, D. C., 1972), p. 2, table 2. A conservative projection of the increase in prices to 1973 brings the estimate for the whole period up to 48 percent. A similar estimate is arrived at from the ratio of the index of nominal cost in 1973, as budgeted on base 1963, to the index of laboratory employment. Both indexes are computed from PMA data. Laboratory employment is taken as the measure of total real input for this purpose.

[5] This is a rough estimate based on private inquiries to manufacturers. The percentage varies inversely with the number of compounds in the developmental stage of research and directly with the absolute size of the discovery program.

To my knowledge, no estimate has previously been made of the share of total pharmaceutical R&D expenditures devoted to discovery research. The reason is that the expenditures per compound are only estimated by the research laboratories after the decision is made to perform clinical tests and toxicology testing begins, which in the industry's terminology marks the beginning of the development part of R&D. The discovery research will synthesize and test many compounds that never reach toxicology testing because they fail to show the desired biological reaction or because toxic effects are found in the early animal studies. The costs of such research are properly charged to the successful product candidates along with those costs that can be directly allocated to them. That discovery costs can constitute a large share of total R&D costs can be seen in the report by PMA that in 1970 its members "obtained, prepared, extracted, or isolated" 126,060 compounds, and tested pharmacologically 703,900 compounds. That developmental research was limited to a small number is shown by the fact that 1,013 compounds were tested clinically. See Pharmaceutical Manufacturers Association, *Annual Survey Report* (1970–71), p. 15.

[6] The share of total developmental cost accounted for by each product class is obtained by multiplying the number of new products in the class by the relative cost and expressing each product as a percentage of the sum of the products. On the basis of Jerome Schnee's estimates of costs of development, the relative developmental costs are as follows: NCE, one dollar; combination drug, thirty cents; dosage form, sixteen cents.

The estimate of the number of drugs in each class is based on de Haen, *Nonproprietary Name Index*. His figure for NCEs is corrected to exclude derivatives, and so forth, as described earlier, and the numbers so excluded are added to his number of new combination of the developmental cost adds $7.5 million to the cost of each NCE, for a total of $24.4 million. Although a company's total R&D cost per NCE before taxes is $24.4 million, a company in fact invests only the after-tax cost, which is approximately half or $12.2 million.

I assume that the expenditures are equally spread over the whole ten-year R&D period. This assumption of an equal distribution over time is conservative and results in overstating the expected rate of return, because the major portion of expenditures actually occurs early in the R&D period. Thus the discovery research, which accounts for 50 percent of total R&D costs, precedes the development period. Clymer, as we have seen, estimates the discovery period to be three to five years. We can combine these estimates with Clymer's estimates of the time distribution of the developmental expenditures for a successful product. On this basis about two-thirds of total expenditures occur in the first half of the R&D period.[7] The evidence thus suggests that the R&D expenditures are concentrated in the first few years of the R&D period and therefore that my assumption of an equal time distribution leads to an overestimate of the rate of return.[8] Our estimate of each of the $c$s in the equation for the expected rate of return thus is $1.22 million ($12.2 million divided by ten).

**Estimating Income.** We must also estimate the anticipated net income per NCE. Average sales in 1972 of the NCEs introduced in 1966–72 were $3 million. The figure is low, first because doctors take as long as two to three years to adjust their

---

drugs. The final number in each class was: NCEs, 86; combination drugs, 280; dosage forms, 154. It should be noted that these numbers include drugs introduced by nonmembers of PMA, while the PMA research expenditure figures include only those of members. Nonmembers have accounted for a larger share of new combination drugs and of new dosage forms than of NCEs. Thus the procedure results in an overestimate of the share of total R&D costs accounted for by combination drugs and dosage forms and, therefore, an underestimate of the cost per NCE. Hence the resulting bias is to overstate the final estimate of the expected rate of return on investment in R&D. See Jerome Schnee, "Innovation and Discovery in the Drug Industry," in Edward Mansfield *et al.*, eds., *Research and Innovation in the Modern Corporation* (New York: W. W. Norton, 1971), pp. 157–86.

[7] The distribution of expenditures over Clymer's twelve-year R&D period (four years for discovery plus eight years for development) is estimated as follows:

| Years | Percent |
|-------|---------|
| 1–4 | 50 |
| 5 | 7 |
| 6–7 | 17 |
| 8–9 | 18 |
| 10–12 | 8 |
| | 100 |

(Based on Clymer, "Changing Costs and Risks of Pharmaceutical Innovation.")

[8] Because of the time value of money, a stream of investment expenditures which is concentrated in the early part of any period is equivalent to a larger expenditure which is spread out more evenly over the whole period. See F. M. Scherer, "Government Research and Development Programs," in R. Dorfman, ed., *Measuring Benefits of Government Investments* (Washington, D. C.: Brookings Institution, 1965), pp. 12–70.

prescribing to new drugs and, second, because very few large-selling drugs were introduced in this period. We should therefore estimate the average sales per NCE in 1972 for a group of NCEs introduced over a period beginning before 1966 and ending before 1972 so as to include in our calculation some drugs whose sales were relatively large. Experimentation with a few periods led to the selection of 1962–68 as the one yielding a relatively high average. Again, the decision is made in such a manner as to result in an overestimate of the expected rate of return. The average sales in 1972 of NCEs introduced in 1962–68 were $7.5 million.[9] In order to include foreign sales in our estimate, on the basis of PMA's estimate for 1972 we can add 47 percent to the estimate of that year's domestic sales, which brings the total to 147 percent of $7.5 million, or $11.0 million per NCE.

We must now calculate the net profit after taxes. Net profit must include the share of total sales spent on R&D, since this expenditure represents new investment. The estimated profit margin, inclusive of R&D expenditures and after taxes, is 15.4 percent of sales. The estimate was arrived at as follows: I used a sample of six firms with over 60 percent of net sales from pharmaceutical products, summed the profits before taxes and R&D expenditures over the six firms, and expressed the sum as a ratio to the sum of net sales (see Table A–1).

The gross margin so computed must be adjusted to exclude the cost of financing the associated investment in plant and equipment, inventories, and receivables. When a new drug is developed and introduced to the market, there must be plant and equipment available to produce it, and funds are also required for working capital.[10] It is estimated that 2.6 percentage points of the gross

---

[9] Limiting the NCEs to those introduced between 1962 and 1968 permitted all of the drugs included to have had ample time to achieve their full sales potential by 1972. Thus 1972 represented the eleventh year of commercial life for the drugs introduced in 1962 and the fifth year for those introduced in 1968. In addition, the selection of this period results in a higher estimate of the expected rate of return than alternative selections, as the following table shows:

| Period of Introduction | Average Sales per NCE in 1972 ($ millions) |
|---|---|
| 1956–66 | 5.3 |
| 1960–68 | 6.3 |
| 1960–69 | 6.2 |
| 1962–68 | 7.5 |
| 1962–70 | 6.8 |
| 1965–69 | 5.6 |

[10] The total investment required for plant and equipment for the six companies in the sample is estimated conservatively on the basis of the book value of plant and equipment after depreciation in 1972. The book value of net working capital was added to obtain the required capital investment. A total for all six companies taken together was obtained. An interest rate of 8 percent was applied to this total to obtain the cost of financing. Not all of this estimated cost of financing could be deducted from the profit margin computed earlier, since the net income figure was net of interest payments. Hence, we subtracted from this estimate of the cost of financing the interest payments that were actually made. The cost of financing so adjusted was subtracted from the profits previously calculated and the result was expressed as a percentage of sales. More details are found in the Appendix.

**Table 1**

## ESTIMATED STREAM OF COST OF R&D AND NET INCOME FOR AN AVERAGE NCE

| Year | R&D Cost (c) ($ millions) | Year | Net Income (y) ($ millions) |
|------|------|------|------|
| 1 | −1.22 | 11 | .47 |
| 2 | −1.22 | 12 | .94 |
| 3 | −1.22 | 13 | 1.40 |
| 4 | −1.22 | 14 | 1.40 |
| 5 | −1.22 | 15 | 1.40 |
| 6 | −1.22 | 16 | 1.40 |
| 7 | −1.22 | 17 | 1.40 |
| 8 | −1.22 | 18 | 1.40 |
| 9 | −1.22 | 19 | 1.40 |
|   | −1.22 | 20 | 1.40 |
|   |       | 21 | 1.40 |
|   |       | 22 | 1.40 |
|   |       | 23 | 1.40 |
|   |       | 24 | .94 |
|   |       | 25 | .47 |

margin is required for these purposes, which leaves a profit margin of 12.8 percent of sales as the return on investment in R&D. When we apply this margin to annual sales of $11.0 million per NCE, we obtain $1.40 million in net profits per year per NCE. This is the estimated value, after sales level off, for each of the $y$s in the equation.[11]

We must now estimate the period during which a company can expect to sell an NCE in reasonably large quantities, and I estimate this commercial life to be fifteen years.

**Calculating the Expected Rate of Return.** The final task is to solve the equation for $i$ and so obtain the expected average rate of return. The estimated stream of $c$s and $y$s for an average NCE is shown in Table 1. The expected rate of return on R&D investment obtained by using this schedule is 3.3 percent.

---

[11] I assume that this leveling off occurs in the third year after introduction (year 13 of Table 1). Some evidence suggests that the period of introduction is longer, especially for widely used drugs. In that case, the short introduction period tends to overstate the rate of return. I should also mention that I assume that sales in the year of introduction (year 11 of Table 1) are one-third of the peak level (year 13 and the following years until the decline sets in) and two-thirds of this level in the year following the introduction. I assume that the decline beginning in year 24 is symmetrical with the growth period after the drug is introduced.

## Table 2
## EXPECTED RATES OF RETURN ON INVESTMENT
## IN R&D IN 1973

| | Estimated Rate of Return on Investment | |
|---|---|---|
| Gross Margin | Commercial life of 15 years | Commercial life of 20 years |
| 15.4[a] | 3.3 | 5.1 |
| 17.5 | 4.6 | 6.3 |
| 20.0 | 6.0 | 7.5 |

[a] This gross margin is based on company reports of profits before taxes plus R&D expenditures as a percentage of total sales. The percentage so arrived at is 30.8, which is then adjusted for taxes by dividing by two. See text and Appendix for additional details.

Before interpreting the significance of this estimate, I will present alternative estimates based on other assumptions regarding the gross margin and the length of commercial life. The objection may be made that the assumed gross margin is based on the total sales of the six companies and that their margins may be lower on nonpharmaceutical products than those on pharmaceutical products. In addition, the commercial life may be longer than the assumed fifteen years.[12] Consequently, I present in Table 2 other estimates based on gross margins (before correction for cost of financing fixed and working capital) of 17.5 percent and 20.0 percent,[13] and an assumed commercial life of fifteen years, as well as twenty years, together with the original estimate.

To determine whether the estimated rates of return are or are not sufficient to encourage the industry to continue investing in R&D, we must set up a standard for evaluation. An often used decision criterion in other industries used to be 10 percent after taxes. Several years ago this was the minimum rate required in farm machinery, textiles, and electrical equipment. The minimum probably has increased with the steep rise in the rate of interest since then. At approximately 10 percent today, it is about what would be required to obtain financing and

[12] The estimated commercial life in 1960 was five years, according to a study by W. E. Cox, "Product Life Cycles and Promotional Strategy in the Ethical Drug Industry" (Ph.D. diss., University of Michigan, 1963), chap. 4. The general opinion as expressed by Clymer, "Changing Costs and Risks of Pharmaceutical Innovation," is that the average life of new drugs has increased since then. Clymer himself assumes a life of fifteen years.

[13] We can see from the following analysis that 20 percent errs on the high side. The Securities and Exchange Commission 10-K reports indicate that the pharmaceutical sales of the companies in our sample account for 70 percent or more of total sales. (The higher this percentage is, presumably the higher is the overall gross margin, since the assumed error is for the gross margin on pharmaceutical products to be understated by the inclusion in total sales of other products.) We can also assume that the after-tax gross margin on sales of nonpharmaceutical products is no less than 10 percent. These estimates yield a maximum estimate of the after-tax gross margin on total sales of 17 percent, but we have seen that the overall margin in fact was 15.4 percent.

includes no allowance for risk. The minimum required rate for the pharmaceutical industry probably should be above that for other industries, because pharmaceutical R&D is more risky than investment in plant and equipment in this and other industries. The probability that a given research project conducted by a specific company will yield a successful product that will generate sufficient sales to recoup the investment plus some profits is small, and the probability appears to have declined since 1960. Thus, the minimum rate of return required for investment in the pharmaceutical industry should be above 10 percent. Nevertheless, in accordance with the rule of caution that we have been following, I will use 10 percent as the criterion.

Thus, the estimates of the expected rates from investment in pharmaceutical R&D are well below the minimum rate required in other industries. Apparently, the combination of current cost of research, of innovation rates, of product prices, and of sales yields a much lower expected rate of return from current investment in research than would be required to maintain such research at the current level. Indeed, the best estimate of the expected rate of return, namely, the one that is based on a 15.4 percent gross margin and a fifteen-year commercial life and equals 3.3 percent, is far below the required minimum. It is of some interest to see how much larger average sales of NCEs would have to be in order for the expected rate of return to reach the 10 percent decision criterion. The same assumptions concerning the gross margin and the commercial life yield a required level of sales of $23.5 million,[14] or 114 percent above the estimated level of $11.0 million.

What are the potential objections to my estimates? One immediately comes to mind, namely, that while the sales of NCEs can be expected to grow with the market as a whole, which has been growing at an average annual rate of 7 percent, I have assumed that the average sales of NCEs will remain at the same level as in 1972. The objection is not as serious as it may appear to be at first glance, because it is the sales of all ethical pharmaceutical products that have grown at the rate mentioned, rather than the average sales of new single entities, and part of the growth in total pharmaceutical sales is due to the introduction of new products that open new markets. It is true that the average sales of NCEs have increased since the early 1960s owing, at least partly if not wholly, to the decline in the number of new drugs per year. It is hazardous, therefore, to predict continued growth in average sales per NCE. For this reason, I have not assumed that average sales of NCEs will continue to grow.

In addition, the error resulting from the failure to provide for future growth of sales may be offset by other errors in the opposite direction that may together

---

[14] At this level of sales the net income (the $y$s in the equation for the expected rate of return) would be $3.0 million. It thus can be seen that the best estimate of the expected rate of return, which is 3.3 percent, is well below even the rate of return available on U.S. Treasury notes. This is true even of the estimate based on the twenty-year commercial life and the 20 percent gross margin.

be of approximately equal magnitude: my disregard of the increase of 6 percent per year in the prices of goods and services consumed in R&D; my omission of the rise in the costs of research due to both the increased difficulty of R&D and the greater regulatory requirements for approval of new drugs; and my disregard of all increases in the associated costs of plant and equipment since the time of construction of the existing units.

Another, more general, objection to the estimates of the current expected return on industry investment in drug R&D is that it may appear to be the result of a fanciful chain of reasoning. Since no one in the industry has reported making estimates of rates of return on R&D investment and the industry has continued to increase its R&D investment despite the low expected rates of return, it may seem that my estimate is wholly imaginary. Yet firms *do* consider the ultimate profitability of R&D expenditures, even if they do not use identical estimating procedures. Also, some financial analysts have recently made bearish forecasts of future industry earnings based on similar appraisals of the effect of the increase in R&D costs and the decline in the number of new drug product introductions.[15]

Moreover, the expected rate of return for the industry as a whole is only one consideration. Individual companies continue to increase their investments for a number of reasons: some firms expect to do better than average on the basis not only of their individual past records but also because of information they have about the prospects for specific research projects they have under way. This would be particularly true for compounds that have reached or gone beyond the stage of clinical trials designed to determine efficacy.[16] Similarly, their hope of a large return may be based on the possibility of a breakthrough in their own or in other laboratories that will inaugurate another stream of innovations. To be able to take advantage of such a breakthrough they must maintain research staffs and programs. In addition, individual companies may be willing to gamble in the hopes of beating the high odds against finding a drug that will have sales as huge as those of Valium.

The foregoing considerations can be summarized with the aid of the economic concepts of the short run and the long run. Pharmaceutical firms will maintain and possibly even increase their R&D expenditures on the basis of short-run expecta-

---

[15] The Futures Group, a consulting firm in Glastonbury, Connecticut, predicts a sharp drop in the average after-tax margin of the industry before 1980 as a result of increased R&D costs and an increased share of sales to hospitals, clinics, and health maintenance organizations (HMOs). No account is taken of the drop in the number of NCEs. See *Chemical and Engineering News*, 4 February 1974, p. 7.

[16] This consideration suggests that the firm's decisions to continue or discontinue research projects that are already under way will depend on information concerning the prospects of success that are specific to the firm rather than on the expected rate of return from investment in R&D in the industry as a whole. But the decision to inaugurate a new line of research may depend more on an evaluation of the prospects of success that gives a great deal of weight to the industry's performance, especially since any new project will take several years to complete and during this period the personnel engaged in the project may turn over. In other words, over a long period, a firm cannot count on doing any better than other firms of the same size, general location, and wealth.

tions. They already have the R&D staff and facilities, and they are not ready to abandon them, particularly if they are optimistic about the projects that they have under way. On the other hand, the estimates that I have made are pertinent to long-run decisions concerning business strategy. Should firms decide not to continue spending such large sums on research as they have in the past, they would in effect be giving up the strategy of increasing sales through innovation. In that case, they will have to develop another strategy, based perhaps on the manufacture and sale of generic products whose appeal will be based strictly on price. Although some firms have moved in this direction, not all firms may be ready to do so.

### The Expected Rate of Return on R&D Performed in 1960

It is reasonable to suppose that the pharmaceutical industry made large R&D investments in the 1960s because the expected rate of return at the beginning of that decade was attractive. To test this hypothesis, I estimated the expected rate of return on R&D for the industry in 1960, based on the number of new single entities appearing during the years 1955–58. Over this period the average annual number of new single entities was 36.5. I group derivatives with the original products and, since the R&D period was much shorter than it is now, I assume it to have been five years. Hence the period in which the research was done for the products emerging in 1955–58 can be estimated from the average expenditures per year in the 1952–55 period, which was $74.8 million. Since this was a period of price stability, it is reasonable to suppose that in 1960 it cost no more to do the required R&D for an NCE than it did in 1952–55. As before, I estimate that discovery research accounted for 50 percent of total R&D costs and that all of this amount is assignable to NCEs. The discovery cost per NCE was thus $37.4 million divided by 36.5 NCEs or $1.02 million per NCE.

The cost of developing an NCE was $285 thousand, and we add this amount to the discovery cost to obtain a total R&D cost per NCE of $1.30 million before taxes. We can now distribute the after-tax cost, $.65 million, equally over the R&D period of five years.[17] (Thus, $.13 million is the value of each of the $c$s in our formula.)

The income from each NCE is calculated as follows: Assuming that the gross margin was the same in 1960 as in 1973, or 15.4 percent, and that the cost of financing plant and equipment and working capital also represented the same

---

[17] I have been told by people who were members of industrial research laboratories at the time that the R&D period was much shorter. Moreover, Schnee ("Innovation and Discovery in the Drug Industry," p. 77) estimates the development period then to have been two years. Sarett's estimate for 1958–62 ("Impact of FDA on Industrial Research and Development") is the same. My estimate, therefore, tends to understate the expected rate of return in that earlier period.

percentage of sales as in 1973, or 2.6 percent,[18] the average sales per NCE in 1960 of those introduced between 1955 and 1958 was $2.2 million. Thus the net income (the $ys$) in the three-year plateau of the total five-year commercial life is estimated at $.28 million.[19] The result is an estimate of an expected rate of return of 11.4 percent. This is considerably larger than the current expected rate, but not very much above the postulated minimum rate of 10 percent required to attract continued investment.[20]

By performing calculations for 1960 similar to those for 1973 summarized in Table 2, alternative estimates for the expected rate of return during 1960 were derived. As Table 3 shows, these alternative estimates of the expected rate of return from investment in R&D in 1960, based on assumed gross margins of 17.5 and 20.0 percent, are substantially higher. These alternative gross margin estimates yield expected rates of return of 14.9 percent and 18.4 percent.

The expected rate of return may have been well above our best estimate of 11.4 percent owing to errors in the lengths assigned to the R&D period and the commercial life. I have suggested that the bias in both cases results in an under-estimate of rate of return. Therefore, the decline in the expected return on invest-ment in R&D may have been larger than the estimates indicated.

---

[18] The cost of financing plant and equipment and working capital probably accounted for a larger proportion of sales in 1973 than in 1960 because of increases in both the cost of construction of plant and equipment and in interest rates relative to the prices of drugs. So the use of 2.6 percent as an estimate for 1960 results in an understatement of the expected rate of return in that year.

[19] The estimated stream of cost of R&D and net income for an average NCE for those years is as follows:

| Year | Net Income ($ millions) |
|---|---|
| 1 | −.13 |
| 2 | −.13 |
| 3 | −.13 |
| 4 | −.13 |
| 5 | −.13 |
| 6 | .14 |
| 7 | .28 |
| 8 | .28 |
| 9 | .28 |
| 10 | .14 |

Cox's study, "Product Life Cycles and Promotional Strategy," from which the estimate of the expected commercial life of NCEs in 1960 is obtained, is based on observations of those NCEs that were introduced in 1955 and 1956. He considered the commercial life of a drug to be terminated when sales declined to 20 percent of peak sales. Cox estimated the average on the basis of the number of years that elapsed following the year of introduction when 50 percent of the drugs introduced had reached this level. Informal oral sources within the industry agree that five years was the expected commercial life at that time. Cox's estimate is for all NCEs, and the commercial life of "important" drugs may have been longer. Since our list of drugs is more selective than Cox's, we may be understating the expected life of drugs in the category with which we are dealing.

[20] Using the same assumptions concerning gross margin, the cost of financing plant and equipment and working capital, and the length of commercial life as for 1960, the estimate of the expected rate of return for 1956 is about the same as in 1960.

74

# Table 3

## ESTIMATES OF EXPECTED RATES OF RETURN FROM INVESTMENT IN PHARMACEUTICAL R&D IN 1960, BASED ON ALTERNATIVE GROSS MARGINS

| Gross Margin (percent of sales) | Expected Rate of Return (percent) |
|:---:|:---:|
| 15.4 | 11.4 |
| 17.5 | 14.9 |
| 20.0 | 18.4 |

**Note:** See text for computation.

The validity of my procedure may be challenged by the apparent inconsistency between the current average rate of return on stockholders' equity after taxes, which is about 19 percent (1971), and the estimate of the expected rate for 1960. Some reasons for the apparent inconsistency are the increase in the commercial life of drugs since 1960 and the growth of both domestic and foreign sales. Between 1961 and 1972, the industry's combined domestic and foreign sales grew by 170 percent. The actual rate of return on investment thus turned out to be greater than the estimated expected rate because of unanticipated changes in the market. Another reason for the apparent inconsistency is that the rate of return on stockholders' equity as reported by companies treats R&D expenditures as a current expense rather than as an investment that is depreciated over time. The effect of treating R&D expenditures as expenses can be seen in the following analysis: Profits $(P)$ equal sales $(S)$ minus costs $(C)$. Treating R&D as expense raises $C$ by the full amount of the R&D expenditures in the current year, so $(S-C)$ is reduced by this amount. But the *rate* of profit is $(S-C)/E$, where $E$ represents stockholders' equity. Treating R&D as an item depreciable over time reduces $(S-C)$ less than treating it as expense does, but it also raises $E$ to the extent that part of R&D remains undepreciated and in stockholders' equity.[21]

Jesse Friedman estimates that capitalization of R&D expenditures would reduce the average rate for a sample of six drug companies from 21.2 percent to 16.8 percent, or by 4.4 percentage points. We can assume that the change for the industry average rate would be approximately the same.[22]

---

[21] The Federal Trade Commission has recognized that the rate of profit of companies that spend large sums on research may be overstated owing to the practice of treating R&D as expense.

[22] Another estimate of the effect of treating R&D as expense is provided by Harry Bloch who puts it at about six percentage points. See H. Bloch, "True Profitability Measures for Pharmaceutical Investment" (Paper presented at the Second Seminar on Economics and Dynamics of Pharmaceutical Innovation, The American University, Washington, D. C., 14–16 October 1973), p. 20, table 7.

Finally, we must inquire why the expected rate of return on investment in R&D declined between 1960 and 1973. The decline is due to the increase in the cost of R&D over this period and the decrease in the number of NCEs. We have seen that in 1960 the cost of R&D per NCE was $1.3 million compared to $24.4 million in 1973. The increase in sales per NCE was substantial, as was the increase in the commercial life of each drug, but the effects of these two changes taken together were insufficient to offset the increase in the cost of R&D.[23]

## Conclusions

Public policy toward the drug industry should be formulated in the context of a broader policy to improve the medical care system. Since drugs are our major and most cost-effective technology, improving that technology by developing new drugs will improve the medical care system, reduce suffering, and lower the cost of disease.

---

[23] The decline in the expected rate of return set in immediately after the 1962 drug amendments rather than gradually over an extended period. Thus, the estimate of the expected rate of return for 1967 is negative. On the basis of Sarett, "Impact of FDA on Industrial Research and Development," I assumed the R&D period to be six years. I had no basis for the estimate of the commercial life, so I assumed that it was ten years, which is intermediate between the five-year estimate for 1960 and the fifteen-year estimate for 1973. The total pretax R&D cost per NCE was estimated at $7.9 million. The estimate was based on the number of new entities appearing in the years 1961–65. The costs of the required research were estimated on the basis of PMA figures on research expenditures during the years 1958–62. To take care of price increases, I estimated the increase in prices of research goods and services between 1960 and 1966 as 20 percent. As before, I assumed that 50 percent of total R&D expenditures was for discovery research, and this part of the total was allocated entirely to the cost of R&D for NCEs. The development costs were distributed between NCEs and other new drugs. The after-tax cost of R&D ($7.9 million times .5) was distributed equally over the six-year R&D period, so each of the $c$s in the formula was estimated at $.66 million.

To arrive at the net income, I first estimated the average sales of NCEs in the United States at $2.7 million, which was the average sales in 1966 of NCEs introduced in the period 1957–64. Alternative average sales figures were as follows:

| Period of Introduction | Average Sales in 1966 ($ millions) |
|---|---|
| 1958–64 | 2.2 |
| 1957–64 | 2.7 |
| 1956–64 | 2.6 |
| 1955–64 | 2.5 |

To arrive at total world sales, I multiplied the domestic sales by 1.33, since according to PMA, foreign sales in 1966 were 33 percent of total domestic sales.

The same margin (15.4 percent), which after correction for cost of financing plant and equipment and working capital becomes 12.8 percent, was applied to arrive at net income. The substitution of alternative gross margins of 17.5 percent and 20.0 percent resulted in very low positive rates of return—1.1 percent and 3.1 percent respectively.

The low expected rate of return on investment in R&D was due to the sharp rise in the cost of R&D following 1962 and the decline in the number of NCEs introduced each year. The rise in the expected rate of return since 1967 is due to the growth in the size of the market and in the commercial life of drugs.

Designers of public policy for the industry should consider the fact that the industry has been society's principal instrument for the discovery and development of new drugs in past decades. Most new drugs originate in the pharmaceutical industry, because the research directed towards the discovery of new drugs is done almost entirely by the industry. Public policies and regulations affecting industry R&D will also affect the rate and volume of new drug discovery and development.

If the drug industry is to maintain or increase its investment in R&D, the rate of return it expects from such investment must at least equal that obtainable from available alternative investments. The minimum expected rate of return from investment in other industries has been about 10 percent after taxes, but the expected rate of return from investment in pharmaceutical R&D is estimated at 3.3 percent. This expected rate of return represents a sharp decline from the levels of 1960. It therefore seems likely that the low level of expected rate of return, and the decline in that rate from the previous high level, will cause investment in pharmaceutical R&D to fall.

These are the primary considerations that must guide the development of public policy. Unfortunately, the debate over alleged monopoly power in the industry has dominated discussion and has largely obscured these considerations from public view.

The industry as a whole has not reduced its R&D expenditures for a number of possible reasons: optimism on the part of firms about the projects that are well along the way in their laboratories; the continued high profits from previously introduced drugs; a reluctance to abandon research, which many members of the industry regard as its justification for existence; the hope of a reduction in the restrictiveness of the FDA in approving NDAs; and the hope of a major discovery. On the other hand, the effect of the low profitability of R&D is already reflected in the decisions of at least two firms (Carter-Wallace and U.S. Vitamin) to reduce their expenditures sharply. So we are beginning to see the effects of the economic pressures we have been considering.

The industry's laboratories have conducted most of the research directly aimed at the discovery and development of drugs, and should these economic pressures lead to the abandonment by the industry of its R&D activities, other newly created organizations will have to undertake them.

What are the possible alternatives? Laboratories sponsored by government agencies are unlikely to be a satisfactory substitute for the present industry laboratories, if one of our objectives is to reduce the cost of drugs. The cost of innovation is likely to be higher when government laboratories do the required research than when industrial laboratories do it. The discipline imposed by profit-and-loss constraints on costs will be absent. The government might contract out research to university, nonprofit private, and industrial laboratories, but research costs are difficult to control even under this type of budgetary control.

Acting against "monopoly" will have serious effects. Since the industry has been and remains the source of new drugs, and since we cannot count on existing nonindustrial organizations to develop them or easily create an equally productive alternative system, policy makers must examine just what these effects of "anti-monopoly" policies against the drug industry will be on new drug development. For example, the enactment of legislation to shorten the life of drug patents, to reduce prices, or otherwise to diminish the profits of the industry would further reduce the expected return from investment in pharmaceutical R&D. It would thereby create great economic pressure on the pharmaceutical firms to reduce their investment in the search for new drugs. This would be most unfortunate. The nation needs new drugs; the evidence of the exercise of monopoly power by pharmaceutical firms is dubious, and in any case the social benefits antimonopoly policies would produce would be very small. Drugs, after all, account for only a small part of the total cost of medical care. The profits earned by manufacturers are an even smaller fraction.

The prospect for the maintenance of drug research appears to be so gloomy as to call for government not merely to desist from policies designed to reduce industry profits but to actively encourage research by the industry. The possible policies to encourage industry research include the acceleration of approval of NDAs by the FDA and the extension of the patent life of new drugs. I do not wish to disparage the concern of policy makers with the possible risks to the safety of patients resulting from hasty approval of NDAs. This paper, however, suggests that there is another important consideration. An unfortunate effect of the delays in regulatory approval of NDAs is to discourage research by reducing its profitability and so to reduce the number of available drugs.

The social and economic benefits from mobilizing the industry's resources in the war against disease and in reducing the costs of medical care are potentially enormous. The development of new drugs in the last three decades has already resulted in great benefits. The potential gains from further advances remain large. To risk such gains for the sake of a dubious argument concerning monopoly is unwise. Our major objective should be to encourage a continued high level of investment in pharmaceutical R&D by the industry. Many current policy proposals are fraught with risks for the achievements of this objective, and thus for the ultimate performance of the medical care system. The welfare of the nation's population requires that policy makers not lose sight of this objective.

## Appendix

The formula used to obtain $y$ was as follows:

$$y = .5\left[\text{profits before taxes} + \text{R\&D} + \left(\frac{.08\ \text{debt}}{\text{debt} + \text{equity}}\right)\left(\frac{\text{working}}{\text{capital}} + \frac{\text{net}}{\text{plant}}\right)\right.$$
$$\left. -.08\left(\frac{\text{working}}{\text{capital}} + \frac{\text{net}}{\text{plant}}\right)\right].$$

Thus, $y$, which is the net income from investment in R&D, equals profits plus R&D expenditures less the cost of financing working capital and plant and equipment after the appropriate adjustment for taxes. The book value of net plant is taken as an estimate of the average investment in plant and equipment required to generate the indicated profits and R&D expenditures. The interest rate is assumed to be 8 percent. Since profits are computed after interest payments, and such interest is already deducted in the term representing the cost of financing working capital and plant and equipment, a further adjustment is needed. We add back into profits the part of the cost of financing working capital and plant and equipment that is financed by debt. The entire expression is multiplied by .5 to adjust for taxes.

Table A–1 reports some of the data used in the calculations. The entries in the formula were represented by totals for the six companies in the sample.

## Table A-1

### FINANCIAL DATA FOR SIX PHARMACEUTICAL COMPANIES, 1972
($ thousands)

| Company | Net Sales | R&D | Profits before Taxes | Gross Plant | Net Plant | Current Assets | | | Current Liabilities | Working Capital |
|---|---|---|---|---|---|---|---|---|---|---|
| | | | | | | Inventory | Accounts Receivable | Other | | |
| Abbott | 521,818 | 31,249 | 60,116 | 340,464 | 230,372 | 113,231 | 112,372 | 67,082 | 129,295 | 163,390 |
| Eli Lilly | 819,718 | 74,287 | 196,361 | 489,639 | 308,215 | 168,626 | 132,604 | 211,187 | 226,928 | 285,489 |
| Merck | 958,266 | 79,665 | 266,456 | 556,183 | 300,041 | 195,724 | 175,880 | 92,712 | 174,409 | 289,907 |
| G. D. Searle | 271,878 | 35,892 | 53,388 | 108,234 | 68,781 | 53,691 | 72,130 | 92,910 | 71,074 | 147,657 |
| Upjohn | 511,337 | 50,276 | 91,456 | 335,158 | 198,575 | 116,690 | 117,435 | 66,051 | 115,091 | 185,085 |
| Syntex | 160,408 | 15,342 | 42,819 | 94,588 | 68,152 | 40,527 | 34,307 | 52,139 | 50,056 | 76,917 |
| Total | 3,243,425 | 286,711 | 710,596 | 1,924,266 | 1,174,136 | 688,489 | 644,728 | 582,081 | 766,853 | 1,148,445 |
| Percent of net sales | 100.0 | 8.8 | 21.9 | 59.3 | 36.2 | 21.2 | 19.9 | 17.9 | 23.6 | 35.4 |

Note: Companies selected on the basis of their being cited in the FDC "Pink Sheet" pharmaceutical index as having over 60 percent of net sales from pharmaceuticals. All companies reported for calendar year ending 31 December 1972 except Syntex whose figures are for year ending 31 July 1973.

Source: Securities and Exchange Commission 10-K reports and company annual reports.

# THE PROFIT RATES
# AND ECONOMIC PERFORMANCE
# OF DRUG FIRMS

*Robert Ayanian*

## Introduction

It has been indicated several times in these proceedings that drug manufacturing firms typically show relatively high rates of return and spend heavily for advertising, research, and development (ARD). There is an interesting and important connection between these two phenomena. Their relationship is often interpreted to mean that the ARD spending rate constitutes an entry barrier that contributes to maintenance of profit rates. An alternative explanation will be offered here in terms of a possible bias in drug firm accounting rates of return—the central topic of this paper. Since a crucial factor for correcting this bias is the rate of depreciation of drug firms' expenditures for ARD, some estimates of this rate will be made. These estimated depreciation rates are used to calculate some corrected rates of return for a sample of six drug firms.

## Barriers to Entry

The more-or-less standard interpretation of the high rates of return in the drug industry is that drug firms are earning monopoly profits and that the heavy ARD expenditures by these firms must be creating barriers to entry into the drug industry. It is reasoned that in the absence of barriers one would expect these high profit rates to attract new firms into the industry. This would result in an increasing supply of pharmaceutical products, tending to lower drug prices, and in increasing demands for resources used in producing pharmaceuticals, tending to raise production costs. In the face of these falling prices and rising costs one would expect the high profit rates to disappear, but this has not happened in the drug industry. Instead one sees persistently high profit rates year after year, giving rise to the view that there exists a monopoly problem here that has not been dealt with by market forces. Such a monopoly situation is generally considered undesirable because its removal would enable consumers to get more for less—and most people prefer more goods for less.

As soon as the issue of monopoly power, together with the possibility of getting more for less, is raised, government is almost certain to enter the picture.

Thus it is that drug firm rates of return are currently an issue of public policy. The importance of the issue stems from the fact that governmental action designed to deal with a monopoly problem is more likely to be destructive if the industry is in fact competitive than if the industry is characterized by monopoly. Since the basis of the monopoly-returns, barriers-to-entry view of the drug industry is the high accounting rates of return within this industry, and since further governmental intervention is being contemplated on these grounds, these accounting rates of return warrant close examination.

### Accounting Bias

It is possible, even likely, that drug firm accounting rates of return are significantly biased upwards by standard accounting procedures that treat ARD expenditures as current expenses. In the case of drug firms, which spend heavily for ARD, this bias can be very large. The key to the bias is the fact that ARD expenditures are in reality investments that yield revenues to the firm over a number of years. These expenditures are investments in an intangible asset: knowledge. This knowledge is comprised of consumers' knowledge of the firm's products, that is, its reputation or goodwill, and the firm's knowledge of technological processes. When these investments are written off as current expenses, a very distorted picture of the firm's rate of return can result. If such a distortion is to be avoided, one must depreciate these investments over their actual lives, just as must be done in the case of tangible assets. A simple example will illustrate this point.

Consider a firm that as of 31 December 1974 has accounting stockholders' equity of $400 and net revenue for the year of $80. Then its accounting rate of return on stockholders' equity is $80 divided by 400, or 20 percent.

Now, suppose that starting 1 January 1965 this firm has made ARD expenditures of $100 at the beginning of each year for ten years, and that each of these expenditures has been written off as a current expense. Then the firm's ARD expenditure history is as shown in the column showing ARD expenditures in Table 1. Let us further assume that the actual life of each ARD expenditure is ten years and that 10 percent of the original expenditure depreciates each year of its life. Then on 1 January 1974 the firm's actual ARD capital is $550, comprised of $100 of 1974 expenditures, $90 of 1973 expenditures, $80 of 1972 expenditures, and so forth, as shown in the column showing undepreciated portion of ARD as of 1 January 1974 in Table 1. The last column of Table 1 shows the firm's end-of-1974 ARD capital, totaling $450. Comparing the 1974 beginning-of-year and end-of-year ARD capital, we see that there has been total ARD depreciation of $100 during the year or $10 depreciation on the expenditures of each of the ten years.

If we are to correct the firm's rate of return for the presence of the ARD asset we must do two things: The firm's net revenue must be recalculated by

**Table 1**

HYPOTHETICAL FIRM ARD EXPENDITURES AND CAPITAL
USING TEN-YEAR, STRAIGHT-LINE DEPRECIATION

| Year | ARD Expenditures on 1 January | Undepreciated Portion of ARD as of 1 January 1974 | Undepreciated Portion of ARD as of 31 December 1974 |
|------|-------------------------------|---------------------------------------------------|-----------------------------------------------------|
| 1974 | $100 | $100 | $ 90 |
| 1973 | 100 | 90 | 80 |
| 1972 | 100 | 80 | 70 |
| 1971 | 100 | 70 | 60 |
| 1970 | 100 | 60 | 50 |
| 1969 | 100 | 50 | 40 |
| 1968 | 100 | 40 | 30 |
| 1967 | 100 | 30 | 20 |
| 1966 | 100 | 20 | 10 |
| 1965 | 100 | 10 | 0 |
|      |     | $550 | $450 |

replacing the firm's current ARD outlays with actual depreciation of its ARD capital; and the end-of-year ARD capital must be added to its accounting stockholders' equity to get the actual stockholders' equity. Thus the firm's corrected rate of return is

$$\frac{\text{net revenue} + \text{current ARD} - \text{ARD depreciation}}{\text{accounting stockholders' equity} + \text{ARD capital}} \cdot$$

In the case of the firm shown in Table 1 we have

$$\text{corrected rate of return} = \frac{80 + 100 - 100}{400 + 450} = \frac{80}{850} = 9.4 \text{ percent.}$$

We see that in this case the accounting rate of return of 20 percent was a tremendous overstatement of the actual rate of return of 9.4 percent.

The equality of current ARD outlays and actual ARD depreciation in this example was merely a coincidence resulting from the constancy of ARD outlays over an immediately preceding time period equal to the life of an ARD expenditure, in this case ten years. That is, when a firm's ARD outlays have been growing over a period of time, its current ARD outlays will exceed the depreciation on its past expenditures, resulting in an increase in its corrected net revenue. To demonstrate this, let us suppose that the above firm began its ARD outlays in 1970 rather than in 1965. In this example, the five years of expenditure is less than the ten-year life of the ARD asset. From Table 1 we can easily calculate the firm's 1 January and 31 December 1974 ARD capital resulting from the five years of expenditure as $400 and $350 respectively. ARD depreciation over the year is $50, or $10 on the expenditures of each of the five years. In this case, the firm's corrected rate of return would be

$$\frac{80 + 100 - 50}{400 + 350} = \frac{130}{750} = 17.3 \text{ percent.}$$

The reason the corrected rate of return did not fall as much here as in the previous example is that the increase in the firm's net revenue tended to offset the increase in the stockholders' equity. It is possible to have a rate of growth of ARD expenditures so high that the increase in net revenue completely offsets, or even dominates, the increase in stockholders' equity, resulting in an unchanged or even increased corrected rate of return. In practice, one seldom meets this situation, so we will not further concern ourselves with it here.

Table 1 can also be used to show the effect of greater or lesser ARD expenditures on the bias in accounting rate of return. In the first example, let us change only the firm's ARD expenditures, which are now only $10 per year over the firm's ten-year expenditure history. Then the firm's ARD capital at the beginning of 1974 is $55, and at the end of 1974 it is $45. There has been $10 ARD depreciation over the year, or $1 on the $10 expenditure of each of the ten years. In this case the corrected rate of return is

$$\frac{80 + 10 - 10}{400 + 45} = \frac{80}{445} = 18 \text{ percent.}$$

As one would expect, the overstatement in accounting rate of return is relatively small when the improperly handled ARD expenditures are small relative to the stockholders' equity.

We have seen what happens to the numbers when we treat ARD expenditures as investment and correct the rate of return for the presence of an ARD capital asset, but what are we trying to accomplish by doing this? What in any case is the desired meaning of rate of return?

Recall that the commonly used rate of return measure is net revenue divided by stockholders' equity. Now the stockholders' equity is simply the firm's net assets, that is, assets minus liabilities. Thus the rate of return is seen to be earnings per dollar invested in the firm and is comparable to an interest rate. Indeed, if stockholders did not have money invested in the firm they could have it earning interest elsewhere. Thus the rate of return can be viewed as the interest stockholders are earning on investment in the firm.

This interest arises as a compensation to investors for forgoing the use of their money for a period of time. That is, when a firm uses this money to purchase resources to produce its products, it does not simultaneously receive payment for the goods it will produce with those resources and subsequently sell.

In the case of durable assets, the receipts may not come for many years. Thus the investor must put out money now in hopes of revenues in the future. Obviously, some prospective revenues in excess of the initial outlay must be offered: the annual compensation per dollar of outlay is interest.

What has all this to do with ARD? Recall that the standard accounting procedure is to treat these outlays as current expenses. By doing so it is implicitly assumed that the period of time between ARD outlays and the receipt of revenues from these outlays is so short that interest on the money invested in these activities may be ignored. The foregoing numerical example shows that if the time-lag lengthens to several years, this implicit assumption is unwarranted; interest on ARD funds may not be safely ignored. Ignoring money invested in ARD may result in attributing sizeable interest payments on these funds to the other assets of the firm, thus making it appear that these latter assets are earning a much higher rate of return than they in fact are. If we are to get a more reliable view of the actual rates of return of firms that invest heavily in ARD, we must correct their measured net revenues by depreciating past ARD expenditures, and we must show the actual amount of money invested in the firms by adding their undepreciated ARD expenditures to their accounting stockholders' equity.

## ARD Depreciation Rate

Making corrections in the hypothetical example was a simple matter. But in attempting to perform these corrections on the accounting of actual firms we encounter a monumental problem: What *is* the annual depreciation of a firm's ARD expenditures? This question may be interpreted in two ways: (1) what does it mean for ARD expenditures to depreciate? and (2) what is the numerical value of whatever is happening?

Clearly nothing physical is happening to the knowledge produced and transmitted through ARD activities, so the analogy with physical capital does not help here. The discussion of the previous section suggests that ARD expenditures depreciate as their revenue producing capabilities diminish, since what we are trying to capture with this concept is the time-lag between the expenditures and the receipt of revenues from them. Thus if a dollar of advertising this year produces x dollars of revenue this year, x dollars next year, and nothing thereafter, we would say that the life of the advertising investment is two years and that its annual depreciation rate is 50 percent. The advertising message might be just as true and widely known two years hence as initially, but if it has stopped producing revenue for the firm it has, for our purposes, completely depreciated.

Obviously, various ARD expenditures should be depreciated at different rates, since they undoubtedly are depreciating at different rates. Unfortunately, the statistical techniques employed below permit estimation of only a single average depreciation rate for composite ARD expenditures. Thus I proceeded on the assumption that all ARD expenditures depreciate at the same, constant rate. In broadest terms, my approach to the depreciation rate estimation problem evolved to using economic theory and the known attributes of a sample of drug firms to infer an *amount* of ARD capital for a firm, and then to determining what ARD depreciation rate, when applied to the firm's past ARD expenditures, produced the inferred amount of ARD capital.

One way of doing this, which was not chosen because of today's political-economic context, would be to assume that firms in the industry are actually earning only competitive rates of return and then to determine what ARD depreciation rates would be required to give the firms in the sample corrected rates of return equal to, say, the median rate of return of the Fortune 500 or some other typical rate. One could then try to judge whether or not these depreciation rates were reasonable or believable (for example, is the required depreciation rate positive or negative?). However, since the presence or absence of monopoly power is precisely what is at issue in the public policy debate, it seemed unlikely to me that results obtained by assuming competitive markets would be well received. Therefore an alternative approach was chosen.

I begin the ARD depreciation rate estimation by assuming that the sales rates of drug firms can be described by an algebraic expression relating a firm's sales rate to its tangible assets, its intangible assets (ARD capital), and all other resources it employs. Then (as derived in the Appendix) assuming certain input proportions and parameters are constant between firms, one can derive an expression for the factor of proportionality between the ARD capital of two firms. In this case, the general expression for the relation between the ARD capital of firm 1, $ARD_1$, and the ARD capital of firm 2, $ARD_2$ turns out to be

$$ARD_1 = \left(\frac{T_1}{T_2}\right) \left[\frac{\left(\frac{S}{T}\right)_1}{\left(\frac{S}{T}\right)_2}\right]^a ARD_2, \qquad (1)$$

where

$T = \$$ tangible assets of a firm,

$S = \$$ annual sales of a firm, and

$a = $ an (unknown) parameter whose value is greater than 1 and dependent on the parameters and assumptions of the original sales description equation. See equation (A–1) in Appendix.

If two firms with equal sales to tangible assets ratios can be found, the expression in the brackets is 1, independent of the value of $a,$ and we have

$$ARD_1 = \left(\frac{T_1}{T_2}\right) ARD_2. \qquad (2)$$

Since $T_1$ and $T_2$ are known to us, we know the ratio of $ARD_1$ to $ARD_2$.

86

If we can find even two firms whose sales to tangible assets ratios are approximately equal, it may be possible to estimate closely the ratio of $ARD_1$ to $ARD_2$ by making informed guesses as to the value of $a$, since with $(S/T)_1/(S/T)_2$ close to one any values of $a$ other than extremely high ones will affect the ratio very little. (This is the procedure followed below.)

With this estimated ratio of $ARD_1$ to $ARD_2$ and two additional assumptions, an estimate of the average ARD depreciation rate for drug firms may be obtained. The first assumption, made for mathematical tractability, is that a fixed proportion of beginning-of-year ARD capital depreciates each year. The second is that the rate of growth of firms' ARD expenditures in the period prior to 1964, for which I do not have data, was the same as during the 1964–73 period covered by my data.

Given these assumptions (the estimated ratio of $ARD_1$ to $ARD_2$ and firms 1 and 2 having differing ARD expenditure histories), there is only one ARD depreciation rate that, when applied to the past ARD expenditures of the two firms, will give each firm an amount of ARD capital such that the estimated factor of proportionality holds. This ARD depreciation rate is my estimate of the general ARD depreciation rate for the drug industry.

The sample for this study consisted of six pharmaceutical manufacturers who provided me with data on their ARD expenditures for the years 1964–73 inclusive. Other data on the firms were obtained from *Moody's Industrial Reports*. The six firms that contributed their data are: Abbott Laboratories, Eli Lilly and Company, Pfizer, Richardson-Merrell, G. D. Searle and Company, and The Upjohn Company.

Two criteria were used to select the pair of firms with which to estimate the ARD depreciation rate: the firms' sales to tangible assets ratios had to be approximately equal and their ARD expenditure growth rates had to differ as much as possible. This latter condition makes the estimated depreciation rate insensitive to minor errors in the estimated ratio of the ARD capitals of the two firms. The two firms in my sample that best fulfilled these criteria were Abbott Laboratories and Eli Lilly and Company.

Since these two firms did not have exactly equal sales to tangible assets ratios, it was necessary to assume some value for the $a$ parameter discussed above in order to estimate the ratio of ARDs. Fortunately, previous work in economics implied some reasonable values for $a$. As discussed in the Appendix, I employed this prior information in two different ways and obtained values of $a$ equal to 2.75 and 3.71. Each of these values was used separately to estimate $(ARD_1/ARD_2)$ and an associated ARD depreciation rate for these firms. The results of these two ARD depreciation rate estimations are as follows:

| Value of a | ARD Depreciation Rate [1] |
|------------|---------------------------|
| 2.75       | 13%                       |
| 3.71       | 9%                        |

[1] $(S/T)_1/(S/T)_2$ for 1971–73 for Abbott Laboratories and Eli Lilly and Company is 1.02774.

These results indicate that (1) the ARD depreciation rate estimate is quite insensitive to the value of the $a$ parameter, at least over this range of values, and (2) the actual depreciation rate of drug firm ARD expenditures appears to be about 10 to 15 percent per year. This latter finding is decidedly at odds with the accounting assumption that the ARD depreciation rate is 100 percent per year.

Before using these ARD depreciation rates to recalculate rates of return for the six drug firms, let us see how sensitive the depreciation rate estimates are to any other errors in the estimated ratios of $ARD_1$ to $ARD_2$. To carry out this sensitivity test, each of the $(ARD_1/ARD_2)$ ratios was decreased 5 percent and the depreciation rate recalculated. Then it was increased 5 percent and the depreciation rate again recalculated. This yields a range of depreciation rate estimates including the estimate that would be obtained using the true ratio, if the true ratio is within 5 percent of either of the estimated ratios. These results are:

| | Estimated Depreciation Rate Using | | |
|---|---|---|---|
| Value of a | 95% of estimated ratio | Estimated ratio | 105% of estimated ratio |
| 2.75 | 28% | 13% | 6% |
| 3.71 | 19 | 9 | 4 |

We see that if the true ratio of $(ARD_1/ARD_2)$ is within 5 percent of either of the estimated ratios, then the depreciation rate estimates we have made do not differ greatly from those that would be obtained using the true ratio. I interpret all this to mean that, if the above procedure is at all reliable, the ARD depreciation rate for drug firms is almost certainly less than 30 percent per year, and it is possibly as low as 5 to 10 percent per year.

### Estimated Corrected Rates of Return

In this section each of the ARD depreciation rate estimates is used to calculate a set of corrected rates of return for the six drug firms in my sample, following the general procedure outlined in the section dealing with accounting bias. The two assumptions regarding ARD capital made in the preceding section—that a fixed proportion of beginning-of-year ARD capital depreciates each year, and that the presample period ARD growth rate was the same as that in the sample period—are continued here.

Table 2 shows the accounting and corrected rates of return for the six drug firms for 1973. We see that the corrected rates of return are considerably below the accounting rates of return for these firms. Indeed, the corrected rates of return are, on average, about four percentage points below the accounting rates. More dramatically, we may say the accounting rates of return are, on average, more than 25 percent higher than the corrected rates of return. If these estimated

**Table 2**

ACCOUNTING AND ESTIMATED CORRECTED
RATES OF RETURN FOR SIX DRUG FIRMS, 1973

| Firm | Accounting Rate of Return | Corrected Rate of Return | |
| --- | --- | --- | --- |
| | | When ARD depreciation rate is 13 percent | When ARD depreciation rate is 9 percent |
| Abbott Laboratories | 14.12% | 11.47% | 11.20% |
| Eli Lilly and Company | 21.30 | 16.45 | 16.00 |
| Pfizer | 15.90 | 13.62 | 13.34 |
| Richardson-Merrell | 13.91 | 12.19 | 12.06 |
| G. D. Searle and Company | 21.94 | 17.72 | 17.23 |
| Upjohn Company | 19.03 | 12.89 | 12.32 |
| Six-firm average | 17.70% | 14.06% | 13.69% |

**Source:** Equation (A–27) and data from firms.

ARD depreciation rates are indicative of the actual rates of depreciation of drug firms' advertising, research, and development expenditures—and I find them believable per se—then the upward bias in these drug firms' accounting rates of return is large.

For comparison purposes I note that a ranking of firms in the 1973 Fortune 500 by accounting rate of return shows the middle 50 percent of these firms to have accounting rates of return between 9.5 percent and 15.4 percent inclusive, with a median rate of return of 12.4 percent. Of course, there is a problem in comparing the corrected rates of return of the six drug firms to the accounting rates of return of firms in the Fortune 500. But the lack of correspondence of the rate of return measures is not likely to be important for two reasons. First, most firms in the Fortune 500 do not have heavy ARD expenditures, so correcting their rates of return would have little, if any, impact on their profit rates. Second, a measure such as the median is not particularly sensitive to changes in the profit rates, since it simply divides the rates of return into two equal groups—those higher than the median and those lower than the median. All of the rates of return in the Fortune 500, for example, could be corrected without affecting the median, as long as none of the rates fell from above 12.4 percent to below 12.4 percent. Thus I think the 9.5 percent to 15.4 percent range reasonably may be used as an approximate range of typical profit rates in 1973.

We see from Table 2 that the corrected rates of return of the six drug firms on average, and most of them individually, were in this typical range for 1973.

Indeed, at the lower depreciation rate, three of the firms have corrected rates of return above the median rate of return of the Fortune 500 and three have corrected rates of return below the Fortune 500 median.

The dispersion of the rates of return is also of interest. In the absence of barriers to entry one expects the flow of resources into and out of various activities to tend to produce equality of profit rates among firms, by altering their costs and revenues. Thus an absence of dispersion of rates of return can indicate an absence of barriers to entry. The reason I say "can" rather than "does" is that the existence of a barrier to entry into an industry does not preclude competition among the firms within the industry. In this case all the firms in the industry could be earning a similar, but monopoly, rate of return. On the other hand, a lack of dispersion of profit rates within an industry in conjunction with an average rate of return similar to that of other industries indicates a general state of competition at both the firm and industry level.

A commonly used measure of dispersion is "variance" (the average of squared differences from the average). Using the variances of the accounting and corrected rates of return we can construct a measure of the proportion of dispersion in the accounting rates of return eliminated by the capitalization of ARD expenditures. This measure is

$$\frac{\left(\begin{array}{c}\text{variance of the}\\\text{accounting rates of return}\end{array}\right) - \left(\begin{array}{c}\text{variance of the}\\\text{corrected rates of return}\end{array}\right)}{\left(\begin{array}{c}\text{variance of the}\\\text{accounting rates of return}\end{array}\right)}.$$

Let us call this measure $P$. Notice that if the variance of the corrected rates of return equals the variance of the accounting rates of return, $P$ equals 0; no accounting rate dispersion has been explained through the capitalization of ARD. If the variance of the corrected rates of return equals zero, that is if the rates are all equal, then $P$ equals 1; 100 percent of the accounting rate dispersion has been eliminated by capitalizing ARD.

In the case of the six drug firms we see from Table 2 that, if the ARD depreciation rate is 13 percent, $P$ equals .51, and if the depreciation rate is 9 percent, $P$ equals .55. Thus, using even the rough adjustment procedures of this paper, over 50 percent of the dispersion in accounting rates of return among these firms has been eliminated as a result of the capitalization of their ARD expenditures. This, combined with the similarity between their corrected rates of return and the mid-range of rates of return in the Fortune 500, is evidence of a generally competitive state of affairs for these firms.

Drawing inferences from a sample of this size on the basis of numbers as contingent as these is difficult. Not only are we confronted with the fact that the corrected rates of return are only rough estimates, but we also do not know to what extent the sample is representative of the industry.

90

On the other hand, we have seen that the corrected rates of return are quite insensitive to the ARD depreciation rate over the range of ARD depreciation rate estimates. In addition, if corrected rates of return are recalculated for each firm using ARD depreciation rates of 28 percent and 4 percent, the extreme estimates shown on page 88, average corrected rates of return of 15.2 percent and 13.2 percent, respectively, are obtained. Each of these average corrected rates of return is within the mid-range of the Fortune 500, indicating that the qualitative conclusions concerning the sample are quite robust. Also, there is some evidence that the sample may be representative of the drug industry in general. Not only are all these firms major drug producers, but their average accounting rate of return in 1973 was 17.7 percent, while the median accounting rate of return of all drug firms in the 1973 Fortune 500 was 18.1 percent. I certainly see no reason to believe that this sample is not indicative of the drug industry in general.

**Summary and Conclusion**

The rates of return of drug firms are of great current interest. Being unusually high relative to those of most other firms, they are evidence of monopoly power in the drug industry. The evidence of this paper points to the conclusion that drug firms, as a group, do not earn unusually high rates of return. The accounting rates of return of drug firms may be significantly biased upwards by accounting procedures that treat advertising, research, and development outlays as current expenses, rather than investments. Correcting the rates of return of a sample of six drug firms by capitalizing the firms' past advertising, research, and development expenditures yields corrected rates of return that are not unusually high. This is evidence that the alleged barriers to entry and monopoly profit rates of the drug industry do not exist.

Another way of stating this conclusion is that scientific research (R&D) and freedom of speech (advertising) are compatible with competitive markets. Stated this way, the conclusion is not surprising. But this statement leaves unclear which—were compatibility not the case—would have to go: the monopoly profits, which in terms of static equilibrium economic efficiency are undesirable, or the advertising, research, and development activities allegedly responsible for the monopoly. My choice for retention would be freedom of speech, scientific research, and governmental nonintervention. A justification of governmental intervention requires more than the mere existence of monopoly profits: instead, the entire package of "goods" and "bads" associated with each state of affairs must be evaluated. Fortunately, in this case there appears to be no conflict between economic efficiency and the existence of advertising, research, and development activities. Thus I see no basis here for further governmental intervention in the drug industry.

## Appendix

**ARD Depreciation Rate Estimator.** Assume that a firm's sales rate can be described as a linear homogeneous Cobb-Douglas function of ARD capital, tangible capital, and all other inputs. Thus

$$S(t) = \beta_0 C(t)^{\beta_1} T(t)^{\beta_2} Z(t)^{\beta_3} \qquad (A\text{--}1)$$

where

$t =$ time,
$S = \$$ sales rate of the firm,
$C = \$$ ARD capital,
$T = \$$ tangible capital, hereinafter referred to as "assets,"
$Z = \$$ all other inputs,
$\beta_i$ ($i = 0 \ldots 3$) are positive constants specific to the industry,

and

$$\sum_{i=1}^{3} \beta_i = 1. \qquad (A\text{--}2)$$

Alternatively assume

$$Z(t) = \gamma T(t) \qquad (A\text{--}3)$$

or

$$Z(t) = \delta C(t) \qquad (A\text{--}4)$$

or

$$Z(t) = \epsilon S(t) \qquad (A\text{--}5)$$

where $\gamma$, $\delta$, and $\epsilon$ represent constants specific to the industry. That is, assume that the ratio of other inputs to assets, or to ARD capital, or to sales is the same for all firms in the industry. Then from (A–1), (A–2), and (A–3), dropping $t$,

$$\frac{S}{T} = \beta_0 \gamma^{\beta_3} \left(\frac{C}{T}\right)^{\beta_1}. \qquad (A\text{--}6)$$

Or from (A–1), (A–2), and (A–4),

$$\frac{S}{T} = \beta_0 \delta^{\beta_3} \left(\frac{C}{T}\right)^{1-\beta_2}. \qquad (A\text{--}7)$$

Or from (A–1), (A–2), and (A–5),

$$\frac{S}{T} = \left(\beta_0 \epsilon^{\beta_3}\right)^{\frac{1}{1-\beta_3}} \left(\frac{C}{T}\right)^{\frac{\beta_1}{1-\beta_3}}. \qquad (A\text{--}8)$$

Now consider two firms, 1 and 2. Under (A–3) from (A–6),

$$\frac{\left(\dfrac{C}{T}\right)_1}{\left(\dfrac{C}{T}\right)_2} = \left[\frac{\left(\dfrac{S}{T}\right)_1}{\left(\dfrac{S}{T}\right)_2}\right]^{\frac{1}{\beta_1}}. \qquad (A\text{--}9)$$

Under (A–4) from (A–7),

$$\frac{\left(\frac{C}{T}\right)_1}{\left(\frac{C}{T}\right)_2} = \left[\frac{\left(\frac{S}{T}\right)_1}{\left(\frac{S}{T}\right)_2}\right]^{\frac{1}{1-\beta_2}}. \tag{A–10}$$

Under (A–5) from (A–8),

$$\frac{\left(\frac{C}{T}\right)_1}{\left(\frac{C}{T}\right)_2} = \left[\frac{\left(\frac{S}{T}\right)_1}{\left(\frac{S}{T}\right)_2}\right]^{\frac{1-\beta_3}{\beta_1}}. \tag{A–11}$$

From (A–9) through (A–11) we see that in the context of this model we may conclude that under any one of three assumptions, (A–3), (A–4), or (A–5), firms with equal sales to assets ratios also have equal ARD capital to assets ratios.

More generally, under (A–3) from (A–9),

$$\left(\frac{C}{T}\right)_1 = \left[\frac{\left(\frac{S}{T}\right)_1}{\left(\frac{S}{T}\right)_2}\right]^{\frac{1}{\beta_1}} \left(\frac{C}{T}\right)_2. \tag{A–12}$$

Under (A–4) from (A–10),

$$\left(\frac{C}{T}\right)_1 = \left[\frac{\left(\frac{S}{T}\right)_1}{\left(\frac{S}{T}\right)_2}\right]^{\frac{1}{1-\beta_2}} \left(\frac{C}{T}\right)_2. \tag{A–13}$$

Under (A–5) from (A–11),

$$\left(\frac{C}{T}\right)_1 = \left[\frac{\left(\frac{S}{T}\right)_1}{\left(\frac{S}{T}\right)_2}\right]^{\frac{1-\beta_3}{\beta_1}} \left(\frac{C}{T}\right)_2. \tag{A–14}$$

Let us write in general

$$\left(\frac{C}{T}\right)_1 = \alpha \left(\frac{C}{T}\right)_2. \tag{A–15}$$

In cases where firms have equal sales to assets ratios, $\alpha$ equals 1.

Letting

$I =$ beginning-of-year ARD expenditures,
$\rho =$ constant annual ARD growth rate, and
$1 - \lambda =$ annual ARD depreciation rate,

it follows that

$$I(t) = I(0)(1 + \rho)^t, \tag{A-16}$$

and

$$C(t) = \sum_{i=0}^{\infty} \lambda^i I(t-i). \tag{A-17}$$

Substituting (A–16) into (A–17) and simplifying yields

$$C(t) = I(t) \left( \frac{1 + \rho}{1 + \rho - \lambda} \right). \tag{A-18}$$

Substituting equation (A–18) for $C_i$ into (A–15), solving for $\lambda$ and simplifying yields

$$\lambda = \frac{\alpha \left( \frac{I}{T} \right)_2 - \left( \frac{I}{T} \right)_1}{\alpha \left( \frac{I}{T} \right)_2 \Big/ (1 + \rho_1) - \left( \frac{I}{T} \right)_1 \Big/ (1 + \rho_2)}. \tag{A-19}$$

Equation (A–19) permits estimation of an ARD retention rate from estimates of $\alpha$ and of firms' ARD to assets ratios and ARD growth rates.

The obvious choice of firms for estimating $\lambda$ is a pair with equal sales to assets ratios, making $\hat{\alpha} = 1$ independent of the $\beta_i$. (The effect on $\hat{\alpha}$ of violation of the $Z$ assumptions, (A–3), (A–4), and (A–5), is considered on pp. 95–96.)

The ARD growth rate, $\rho$, can be estimated as follows:
Rewrite equation (A–16) as

$$I(t) = I(-1)(1 + \rho)^{t+1},$$

then

$$\ln I(t) = \ln I(-1) + [\ln(1 + \rho)](t + 1). \tag{A-20}$$

Estimating (A–20) via *OLS* yields $\ln(1 + \rho)$ and $\ln I(-1)$ estimates as slope and intercept respectively. The values for $\hat{\rho}$ obtained from the expressions $\hat{\ln}(1 + \rho)$ can then be used with $\hat{\alpha}$ and firms' ARD to assets ratios in (A–19) to obtain $\hat{\lambda}$.

Inequalities among firms' sales to assets ratios present a problem in estimating $\alpha$. From equations (A–12) through (A–14) we see that under (A–3), (A–4) or (A–5) when firms' $(S/T)$ ratios are not equal their ratio must be raised to some power greater than one to obtain $\alpha$. Determination of the correct exponent was obviously impossible. This problem was dealt with in the following manner.

Numerous Cobb-Douglas aggregate production function studies have found the exponents of capital and labor to be about .25 and .75 respectively. I employed this information in two different ways. The first way was to assume that $\beta_2 = (1/3)\beta_3$; the second was to assume that $(\beta_1 + \beta_2) = (1/3)\beta_3$. In both instances I also assume that $\beta_1 = \beta_2$. Given (A–2), the assumed exponents were thus $\beta_1 = \beta_2 = .2$ and $\beta_3 = .6$ in the first case, and $\beta_1 = \beta_2 = .125$ and $\beta_3 = .75$ in the second case. I further assumed that assumptions (A–3), (A–4), and (A–5)

94

were equally probable and that one of them must hold. Then the expected value of the exponent of the ratios of $(S/T)$s in equations (A–12) through (A–14) is 2.75 under the first assumptions about the $\beta_i$, and 3.71 under the second. The expression $\alpha = [(S/T)_1/(S/T)_2]^a$ was evaluated using $a = 2.75$ and $a = 3.71$ to obtain two $\hat{a}$s with which to estimate two $\hat{\lambda}$s for the firms. While somewhat arbitrary, these procedures undoubtedly reduced the expected error in $\hat{\alpha}$, and thus in $\hat{\lambda}$, relative to, say, letting $a = 0$ or $a = 1$.

**The Z Assumptions.** If assumption (A–3), (A–4), or (A–5) does not hold for the two firms used in estimating $\lambda$, then $\alpha \neq 1$ when the firms have equal sales to assets ratios. For example, let us replace (A–3) by

$$Z_1(t) = \gamma_1 T_1(t)$$

and

$$Z_2(t) = \gamma_2 T_2(t). \tag{A–21}$$

Then

$$\left(\frac{S}{T}\right)_1 = \beta_0 \gamma_1{}^{\beta_3} \left(\frac{C}{T}\right)_1^{\beta_1} \tag{A–22}$$

and

$$\left(\frac{S}{T}\right)_2 = \beta_0 \gamma_2{}^{\beta_3} \left(\frac{C}{T}\right)_2^{\beta_1}. \tag{A–23}$$

Specifying $(S/T)_1 = (S/T)_2$ we see that this can be true if

$$\frac{\left(\dfrac{C}{T}\right)_1}{\left(\dfrac{C}{T}\right)_2} = \left(\frac{\gamma_1}{\gamma_2}\right)^{\frac{\beta_3}{\beta_1}}. \tag{A–24}$$

One virtue of (A–24) is that as a matter of chance it seems unlikely to happen. This is in contrast to (A–3) which we would expect to hold if firms faced the same relative factor prices for these inputs. If (A–24) did occur, proportional differences in the firms' $(C/T)$ ratios could be greater than, less than, or equal to the proportional differences in their $(Z/T)$ ratios depending on whether $\beta_3$ was greater than, less than, or equal to $\beta_1$ respectively.

Repeating this analysis by relaxing assumption (A–4) yields

$$\frac{\left(\dfrac{C}{T}\right)_1}{\left(\dfrac{C}{T}\right)_2} = \left(\frac{\delta_1}{\delta_2}\right)^{\frac{\beta_3}{1-\beta_2}}. \tag{A–25}$$

In this case proportional differences in the $(C/T)$ ratios are unambiguously scaled down from the proportional difference in the $(Z/C)$ ratios.

Relaxing (A–5) and repeating the above procedure yields

$$\frac{\left(\frac{C}{T}\right)_1}{\left(\frac{C}{T}\right)_2} = \left(\frac{\epsilon_1}{\epsilon_2}\right)^{\frac{\beta_3}{\beta_1}},$$ (A–26)

which is analogous to (A–24). Equations (A–24), (A–25), and (A–26) indicate that if assumption (A–3), (A–4), or (A–5) is even approximately correct the ratio of the $(C/T)$ ratios may not differ greatly from one when the $(S/T)$ ratios are equal. They will differ greatly only under (A–21) or its analog for assumption (A–5) and $\beta_3$ close to one.

**Estimated Corrected Rates of Return.** The depreciation rate estimates in Table 2 were used to estimate corrected profit rates for 1973 for the six firms in my sample. Corrected firm rates of return were estimated as

$$\frac{\text{(net revenue)} + I - (1 - \hat{\lambda})\hat{C}}{\text{equity} + \hat{\lambda}\hat{C}}.$$ (A–27)

Rather than using equation (A–18) to estimate $C$, a somewhat more accurate expression employing my $(k + 1)$ actual ARD observations and imputing the sample period ARD growth rate to the presample period was used. Recall that $C(t)$ is defined, from (A–17), as

$$C(t) = \sum_{i=0}^{\infty} \lambda^i I(t - i).$$

Writing this in two parts we have

$$C(t) = \sum_{i=0}^{k} \lambda^i I(t - i) + \sum_{i=k+1}^{\infty} \lambda^i I(t - i).$$ (A–28)

Imputing the sample period $\rho$ to the presample period, (A–28) becomes

$$C(t) = \sum_{i=0}^{k} \lambda^i I(t - i) + \lambda^{k+1} I(t - k - 1) \left(\frac{1 + \rho}{1 + \rho - \lambda}\right)$$ (A–29)

which was used in (A–27) to estimate corrected rate of return. The growth rate $\rho$ was estimated from (A–20). The term $I(t-k-1)$ is the same as $I(-1)$ in equation (A–20), so it was obtained from the intercept estimate in that regression.

# PROFITABILITY MEASURES IN THE PHARMACEUTICAL INDUSTRY

*Thomas R. Stauffer*

## Introduction

In this paper we shall develop a financial model for a growing pharmaceutical firm and then fit that model to empirical data on some six firms in order to derive a better estimate of economic or financial profitability for those firms. It is shown that rate of return as conventionally computed by accountants—net income divided by net assets—is seriously in error, generally having an upward bias and thus overstating the economic rate of return of the firms. While it may be shown that such discrepancies are inherent in the accountants' measure of profitability and return to capital, the discrepancies are particularly large for discovery-intensive industries such as pharmaceuticals.

**The Pharmaceutical Industry.** The conspicuously high book profitability of the pharmaceutical industry in the United States has attracted persistent attention and adverse criticism in recent years. It is appropriate that we examine pharmaceuticals here in order to establish whether these reported corporate rates of return accurately reflect the industry's return on capital. One is hard pressed to identify any other industry for which the question of profitability has evoked so vehement a discussion in recent times. A Department of Health, Education, and Welfare (HEW) task force perceived this unusual intensity of concern and noted in its report: "This controversy and debate apparently stem from many factors, some that relate to the nature of the industry itself and some to the nature of the economic, social, and political environment in which it functions." [1]

Since the pharmaceutical industry, compared with most industries, is characterized by high levels of both advertising and R&D activity, our theoretical models would predict that its conventional accounting profitability might seriously overstate the real rate of return. It is therefore of especial relevance to establish whether the real economic rate of return in the pharmaceutical industry is indeed abnormally high or whether the high book rates of return simply reflect an accounting anomaly.

Various stages of this research were supported by the Ford Foundation, SmithKline & French Laboratories, Pfizer, Inc., and Eli Lilly and Company.

[1] U.S., Department of Health, Education, and Welfare, *The Drug Makers and the Drug Distributors* (Washington, D. C.: Government Printing Office, 1968), p. 2.

Partisans of both sides have focused their attention upon the special roles of research and sales promotion. In connection with research, it was argued that unusually high profits were necessary in order to reward the companies for the risks of failure and to finance the new research effort. Counterarguments, however, pointed to the stability of profits in most pharmaceutical firms as *prima facie* evidence of minimal risk, at least in the sense that stochastic effects had been effectively damped through diversification of research effort.[2]

However, for all of the passion with which rates of return have been discussed in connection with the pharmaceutical industry, comparatively little attention has thus far been given to the relationship between the economic return and the book yield. The sole exceptions, until very recently, have consisted of a few, almost isolated efforts that were directed toward capitalizing R&D expenditures and showing that such capitalization results in a decrease in the book profitability. Rosalind Schulman[3] examined data for a single firm and for the aggregate industry for a single year and showed that the apparent rate of return dropped by about one-fourth in both cases when R&D was capitalized instead of expensed. Vernon Mund, in a paper presented at the same seminar, attempted to relate the time cost of investing funds in R&D, allowing for the associated long lead-time, to the profit margin on sales needed to yield a 13 percent return on capital. He concluded that the observed profit margin on sales in the pharmaceutical industry was probably not equivalent to a discounted cash flow (*dcf*) rate of return of as high as 13 percent. Mund, however, stopped short of pursuing his analysis to develop internally consistent estimates of the economic rate of return.[4]

---

[2] Ibid., pp. 45–50, contains a capsule treatment of the argumentation.

[3] Panelist comments in J. D. Cooper, ed., *The Economics of Drug Innovation* (Washington, D. C.: The American University, 1970), pp. 213–21. Schulman's analysis comprised a purely *pro forma* accounting capitalization. A variant on this procedure was proposed by M. H. Cooper and J. E. S. Parker, "The Measurement and Interpretation of Profitability in the Pharmaceutical Industry," *Oxford Economic Papers*, n.s., vol. 20, no. 3 (Nov. 1968), pp. 435–41. They examined the ratio of cash flow plus interest to total assets plus depreciation reserves. The fallacy in this approach was analyzed earlier in this paper.

[4] V. A. Mund, "The Return of Investment of the Innovative Pharmaceutical Firm," in Cooper, ed., *The Economics of Drug Innovation*, pp. 125–38. Orace Johnson, "A Consequential Approach to Accounting for R&D," *Journal of Accounting Research*, vol. 5, no. 2 (Autumn 1967), pp. 164–72, argues that it may be of little consequence whether R&D is expensed or amortized using different schedules, although his argument also is confined to purely accounting manipulations. The accountants' arguments for and against capitalizing R&D are summarized effectively in Allan R. Drebin, "Accounting for Proprietary Research," *Accounting Review*, vol. 41, no. 3 (July 1966), pp. 413–25. The literature otherwise is extensive and not particularly rewarding. Another line of analysis needs to be cited: some investigators have accepted the book rates of return as an accurate measure of the financial performance of the pharmaceutical industry and then justify the high level of profitability with reference to special structural attributes of industry. G. R. Conrad and I. H. Plotkin, *Risk and Return in American Industry* (Report to the Pharmaceutical Manufacturers Association, Arthur D. Little, Inc., 1967), demonstrated that high book rates of return were correlated with high "risk," where they employed an interspatial risk measure, as contrasted with the more common intertemporal measure.

The model developed here attempts to go further than merely manipulating the firm's accounts in order to obtain a different accounting measure—further, that is, than the procedure of capitalizing the otherwise expensed outlays such as R&D or advertising and then amortizing them as pseudo-capital items. While it can be shown quite generally that such accounting adjustments may often reduce the magnitude of the bias in accounting measures of economic profitability, it also may be shown with equal generality that such manipulations will not eliminate that bias and, in some instances, may actually increase the error.

This analysis treats the firm as the aggregation of a number of projects of various ages and thus tries to reproduce the financial substructure of the firm. It is based on flows of cash in and out, allowing for timing, and is more basic than accounting conventions.

The research reported here is but one part of a more comprehensive study intended to produce a fully comparable set of estimates of the rates of return for diverse industries. Since all industries exhibit to various degrees the same intrinsic biases in their measured rates of return, corrected rates of return for any one industry cannot be unequivocally interpreted until comparably corrected values are available for a representative sample of industries. Nonetheless, we shall see that the correction to the rates of return for most pharmaceutical firms may be quite large. Since preliminary empirical work (not reported here) also indicates that the appropriate corrections for most industries prove to be small or even negligible, one may conclude with some certainty that the divergence between the real rates of return for pharmaceutical firms and those for the rest of manufacturing industry is much less than naive comparisons might indicate.

This study will first illustrate, using unrealistically simple examples, the magnitude of the error in accounting rates of return which can arise due either to time-lags—gestation periods or inventory holding periods—or to the expensing of quasi-capital outlays, such as advertising or R&D. These heuristic examples emphasize the existence of at least potentially serious biases and thus point the way to the more detailed analyses. We will then describe qualitatively the financial model for a pharmaceutical firm. The detailed mathematical formulation of this model is relegated to the Appendix. The study concludes with the results of applying that model to those six firms for which the necessary data is available publicly.

**Heuristic Analysis of Biases in Profitability Measurement**

Two features of the pharmaceutical industry suggest a priori that the reported rates of return for firms in that industry may be biased. The first is the fact that R&D outlays, which are a major fraction of the firms' annual budgets, are expensed against current income, rather than being capitalized. It is known, if only from precedents in the oil and gas industry, that the two accounting options (expensing or capitalizing quasi-capital outlays such as R&D or oil exploration) lead to quite different numerical values for the rate of return for the same firm. Therefore one must ask which accounting option and hence which rate of return is correct—indeed, one might ask whether both might be incorrect.

The second source of potential discrepancy in rate of return measurement for a pharmaceutical firm is more subtle and elusive but nonetheless real and rather large. There are significant time-lags between the expenditure of an R&D dollar and the first sales receipts generated by a new product. Such lags obviously entail potentially important financial opportunity costs, yet they do not appear explicitly anywhere in the firm's accounts. We shall illustrate this effect below, but an analogy from the electric power industry is suggestive. Utilities are compensated for similar lags—the period of several years during construction of major facilities—by charging a return on their funds tied up in work under construction. The conventional accounting procedures, however, applied to pharmaceuticals, in no way recognize this time-lag effect, so that the firm's profitability is overstated. The error is proportional in some sense to the length of the time-lag that is ignored.

Let us illustrate this latter, time-lag effect by comparing the real and accounting rates of return for three different distilleries, which differ only in their inventory holding periods. This is the pure time-lag case and illustrates the effect in its simplest form. The first firm holds its whisky in bond for only one year, while the other two hold their inventories for eight and twelve years, respectively. The assumptions and results are displayed in Table 1, where in each instance the annual revenue has been so determined that it will yield the firm a *dcf* rate of return exactly equal to 10 percent. However, even though the financial rate of return of each firm is exactly the same, the accounting rates of return, as defined by the ratio of net income to net assets, are markedly different. Firm A, for which

## Table 1

### COMPARATIVE BOOK RATES OF RETURN: TIME-LAG EFFECT

| Firm | Inventory Lag (years) | Annual sales [a] ($ thousands) | Inventory Value, 1 January ($ thousands) | Net Profit [b] ($ thousands) | Accounting Rate of Return (percent) |
|------|------|------|------|------|------|
| A | 1 | 1,100 | 1,000 | 100 | 10.0 |
| B | 8 | 2,144 | 8,000 | 1,144 | 14.3 |
| C | 12 | 8,000 | 12,000 | 2,138 | 17.8 |

Note: Laid-down inventory costs are $1 per barrel; annual sales are one million barrels in each case; all other costs were omitted for clarity.

[a] Sales revenue per barrel equals $(1.1)^N$, or in other words, the gross revenue needed to yield a *dcf* rate of return of 10 percent in all three cases.

[b] Equals annual sales minus costs of withdrawals from inventory ($1 multiplied by one million barrels).

the inventory holding period is one year, does exhibit an accounting rate of return of precisely 10 percent. For firms B and C, with inventory holding periods of eight and twelve years, respectively, the book rates of return are biased upward. Where the inventory holding periods are longer than one year—eight years for firm B and twelve years for firm C—the rates of return that would be determined from the firms' accounting records are 14.3 and 17.8 percent, respectively. Thus, the positive bias in the reported rate of return, as derived from accounting data, is 4.3 and 7.8 percentage points, and this intrinsic discrepancy is attributable to the longer inventory lead period. An analogous error arises for pharmaceutical firms due to the lag between the R&D program outlays and any revenues generated by new products.

A further discrepancy in accounting measures of rates of return can be demonstrated when a firm expenses part of its noncurrent expenditures. An outlay such as R&D or oil exploration is ordinarily expensed against current income. This is consistent with the accountants' argument that there is no objective means of determining the contribution of such expenditures to the asset value of the firm, assuming that a dry hole or an unsuccessful research project is of dubious value. On the other hand, unsuccessful exploration or R&D is an unwelcome but integral part of the process of obtaining successes, whether they be producing wells or new products. Therefore, one may cogently argue that all exploration or R&D outlays in a given period must be charged against the future income streams generated by the fraction of the expenditures that are successful. This practice of capitalizing such outlays and amortizing them against future income is observed among a number of oil and gas companies. It reflects an interpretation of the firm's accounts that does less violence to economic principles, since the outlays are clearly incurred in one period, not to sustain output in that accounting period, but to create new output in future accounting periods.

The debate over proper accounting treatment of quasi-capital outlays has long flourished in the accounting literature, and we wish to note only that the choice of accounting technique leads to numerical results for the rates of return in certain industries which are irreconcilably different. Thus, whatever the merits of the accounting procedure, the results must be used with caution. Let us consider the case of a firm investing in identical projects year after year, for which the real *dcf* rate of return is always exactly 10 percent. The real rate of return for that firm is also 10 percent. Let us now examine the accounting rate of return of such a firm, assuming growth rates of both zero and 6 percent per annum and using three accounting alternatives for each: zero percent, 25 percent, and 50 percent, respectively, of outlays are expensed rather than capitalized. Since the real rate of return is, by construction, exactly 10 percent in all six cases, we can illustrate neatly the discrepancy due to expensing versus capitalizing.

The results, shown in Table 2, indicate the divergence between the economic rate of return, which by construction is precisely 10 percent, and the accounting

## Table 2

### COMPARATIVE BOOK RATES OF RETURN: CAPITALIZATION VERSUS EXPENSING

| Growth Rate of Firm | Fraction of Noncurrent Outlays That Is Expensed | | |
|---|---|---|---|
| | 0 percent | 25 percent | 50 percent |
| 0 percent | 12.2 | 16.2 | 24.3 |
| (Error) | (2.2) | (6.2) | (14.3) |
| 6 percent | 10.7 | 12.3 | 15.4 |
| (Error) | (0.7) | (2.3) | (5.4) |

**Note:** The error is the difference between the computed rate of return in each case and the true rate of return of 10 percent. Cash flow from each investment project is constant for its ten-year life.

rate of return under the various conditions. The error in the accounting rate of return varies between 0.7 percentage points, in the case of 6 percent growth and full capitalization, and as much as 14.3 points, with zero growth and one-half of the outlays expensed.

It is to be emphasized that this very simple example demonstrates that expensing increases the error in the rate of return as defined by accountants. Moreover, the error in the reported rate of return (defined as the difference between the economic rate of return [*dcf*] and the accounting measure) is intrinsic. Regardless of the merits or demerits of the arguments advanced by the several schools of accountants, or the conclusions of the Financial Accounting Standards Board, the discrepancy between the two rates of return persists, and it is greatest when such quasi-capital outlays are expensed against current-period income.

The methodology to be developed below circumvents the question of which accounting practice or method is correct. Instead, we proceed directly to derive an estimate for the underlying economic rate of return for a firm, using the financial data for the firm no matter which set of accounting rules the firm may use—provided only that the accounts are consistent. The preceding discussion serves only to highlight the existence and magnitude of the biases in conventionally measured rates of return.

### Financial Model of a Pharmaceutical Firm

The phenomena described heuristically in the preceding section—time-lags and accounting practices—have a material impact on the measured rates of return of pharmaceutical firms. In order to eliminate the effects of such sources of bias, we must first specify a financial model for a pharmaceutical firm.

**Elements of the Model.** This model assumes that we can identify the time pattern of funds associated with a single product and then add up the individual projects in order to simulate the performance of the firm. Turning to the first step, simulating the full-cycle process of developing and marketing a new product, we must trace four separate flows of funds that are associated with the discovery, development, and manufacture of any successful product. These outflows must be related to the subsequent inflows of cash from the sales of that product.

*R&D expenditures.* These include not only the outlays which are directly attributable to those chemical entities that ultimately reach the marketplace, but also those outlays on other chemical entities that are abandoned during the development process. The expenditures on basic research (see Figure 1) are not identifiable with any specific new drug product but must also be incorporated, duly allowing for the fact that such basic research necessarily pre-dates expenditures on the identifiable development projects.

*Fixed and working capital.* Expenditures for facilities will be required both to support the research effort and also to manufacture and distribute the products which emerge successfully from the development process and which are launched onto the market after receiving regulatory clearance. Working capital will be needed for both stages.

*Sales revenues.* Once a product is marketed, it will generate a pattern of gross sales revenues that will depend upon its price, its speed of penetration into the market, and the comparative success of competing products or alternative therapies.

Since some new products fail ignominiously in spite of manufacturers' hopes, while others vary markedly in their degree of success, it is necessary to use a market or sales-weighted average in order to measure the time pattern for the sales revenues generated by the representative drug product.

*Advertising, manufacturing, and sales promotion costs.* Once a product is ready for release, expenditures for advertising and promotion begin, and these will continue during much or all of the market life of the product. The type of outlay and the level of expenditure may differ when a product first breaks into the market from the expenditures later, when it is sustained in the face of new contenders.

This sequence of expenditures is shown schematically in Figure 1. The sales relate to a single archetypal new product, and the investment in fixed and working capital comprises the incremental outlays needed to increase production facilities for the new product. Similarly, the advertising and manufacturing costs and outlays are specific to the new product. The research expenditures, however, involve three different categories of costs, two of which are not specific to the new product. These latter terms of cost must be allocated to the successful products. Insofar as that allocation is meaningful, we can obtain a conceptually consistent financial model for the full cycle of the research-development-production-marketing process. The firm then is interpreted as the sum of these product cycles, and the model can

**Figure 1**

## DRUG PRODUCT EXPENDITURES AND RECEIPTS

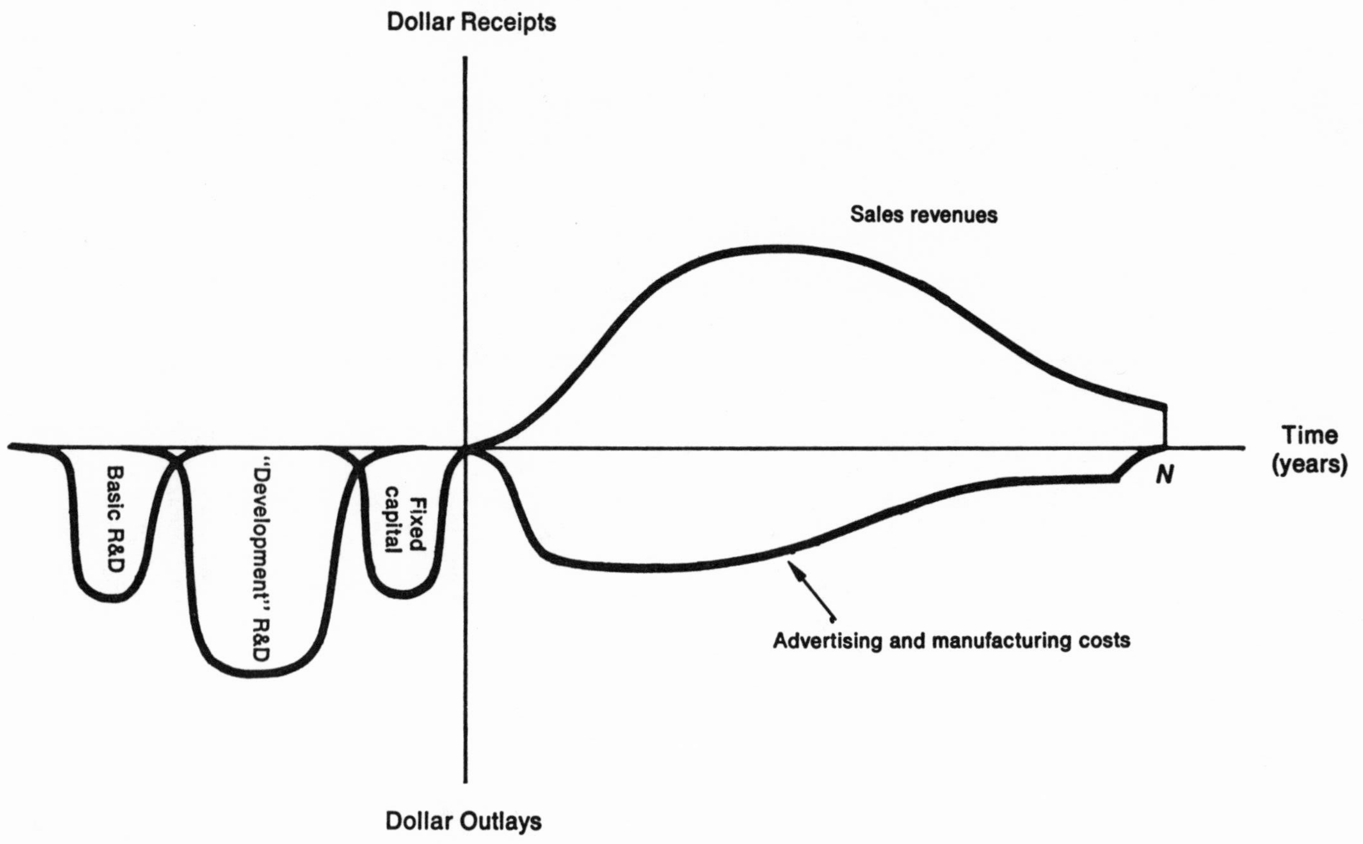

then be fitted to empirical data for the firm in order to derive the economic rate of return, which is equivalent to the reported, accounting rate of return. The mathematical formulation of this model is presented in the Appendix. We discuss the financial assumptions more fully in the following sections.

**R&D Expenditures.** Modeling of the financial flows within the R&D stage involves three analytical steps of increasing conceptual difficulty:

(1) Identification of the R&D expenditures specific to each particular product which ultimately reaches the market. The duration and time pattern of these outlays can be established empirically through surveys, but not from material presently in the public domain.

(2) Allocation on some rational basis of the generally much larger sums associated with unsuccessful products to that small fraction of R&D projects which does prove successful. Since the a priori probability of success for R&D ventures, like that for oil wells, is low, the allocated amounts exceed the direct outlays. Yet, such allocation is indispensable, since the successes must, on the average, pay not only for themselves, but also for their companion failures.

(3) Estimation of the expenditure on basic research, which we define for the purposes of this financial analysis as research that pre-dates the first clinical testing of a product or the development of methodological techniques not specific to any given product. Since the payoffs from such expenditure programs are ordinarily in the remote future and diffuse in their impact, allocation of basic research is particularly difficult, and the appropriate lag time cannot be specified with any precision.

The time pattern of development expenditures, items (1) and (2), can be estimated, at least in principle, through introducing two assumptions: First, the pattern of spending on unsuccessful products parallels that for ultimately successful products up to the point at which the development project is abandoned. The expenditure on a project which lasts only $x$ years is the full-cycle pattern truncated at year $x$. Second, there exists a stable *survivor function*, that is, a year-to-year probability that any R&D project viable at the beginning of a year survives through the beginning of the succeeding year. This is equivalent to assuming that the attrition rate for R&D projects is constant both over time and across different therapeutic categories. Let the pattern of expenditure on the typical successful product be as shown in Figure 2–A, and let the survivor function (equal to unity minus the cumulative attrition rate) be as shown in Figure 2–B. The pattern of expenditure allocable to each surviving successful product is the product of the curves in Figures 2–A and 2–B, divided by the reciprocal of $P_f$ (the fraction of all R&D projects taken into man which finally reaches market). The resultant pattern is displayed in Figure 3. Under the assumptions of stability and congruence mentioned earlier, this would be the equilibrium time pattern for the R&D outlays that are financially associated with each new product that is finally marketed.

### Figure 2–A

**R&D SPENDING PATTERN: SUCCESSFUL DRUGS**

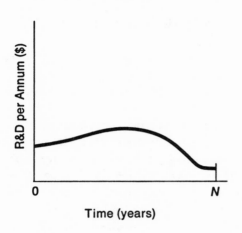

### Figure 2–B

**R&D PROJECT ATTRITION RATE**

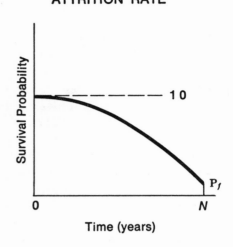

### Figure 3

**FINANCIAL EQUIVALENT R&D SPENDING PATTERN**

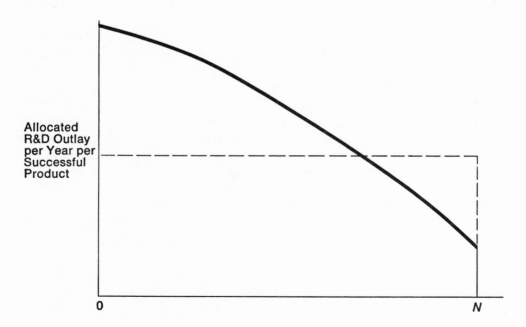

**Note:** Spending pattern normalized for each successful product.

106

Once again, in the absence of definitive empirical studies permitting delineation of the curves in Figures 2–A and 2–B, we have been obliged to make a simplifying assumption and have presumed that the profile for the R&D spending is rectangular, that is, constant over the R&D lead period of $N$ years, as depicted by the dashed curve in Figure 3. A more elaborate analysis can demonstrate that this assumption leads to a systematic underestimate of the magnitude of the correction to the accounting rate of return.

Further, in this version of the model we have not differentiated between basic research and development expenditures. Since any fraction of the total R&D outlays that comprised basic research would occur prior to the reference year 0, this omission introduces a bias in the same direction. Both simplifications, therefore, impart upward biases to the final estimate for the economic rate of return.

**Fixed and Working Capital.** Incorporation of depreciable and working capital into the model is quite straightforward. It is assumed that the only capitalized outlays are for manufacturing and distribution facilities, and these are made one year prior to the beginning of sales from the new product. Straight-line depreciation is used both for tax purposes and for corporate accounting. Similarly, working capital is required only for the manufacturing and sales stages. Working capital is injected at the beginning of the first year of sales and the entire amount is recovered $N$ years later when the product has reached the end of its economic life.

This assumption obviously ignores the significant fixed capital that is tied up in research and development laboratories and the working capital committed to the initial part of the full-cycle development-production-marketing process. The requisite data for allocating R&D to the several stages are not available, and the choice among the various methods for weighting shares of working capital is almost arbitrary. This effect is not inconsequential, but omitting this additional complication also contributes to overstating the final estimate of the financial rate of return, so that at least the direction of the error is known.

**Sales Revenues.** The time pattern for the gross cash flow generated by new products, $K(t)$, plays a crucial role in the analysis, since the estimate of the real rate of return is sensitive to the functional form of the revenue stream. Generally speaking, the more the receipts are skewed toward the early years, the smaller the error in the accounting rate of return. Conversely, the longer the economic life is, or the more the revenues are skewed toward the later years of the product's market life, the greater is the discrepancy between real and reported rates of return.

In principle it would be necessary to estimate both the time profile of the sales receipts and also the market life itself. Thus far, this has not proved to be workable, and the material on market lives available to date is either in error or misleading. Instead, we have surveyed the actual sales histories, over a sixteen-year period, for a large number of drugs in order to assess qualitatively what patterns, if any, might be adduced. The *qualitative* results were unequivocal: (1) Any drug product that was economically significant exhibited a lifetime of at least fifteen years, possibly considerably longer. (2) Sales revenues for such products generally rose steadily for four to ten years, often longer, before any plateau was observed. (3) Only in certain special cases, such as some oral contraceptive products, was the classical product life-cycle phenomenon found. Consequently, it was concluded that the most representative revenue pattern for significant products was a slowly rising ramp, followed by a plateau, which was in turn followed by a steady decline in sales (Figure 4). A full-scale statistical analysis of the market data is yet to be completed, so that this assessment is still impressionistic.

The sample was quite comprehensive, however, so that the qualitative result is well substantiated. The survey covered the products responsible for 51 percent of the sales volume of prescription drugs (new prescriptions) for the period 1955–70. There were two criteria for including a drug in the survey: (1) The therapeutic category constituted at least one percent of total pharmaceutical sales during the period, and (2) the product was one of the four leading products in its therapeutic category either in 1960 or 1970.

Many of the smaller-volume drugs exhibited the same sales pattern, but the survey was not expanded to cover more than 51 percent of all sales, because the number of compounds proliferated rapidly. All data were taken from the *National Prescription Audit* of R. A. Gosselin & Co. One known source of bias is the use of sales figures for new prescriptions, omitting refills, which would be important for some categories, such as oral contraceptives or diabetic therapies.

Hence, until the sales data have been analyzed fully, in the mathematical formulation of the rate of return model (see Appendix) we have assumed that product sales reach a constant level in the first year after market introduction and remain at that same level for fifteen years, at which point the product is presumed to be withdrawn from the market. The latter assumption is obviously a very poor proxy for the sales pattern illustrated in Figure 4. This choice, however, is useful

**Figure 4**

REVENUE PATTERN FOR SIGNIFICANT DRUG PRODUCTS

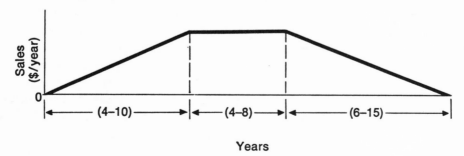

Years

in the restricted sense that it introduces a known upward bias in the estimated economic rates of return; use of a function like that in Figure 4 would yield a lower value for the real rate of return. In the absence of any better measure for the shape of the revenue stream, $K(t)$, the rectangular profile was chosen because a bias of known sign but unknown magnitude was preferable to a bias for which both sign and magnitude were unknown. The corrections to the accounting rates of return are therefore understated.

Net sales receipts in this context are defined as gross sales, reduced by returns, cash manufacturing and distribution costs, and corporate overheads. Specifically, R&D charges and advertising or promotional costs are not deducted from the sales receipts in this formulation. Both R&D and selling costs are instead handled explicitly as in the earlier sections.

**Advertising and Sales Selling Costs.** It was assumed that advertising expenditures and sales revenues are linked via a modified Koyck equation:

$$\text{sales } (t) = \rho \text{ advertising } (t) + \lambda \text{ sales } (t-1).$$

The sales level in any year equals a constant $(\rho)$ times the advertising and promotional outlay plus a decay constant $(\lambda)$ times the prior year's sales. The second term describes the inertial effect of earlier advertising programs. This is equivalent to postulating that there is an increase of $\$\rho$ in sales in the first year in response to an incremental dollar's worth of promotional activity. Thereafter, if no further advertising expenditure is made, sales will decline exponentially, each year's level being $100\lambda$ percent as much as the prior year $(\lambda < 1.0)$. An alternative interpretation of this assumption is that a steady level of advertising expenditures, equal to $\$(1-\lambda)$, will be needed in each subsequent year in order to sustain the initial growth in sales $(\rho$ dollars per year).

In addition, it is assumed that per-unit cash costs for manufacturing and distribution, excluding R&D and advertising expenses, are constant. Derivative evidence on the manufacturing processes themselves suggests that this is not too unreasonable, but fortunately the results are insensitive to this particular assumption. Such an assumption is useful, however, because when cash costs per unit are constant, the time pattern for the gross cash flow is identical with that for gross sales. That permits us to use the empirical results on sales trends to obtain directly the shape of the cash flow profile associated with the typical drug, whereas no data is available permitting direct estimation of the cash flow generated by a new product.

The assumed functional relation between sales and advertising, while plausible in its general features, is clearly grossly oversimplified, if not arbitrary, although it has been widely used in other economic analyses. That choice has been included, *faute de mieux*, in the detailed mathematical model described in the Appendix with no illusion as to its accuracy. The contribution of advertising to the rate-of-return discrepancies for the cases analyzed here is modest, so the overall conclusions are not affected by the imprecision in the economic description of advertising. It is useful to include even this crude model for sales response to advertising in order better to illustrate the direction of the necessary corrections, but it is important to note the caveat that, in other applications where advertising plays a more important role in the financial results, the estimates for the real rates of return might prove quite sensitive to the particular specification of the advertising-sales-response function.

## Estimated Rates of Return for Certain Pharmaceutical Firms

The financial model described in the preceding section was applied to a small set of pharmaceutical firms, and the resulting estimates of the financial or economic rates of return for those firms are displayed and compared with their reported accounting profitability in Table 3. The six firms are the only ones for which the annual R&D outlays could be obtained from the Compustat tape for a long enough period prior to 1971 to permit reliable calculations. In the absence of that data for the remaining firms in the industry, no calculations are possible, but these results are indicative of the discrepancies that one might expect more generally for the entire sample of pharmaceutical firms or for the industry (Standard Industrial Classification 283) as a whole.

The estimated financial rate of return is less than the reported accounting rate of return for five of the six cases, while for firm C the book profitability understates the real economic rate of return by 2.3 percentage points. For the more frequent cases where the discrepancy between the accounting rate of return and the estimated financial rate of return is positive, the magnitude of the error exhibits

## Table 3
### ESTIMATED FINANCIAL RATES OF RETURN

| Firm | Period | Accounting ROI (percent) | Accounting ROI (percent) | Discrepancy (percentage points) |
|------|--------|--------------------------|--------------------------|---------------------------------|
| A [a] | 1963–72 | 17.5 | 15.0 | +2.5 |
| B [a] | 1953–72 | 20.1 | 16.4 | +3.7 |
| C | 1955–72 | 9.8 | 12.1 | −2.3 |
| D | 1953–72 | 29.4 | 21.2 | +8.2 |
| E | 1959–72 | 20.4 | 16.3 | +4.1 |
| F | 1958–72 | 13.3 | 13.1 | +0.2 |

[a] Effect of advertising included; advertising expenditure data is unavailable for other firms.

no obvious pattern, varying from 0.2 points out of 13.1 for firm F to 8.2 points out of 21.2 for firm D.

It is to be noted that some correction to the accounting measure of profitability is necessary in all cases and that the correction is significantly large in all but one instance. Such a discrepancy will always arise; this can be demonstrated quite generally and follows from the theoretical appendix to this paper. The magnitude of the discrepancy, however, depends intimately upon the specific parameters of each example. Even though detailed calculations are necessary for each example, certain general relationships between real and accounting rates of return can be isolated:

(1) The error is positive if the growth rate is less than the firm's accounting rate of return, and conversely.

(2) The error is approximately proportional to the ratio of annual R&D outlays to the firm's net assets.

(3) The error is reduced in such measure as the firm's compound rate of growth over any period is close to its book rate of return for that same period.
Thus the upward revision of the book rate of return for firm C can be shown to be a consequence of the first effect, for its growth rate was 25 percent per annum. Similarly, the very small correction required for firm F, in spite of its high level of R&D activity, results from the fact that its rate of return was very close to its growth rate—13.1 percent and 13.6 percent, respectively.

The estimated discrepancies in the book or accounting rates of return depend upon certain of the assumptions which were embedded in the financial model of the pharmaceutical firm. The empirically important assumptions are listed in Table 4, and it is indicated whether modification of each assumption contributes to a positive or negative bias in the estimated financial rate of return. For example,

## Table 4
### SENSITIVITY TO CENTRAL ASSUMPTIONS

| Assumption | Value | Impact [a] |
|---|---|---|
| R&D gestation lag ($\mu$) | 4 years | Positive, if longer / Negative, if shorter |
| Time pattern for R&D spending | Level | Positive |
| Expenditures for basic R&D | None | Positive |
| Time pattern for gross sales [$K(t)$] | Constant for 15 years | Positive |
| Sales decay rate (advertising efficacy) | $\lambda = 0.7$ | Positive, if less / Negative, if larger |

[a] Plus means the correction is understated, so that the estimated financial rate of return is overstated. The direction of the bias is reversed if the firm's growth rate exceeds its reported rate of return.

the weighted-average gestation lag for pharmaceutical R&D was inferred from external evidence to be about four years. If a better value for that parameter were higher, say six years, then the rate of return estimated in Table 3 is too high, and the real financial profitability is in fact still lower. Conversely, if the gestation lag is in fact shorter than four years, then the estimated financial rate of return is too low.[5] No comprehensive survey has yet been carried out to determine R&D lag times or to estimate any shift in those lags over the last twenty years or so. Hence, the R&D gestation period could only be assumed, based upon statistically undocumented discussions, and the results remain uncertain to that extent.

On the other hand, the other assumptions consistently result in an overstatement of the financial rate of return. The R&D spending pattern has been assumed to be constant; because of steady attrition during the R&D process, the actual spending attributable to successful products would be skewed toward the earlier years of the R&D program, as shown schematically in Figure 3. Omission of this effect leaves a positive bias in the estimated financial rate of return.

Similarly, the sales revenue stream for successful products has been taken to be constant for fifteen years. The survey revealed a rising pattern of sales for almost all therapeutic categories—a revenue pattern akin to that in Figure 4—so that the assumed level-time profile for the revenue introduces a serious upward bias in the estimated financial rate of return. The sales decay rate $(\lambda)$, which measures the inertial efficacy of advertising, was assumed to be 0.7, a value which has no empirical support whatsoever. If the proper value is less, then the rates of return for firms A and B are somewhat overstated. If the value of $\lambda$ equals 0.2, instead of 0.7, then the estimated financial rates of return do not change for firm A but decline by 0.4 percentage points for firm B.[6]

## Conclusion

Although the empirical work in estimating economic rates of return for all industrial firms in general and pharmaceutical firms in particular is still incomplete, three results may be proposed with some confidence: (1) The accountant's measure of rate of return is seriously in error for most pharmaceutical firms; (2) the bias in the accounting rate of return is generally positive (in other words, the real rate of return is overstated); (3) the magnitude of these discrepancies is small for most industries other than pharmaceuticals, oil producing companies, and a few other

---

[5] The sign of the correction is reversed for those rather rare cases where the rate of growth exceeds the rate of return. Hence, this argument is reversed for such anomalous cases.

[6] No correction for inflation has been incorporated in this analysis, but a comprehensive treatment will appear in a forthcoming study. Even in the simplest case of a constant rate of inflation, the correction to the rate of return in order to eliminate inflation will be greater than the inflation rate itself for discovery-intensive industries such as petroleum, pharmaceuticals, or chemicals. *Ceteris paribus* this will reduce the dispersion in inter-industry rates of return.

"discovery intensive" industries. Thus the inter-industry dispersion in real rate of return is *less* than that for accounting rates of return.

Several effects have not been incorporated into the present model. Inflation has been ignored; preliminary computations indicate that the inflation-induced bias in the rate of return is not simply equal to the rate of inflation itself, but rather is a more complex function of the growth rate, the rate of inflation, and the real rate of return. The bias due to inflation, therefore, will be greater than the rate of inflation by an amount related to the underlying error in the rate of return itself and thus will be relatively larger for "discovery intensive" firms or for those industries characterized by very long product lives or long inventory holding periods.

Empirically, the assumption that both the time patterns for R&D spending and sales revenues for each product are constant annual amounts is decidedly unrealistic. Qualitative evidence suggests that both time patterns are markedly skewed so that the simple version of the model understates the necessary correction of the accounting rate of return and still tends to overstate the real rate of return. More comprehensive empirical studies of R&D spending patterns, the attrition rates for new products during the development cycle, and the market performance of successful versus unsuccessful products are needed.

Finally, this model contains no component for market risk, which varies considerably from one industry to another. However, this effect may be less important for the pharmaceutical industry than one might have thought.

The identifiable omissions all result in an understatement of the bias in reported rates of return, but major empirical effort will be needed to obtain more precise estimates of the real rates of return. One can predict that these will be still lower (except in certain known instances) than those calculated using the techniques described here. The additional research is probably warranted.

## Appendix

**Derivation of Rate of Return Equations.** The equation for the accounting rate of return for a steadily-growing pharmaceutical firm is derived below. The analysis involves two steps: First, we determine the time sequence of the flows of cash into the development and manufacture of a new drug product (outflows) and the ensuing time pattern of gross receipts from its sales after development (inflows). These flows permit us to define an internal rate of return (*dcf* rate of return) for each such successful project. The second step consists of describing the firm as the sum of such projects over time, where current income in any year derives from a prior history of projects of different vintages, while current R&D outlays reflect the expenditures for future projects that are in different stages of advancement. Insofar as the firm can realistically be modeled as the sum of identical projects of different vintages, it is possible to develop equations in which the real rate of return is defined implicitly in terms of financial parameters, including the accounting rate of return itself. These equations can be solved, using observed values of the parameters, to yield an estimate of the real rate of return for the firm.

*Financial model of successful new products.* We focus first on a single new product and identify the flow of revenue from that product, once marketed, and also the streams of prior outlays which are directly related to that product (manufacturing facilities and direct R&D funding), or which are allocated to it (appropriate shares of basic research and a pro rata burden of unsuccessful R&D projects). The stream of outlays and net receipts is diagramed in Figure 5:

### Figure 5
### DRUG OUTLAYS AND RECEIPTS

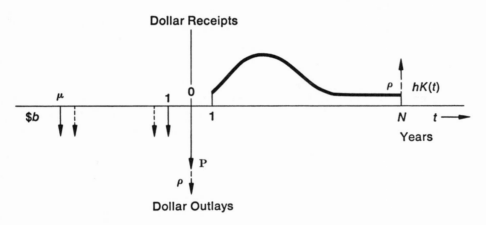

The present value of the cash flow generated by market sales of the new product, discounted at $r$, is

$$\text{present value of cash receipts} = \sum_{i=1}^{N} \frac{hK(i)}{(1+r)^i} = hk(r), \qquad (1)$$

where

$N$ = economic lifetime of the product,
$h$ = scale factor such that the internal rate of return equals $r$ (defined below),
$K(t)$ = time pattern of gross cash flow, before deduction of advertising or R&D costs,
$k(r)$ = present value of $K(t)$, discounted at $r$.

Similarly, the present value of the premarketing expenditures, compounded forward to the beginning of year 1 becomes

$$\text{present value of outlays} = \left( \rho - \frac{\cdot \rho}{(1+r)^N} \right) + P + b \sum_{i=1}^{\mu} (1+r)^i, \qquad (2)$$

114

where

$\rho$ = additional working capital,

P = additional investment in fixed assets,

$b$ = annual R&D outlay required to generate one new successful product,

$\mu$ = duration of R&D program associated with successful new project; includes allocated share of R&D expenditures on unsuccessful projects and basic research.[7]

Equation (2) can be rearranged:

$$\text{outlays} = \rho r S(N,r) + P + b(1+r)^{\mu+1}S(\mu,r) \tag{3}$$

where

$$S(i,x) = \frac{1}{x}\left[1-(1+x)^{-i}\right].$$

If the present values of receipts and outlays are to be equal—the condition that the real rate of return $r$ be realized on each full-cycle project—then equations (1) and (3) must be equal:

$$hk(r) = P + \rho r S(N,r) + b(1+r)^{\mu+1}S(\mu,r) \tag{4}$$

from which we have the definition of the scale factor,

$$h = \frac{1}{k(r)}\left[P + \rho r S(N,r) + b(1+r)^{\mu+1}S(\mu,r)\right]. \tag{5}$$

*Specification of the firm.* Let us assume that the firm consists of the sum of such identical, vintaged projects, new ones being added each year and other products being dropped once they are $N$ years old. We further assume that the firm is growing at the constant rate $g$, which can be specialized to the static case if $g$ is set equal to zero.

In any year the cash flow from products introduced that year and in all prior $N-1$ years is

$$\text{cash flow} = h\sum_{i=1}^{N}\frac{K(i)}{(1+g)^{i-1}} = (1+g)hk(g). \tag{6}$$

The net value of fixed assets at the beginning of the year is the value of the investment in plant, property and equipment added in the current year, plus the depreciated balances of the fixed investments added in each of the $N-1$ prior years. Under the assumed growth condition, if \$P are added in year $t$, then \$P$(1+g)^{-i}$ were added $i$ years before, and the undepreciated balance for assets added $i$ years before equals \$P$(1+g)^{-i}[1-(i/N)]$. The value of the beginning-

---

[7] The time pattern of R&D outlays has been assumed here to be rectangular, that is, constant for the period of $\mu$ years. Available evidence suggests that the expenditure pattern should be skewed toward the earlier years, but comprehensive data is still lacking.

of-the-year net fixed assets for the growing firm as recorded in its accounts (assuming straight-line depreciation) [8] is

$$\text{net PP\&E} = P\left[1 + \frac{\left(1-\frac{1}{N}\right)}{(1+g)} + \cdots + \frac{\left(1-\frac{i}{N}\right)}{(1+g)^i} + \cdots + \frac{\frac{1}{N}}{(1+g)^{N-1}}\right] \cdot \quad (7)$$

$$= P\left[1 + \sum_{i=1}^{N-1}\left(\frac{1}{1+g}\right)^i - \frac{1}{N}\sum_{i=1}^{N-1}\frac{i}{(1+g)^i}\right] \quad (8)$$

A final rearrangement of terms yields the expression for the net fixed assets for the beginning of the year:

$$\text{net fixed assets} = \frac{(1+g)}{g}\,P\left[1 - \frac{S(N,g)}{N}\right] \quad (9)$$

since

$$\sum_{j=1}^{t}\frac{t}{(1+g)^i} = \frac{1+g}{g}\left[S(t,g) - \frac{t}{(1+g)^{i+1}}\right]. \quad (10)$$

The working capital is recovered at the end of each project and can be recycled into a new product. Hence the net additions to the firm's working capital in each year are the difference between the gross sum needed for the new products and the amount of working capital that is recovered from the products introduced $N$ years earlier:

$$\text{working capital} = \rho\left[1 + \left(\frac{1}{1+g}\right) + \cdots + \left(\frac{1}{1+g}\right)^{N-1}\right] \quad (11)$$

or

$$\text{working capital} = (1+g)\rho S(N,g). \quad (12)$$

The value of the beginning-of-year net assets for the firm equals the total of net working capital [9] and net fixed assets:

$$\text{net assets} = (1+g)P\left\{\frac{1}{g}\left[1 - \frac{S(N,g)}{N}\right] + \frac{\rho}{P}S(N,g)\right\}. \quad (13)$$

Turning now to the income account, we find that the annual depreciation charge is the sum of the charges for each of the fixed investments made in the $N-1$ prior years, plus that from the current year:

$$\text{depreciation} = \frac{P}{N}\left[1 + \frac{1}{1+g} + \cdots + \left(\frac{1}{1+g}\right)^{N-1}\right] = (1+g)\frac{P}{N}S(N,g). \quad (14)$$

Conversely, the R&D outlays in the current year relate to products which will appear on the market over $\mu$ future years. The outlays on each of the prospective projects are assumed to be related to the anticipated growth of the firm: $b$ dollars

---

[8] The equations are readily generalized for any other depreciation schedule.

[9] Net working capital is defined empirically as current assets plus trade investments minus current liabilities plus short-term debt included in current liabilities.

were needed in year $-1$ to introduce the new product in year $0$. Hence, in the current budget are $\$b(1+g)$ for next year's products, $\$b(1+g)^2$ for those for the year after, and so on:

$$\text{R\&D} = b\,[(1+g) + \cdots + (1+g)^\mu] \tag{15}$$

which, upon regrouping of terms, becomes

$$\text{R\&D} = (1+g)^{\mu+1}bS(\mu,g). \tag{16}$$

The firm's net accounting income equals its cash flow less the depreciation charges and less the expensed outlays for R&D (interest is not deducted but included as part of the return to total capital employed):

$$\text{net income} = (1+g)hk(g) - (1+g)\frac{\text{P}}{N}S(N,g) - (i+g)^{\mu+1}bS(\mu,g). \tag{17}$$

The accounting profitability of the firm $R^{acc}$ is conventionally defined as the ratio of net income to net assets; if we divide equation (17) by (13) and substitute the expression for $h$ from equation (5) we obtain

$$R^{acc} = \frac{\dfrac{k(g)}{k(r)}\left[1 + \dfrac{\rho}{\text{P}}S(N,r) + \dfrac{b}{\text{P}}(1+r)^{\mu+1}S(\mu,r)\right] - \dfrac{S(N,g)}{N} - (1+g)^\mu \dfrac{b}{\text{P}}S(\mu,g)}{\dfrac{1}{g}\left[1 - \dfrac{1}{N}S(N,g)\right] + \dfrac{\rho}{\text{P}}S(N,g).} \tag{18}$$

It is more convenient to regroup terms so that the contribution due to the R&D outlays is exhibited explicitly:

$$\begin{aligned}
R^{acc} = \frac{1}{Q}&\left\{\left[1 + \frac{\rho}{\text{P}}S(N,r)\right]\frac{k(g)}{k(r)} - S(N,g)\right\} \\
+ \frac{1}{Q}&\left[\frac{k(g)}{k(r)}\frac{b}{\text{P}}(1+r)^{\mu+1}S(\mu,r) - \frac{b}{\text{P}}(1+g)^\mu S(\mu,g)\right]
\end{aligned}$$

where

$$Q = \frac{1}{g}\left[1 - \frac{1}{N}S(N,g)\right] + \frac{\rho}{\text{P}}S(N,g). \tag{19}$$

The ratio $\rho/\text{P}$ which appears in the first term above is not empirically observable. However, from financial data on a firm, the ratio of working capital to net fixed assets ($\alpha$) can be determined. This observable quantity ($\alpha$) can be defined in terms of equations (9) and (12):

$$\alpha = \frac{\text{working capital}}{\text{net fixed assets}} = \frac{\rho S(N,g)}{\text{P}\dfrac{1}{g}\left[1 - \dfrac{1}{N}S(N,g)\right]}, \tag{20}$$

whence

$$\left(\frac{\rho}{\text{P}}\right) = \frac{\dfrac{\alpha}{g}\left[1 - \dfrac{1}{N}S(N,g)\right]}{S(N,g)}. \tag{21}$$

117

Thus, knowledge of the growth rate $g$ and the product lifetime $N$, together with empirical measurement of $\alpha$ yields a value for $\rho/P$.

Similarly, $b$ (the annual R&D outlay per new product under development) is not directly observable, although the total annual R&D outlay on all projects is usually reported. The ratio $b/P$ which appears in the second term of equation (19) can be related to a measurable function $\beta$ (the ratio of annual R&D expenditures to the beginning-of-year net assets), which in turn is directly measurable. Beta equals the ratio of equations (16) and (13):

$$\beta = \frac{\text{R\&D}}{\text{net assets}} = \frac{b}{P}\frac{(1+g)^\mu}{Q}S(\mu,g).\tag{22}$$

Regrouping terms and substituting equation (22) into (19) we obtain the following pair of equations which implicitly relate the unknown economic accounting rate of return $R^{acc}$:

$$R^{acc} = \frac{\left[1+\frac{\rho}{P}S(N,r)\right]\frac{k(g)}{k(r)}-S(N,g)}{Q}$$

$$+\beta(1+g)\left[\frac{k(g)(1+r)^{\mu+1}S(\mu,r)}{k(r)(1+g)^{\mu+1}S(\mu,g)}-\left(\frac{1}{1+g}\right)\right]\tag{23}$$

and

$$\frac{\rho}{P} = \alpha\frac{\frac{1}{g}\left[1-\frac{S(N,g)}{N}\right]}{S(N,g)}.\tag{24}$$

Two additional effects must be considered: income tax liabilities and the impact of advertising outlays. The latter play a role analogous to that of R&D, since advertising expenditures are expensed against current-period income even though the residual effect of any advertising program, if successful, is to generate sales revenues in future periods as well. Advertising, too, is a quasi-capital outlay conceptually, even though accountants insist that it be expensed against current income. Taxes may also affect the interpretation of accounting profitability, since they alter the timing of net expenditures and net receipts. The results of including both effects are stated below without proof and are incorporated into a final, general equation for the accounting rate of return which embodies income taxes, both depreciable and nondepreciable capital, R&D outlays, and advertising:

$$R^{acc} = \left\{\begin{array}{l}\frac{1}{Q}\left\{\left[1+\frac{\rho}{P}S(N,r)\right]\frac{k(g)}{k(r)}-S(N,g)\right\}\\[2mm]+\frac{T}{Q}\left[d(g)-d(r)\frac{k(g)}{k(r)}\right]\\[2mm]+\beta(1-T)(1+g)\left[\frac{k(g)(1+r)^{\mu+1}S(\mu,r)}{k(r)(1+g)^{\mu+1}S(\mu,g)}-\left(\frac{1}{1+g}\right)\right]\\[2mm]+z(1-T)(1+g)\left[\frac{k(g)(1+r-\lambda)S(N,r)}{k(r)(1+g-\lambda)S(N,g)}-\frac{1}{1+g}\right],\end{array}\right.\tag{25}$$

where

> $z$ = ratio of annual advertising outlays to beginning-of-year net assets,
> $\lambda$ = decline parameter for sales *without* advertising,
> $d(x)$ = present value of depreciation schedule, discounted at $x$,
> $T$ = rate of corporate income tax.

The preceding equation assumes that the firm uses the same accounting definitions for its reports to its stockholders as for tax purposes. It also implies the choice of a quite specific model for the response of sales revenues to incremental advertising outlays. Although widely used elsewhere, this advertising-sales model is rationalized principally because it is mathematically tractable and not because of any compelling empirical justification.

The underlying relationship is:

$$\text{sales } (t) = \rho \text{ advertising } (t) + \lambda \text{ sales } (t-1). \tag{26}$$

Here $\rho$ measures the response of sales to an incremental advertising expenditure in the same period, and $\lambda$ is the fraction of the incremental sales that persists in each succeeding period. More sophisticated models exist, but even this simplest version lends itself poorly to statistical estimation, and the "correction" for advertising in this analysis is acknowledged to be imprecise.

# COMMENTARIES

*Frederic M. Scherer*

When three economists agree on *anything* in these unsettled times, one must suspect that the selection procedure was other than random. Nevertheless, it is not altogether surprising that all three authors found accounting profit rates to be overstated in an industry like drugs, with very high R&D and advertising outlays and substantial R&D-to-marketing lags. The key questions are quantitative: How large is the bias, and how much more serious is it for pharmaceutical firms than for other industries in the U.S. economy?

When these comments were revised, I had still not seen the official version of Dr. Stauffer's paper. Maybe "not seeing is believing," but from his initial outline and his oral presentation, I find Stauffer's contribution to be the soundest theoretically and empirically of the three papers before us. My main criticism is that the analysis is based upon a very limited and perhaps not representative set of data—Mr. Clymer's *pro forma* estimates of new-chemical-entity R&D outlays for SmithKline & French. Stauffer seems unaware of Edwin Mansfield's impressive empirical work on drug R&D costs and timing.[1] Even though the Mansfield evidence may be obsolete because it largely pre-dates the 1962 FDA amendments, it would at least have demonstrated that expenditures and time-lags are much smaller for compounded products and alternate dosage forms than for new chemical entities. If my understanding is correct, Stauffer has applied the assumptions for new chemical entities to all pharmaceutical company profits (including profits from proprietary and licensed drug products as well as nondrug items). This almost certainly implies an overcorrection for the accounting profit biases.

The Ayanian paper is extremely weak, combining flimsy evidence with a theoretical procedure of dubious validity. The analysis assumes a "production function" specified in dollar outlay terms, and not the physical input format used in orthodox production function theory. To carry out his corrections on $\alpha$, Ayanian uses exogenously estimated values of the "labor" elasticity for traditional production functions, erroneously implying that "labor" and "all other inputs"

---

[1] E. Mansfield *et al.*, *Research and Innovation in the Modern Corporation* (New York: Norton, 1971), chap. 4.

(including raw materials outlays) are identical. But most important, the key to Ayanian's whole estimation technique is equation (A–19):

$$\lambda = \frac{\alpha \left(\frac{I}{T}\right)_2 - \left(\frac{I}{T}\right)_1}{\alpha \left(\frac{I}{T}\right)_2 \bigg/ (1 + \rho_1) - \left(\frac{I}{T}\right)_1 \bigg/ (1 + \rho_2)}$$

Suppose two firms selected for comparison happen to have identical ARD growth rates—a not implausible possibility. Then $\rho_1 = \rho_2 = \rho$, and the equation collapses to $\lambda = 1 + \rho$. The retention rate is greater than one, which means that the value of an advertising or R&D outlay necessarily appreciates over time. A corollary is that Ayanian can only get sensible results by taking companies with unequal growth rates and plugging them into the formula in the "right" order. It is all rather bizarre and not to be taken seriously.

Professor Schwartzman deserves a "nice try" award for attempting to squeeze interesting implications out of aggregate data on R&D outlays, the number of new chemical entities, and profit margins. The most suspect part of his analysis is the gross margin or R&D quasi-rent estimate, which lumps together results for truly new products with imitative drug and even nondrug product returns and which ignores the likelihood that the ratio of promotional outlays (excluded from the margin) to sales is an increasing function of the gross margin *before* promotional costs.[2] Correcting for these two shortcomings would increase the margins and hence the indicated returns—I suspect substantially. Suppose Schwartzman is, nevertheless, correct in his conclusion that the average return on recent new-drug R&D has been below the cost of capital. The main policy inference he draws is that we ought to ease up on (or perhaps not tighten) antitrust policy toward the pharmaceutical industry. Yet it was surely not antitrust that raised new chemical entity development costs from half a million dollars (the Mansfield-Schnee estimate) to upwards of $7.5 million. One ought to keep one's beams and motes straight.

More important, if drug R&D is about to stagnate, where will the cuts come? It is not enough to look at averages; what matters is what happens at the margin. On that Schwartzman provides no insight. In my judgment, two main classes of drug developments are likely to be affected disproportionately by the actual rise in R&D costs and by a possible (but by no means historically observable) antitrust-induced fall in returns. One is marginal improvements on already available and effective drugs; the other is significant advances toward combatting diseases of very low incidence. I suspect the incentive to develop new entities that are potentially effective against previously untreated diseases of high incidence will be impaired very little by a general R&D cost rise. The social losses attributable

---

[2] See, for example, R. Dorfman and P. O. Steiner, "Optimal Advertising and Optimal Quality," *American Economic Review*, vol. 44 (December 1954), pp. 835–36.

to discouraging the development of marginal improvements over existing drugs must be modest at best. Breakthrough drugs with only small markets pose the toughest incentive problem. In their case, special remedies may be needed—for example, government subsidies for preliminary clinical screening, streamlined new drug approval procedures, and perhaps even *ad hoc* patent-life extensions. A general relaxation of antitrust to deal with special cases such as these seems on the other hand to be totally unwarranted.

## Edmund W. Kitch

These papers suggest that the profits of leading pharmaceutical companies have not been as high when properly measured in terms of return on investment as many had previously assumed on the basis of conventional accounting reports. These findings may serve to deflate the emotional appeal of attacks on the present structure of the drug industry. Critics of that industry have focused on high book rates of return to argue that the industry is not competitive. However, in my view, the level of profitability experienced by particular firms in the industry is not necessarily related to the issue of whether the industry is appropriately competitive.

First, sustained high profits by a particular firm may be consistent with competition and may be explainable by a number of alternative hypotheses— that the firm has superior management, or that an expanding industry must offer superior returns in order to attract capital from other investment sectors. Conversely, "normal" profits can be perfectly consistent with a noncompetitive industry. Critics of the industry's structure have tended to focus on the role of patent and trademark laws. They have argued that these laws make the industry less than optimally competitive.

It has been argued that patents and trademarks may serve to induce excessive investment in research and advertising. Conversely, it had been argued that competition and weaknesses in the patent and trademark laws do not induce sufficient investment in advertising and research. If you listen for the implicit assumptions of some of the positions advanced here today, you will find that both arguments have been assumed.

The critics have generally taken the position that these laws induce excessive investment. However, whether or not the patent and trademark laws are desirable, they would not necessarily result in a higher rate of return to the firms in the industry, but only induce additional investment. Indeed, what these papers are saying is that when we take that investment into account, the firms have not done as much better than other firms as we might have thought from an examination of the accounting reports.

The critics of the industry who focus upon research investment in "me-too" drugs and complain about excessive and, in their view, propagandistic promotional activities really believe that the industry is making excessive investment in these activities, that at least part of this investment is socially undesirable, and that laws should be changed to remove the incentives for these activities or to prohibit them. No matter what the real rate of return of the firms, these issues of public policy remain.

I cannot in the brief time here discuss the technical complexities of the issues that, in my view, these questions present. I do think that if one takes a larger view of the general functions of the patent and trademark laws, it is really incontrovertible that if we expect private firms subject to competition to continue to be important providers of research and of product information, the incentives provided by these laws are essential, no matter what particular problems there may be with the details of those laws.

Indeed, I rather suspect that the most vocal critics of the drug industry are implicitly assuming that it would be preferable for the government to provide— either through its own agencies or by direct subsidy—the research which the industry now provides and for the government, not the industry, to ·provide "desirable" information about drug products. The issue then becomes whether there will be a significant loss in efficiency and accuracy if the government or entities created by it are the exclusive institutional source of these services. My own judgment is that we have reason to fear a loss rather than a gain in social benefits.

. I will discuss one concrete problem. Current, quite popular, proposals that drugs be prescribed only on a generic basis and not on a brand-name basis assume the feasibility of laying down standard specifications for the manufacture and distribution of drugs that, when met, will give us indistinguishable products that can be selected purely on a price basis. Now under those conditions it is important to notice that the positive incentive for all producers is to meet and not to exceed the government standards—meet and not exceed at all, because that will be the condition under which they will win the price competition. The problems presented are similar to those presented by competitive bidding in government procurement. Under competitive bidding the government sets down specifications for products and then takes the lowest of competitive bids. Competitive bidding works very well for the acquisition of certain kinds of commodities but very poorly for the acquisition of certain other kinds. I have never heard, for instance, that the government has any trouble acquiring nails sufficient for its needs. On the other hand, the Department of Defense has had great difficulty in procuring complex weapon systems.

I have heard it said that the government has difficulty buying reliable elevators because it is not able to write specifications that exclude from the list of eligible bidders those firms which make unreliable elevators. I do not know why that is, but if you cannot write specifications that truly give you control over all the quality parameters of a drug, and if you impose a rule of purchasing that eliminates the incentive to exceed the specifications—indeed, creates an incentive not to exceed the specifications—then you are in for serious trouble. As a layman, I have the notion that some drugs are a very complicated matter. There may be some drugs for which quality can be specified, and others for which it cannot.

I am concerned that necessary discriminations will not be made and that government specifications will become the sole standard of quality. I say government, but I assume there will be a prestigious committee of very well informed men chosen to set standards; I assume that the best information available will be brought to bear on the problem, though it may not be. But the resulting standards may not in all cases be adequate. If the kind of flexibility and incentives that trademark law creates for firms to do better than what is required and better than their competition is eliminated, we will lose something that eventually may turn out to have been very valuable.

From my perspective as a lawyer with a particular interest in regulation, there is another aspect of these papers that requires comment. I am accustomed to discussion of rate of return in the context of regulatory pricing decisions. "Should firm Y get a price increase?" is a question that is answered under traditional utility regulation by examining the question of whether its rate of return is sufficient. Now I will hypothesize that a drug pricing commission exists and has the problem of pricing drugs for the American people. This is not entirely a hypothesis because of the important role of the government as a direct purchaser of drugs and as an insurer whose coverage includes the cost of drug purchases. Because of these government roles, the problem of drug pricing is becoming a problem of public policy. These papers, read in that context, suggest that the returns of drug companies are not much different from those of a lot of other companies and, therefore, that their prices are about "right."

Let me suggest, however, that there are serious problems that would make direct regulation of drug prices quite foolish. For purposes of discussing these problems, I will first eliminate the problem of exclusive trademark and patent rights by discussing the pricing of generic drugs—identical drugs manufactured by several different firms. The first regulatory problem will be how to allocate the joint production costs of several of these products. I will assume that some arbitrary but simple formula such as percentage of gross revenues can be used for this purpose.

The next problem will be whether to price the drug on an industry-wide cost basis or on a firm-by-firm basis. If an industry-wide basis is used, the price will be based on the industry's average cost. This means that firms with above-average costs will be unable to profit from making the drug. They will withdraw from the market, reducing total output and lowering the average cost and the regulated price. If this regulatory logic is followed to its bitter end, there will be only one firm producing the drug. Competition will have been eliminated in the interest of regulation. If the drug's price is regulated on a firm-by-firm basis, the price will vary from firm to firm. The lowest-cost, most efficient firm will have the lowest price. In this situation, the regulator will have to decide who will have the privilege of buying from the lowest-cost firm and who will have to buy from the higher-cost firms; or a system of offsetting payments between purchasers can be set up so that all of them pay the same price, while sellers receive different prices. Under this system of regulation, the lowest-cost producer would have no incentive to control his costs. Indeed, he would have an incentive to raise "costs" to the level of the highest-cost producer in the market. This would represent a serious social loss.

These problems are compounded when trademarks and patents are considered. Is the investment expenditure lying behind these rights to be treated as a cost, and if so, how? Unless the regulator wishes to nullify these rights, he must recognize the expenditure as either an investment or a cost. If he does, firms will be able to raise their allowed prices by increasing these expenditures.

In the long run the regulator must allow prices that enable the firms to attract investment capital, and the firms can keep their rate of return within permissible limits by expanding investment. Therefore, firms will invest until the regulated price reaches the market clearing price. This set of conditions is less attractive from any point of view than the set we now have. It provides neither incentives for efficiency, nor drugs at true cost, nor the proper level of investment. It is a regulatory regime that is very likely to arise.

A firm-by-firm approach to pricing would be a bizarre arrangement, but it is one we are quite capable of adopting. We have already imposed it on the oil industry. Oil companies that produce a large percentage of their output from American domestic reserves (something we wish to encourage our oil companies to do in order to decrease our dependence on foreign supplies) now find that, under the regulatory formula applicable to their companies, they have the lowest prices. Their markets are disrupted. When they open their stations, lines form, and they have great trouble keeping their stations open. They are really quite embarrassed by the fact that they have the lower prices, and they have very strong incentives to increase the percentage of foreign crude that they acquire and market, in order to raise their prices; that is, they have incentives to become in a very real sense less efficient.

Some may look at these three papers and say, "Aren't the economists wonderful? They are such wizards with figures." Although it is true that there are a few figures in the calculations based on little more than guesswork, the calculations are a formidable *tour de force*. "Here is the true rate of return," some may say, "and given this advanced economic methodology, we now know enough about this industry to regulate its prices." That would be an unfortunate conclusion to draw from these papers, which are in fact directed to quite a different kind of question.

## Martin J. Bailey

I would like to discuss a few high points of a theme that runs through all these papers. This theme is that there is a bias in accounting rates of return. Professor Ayanian was especially helpful in clarifying just what that means in both his paper and his extemporaneous remarks. After emphasizing certain of his points, I will cast the issues involved in a slightly different perspective.

Suppose we say that $\pi$ is profits (or net income flow of the firm), $E$ is equity capital, and the superscript star (*) means "true" values as distinct from accounting values, and also that P is the growth rate of capital, as an annual fraction. If, for example, capital were growing at 10 percent a year, P would be .10.

Now, a general finding that comes out of Professor Ayanian's paper, and also Stauffer's, is that either we have $\pi/E$, the accounting rate of return, greater than $\pi^*/E^*$, the true rate of return, which in turn is greater than the growth rate expressed as P/1 + P, or else we have the opposite set of inequalities:

$$\frac{\pi}{E} \leqslant \frac{\pi^*}{E^*} \leqslant \frac{P}{1 + P}.$$

The inequalities can have only one sequence, or its exact opposite. (The term 1 + P in the denominator is an adjustment from continuous compounding, which you hear about from savings and loan associations these days, to a straight annual rate of return; it is not much of an adjustment.)

Now, if you study that result, you can see that Professor Stauffer was saying that accounting practices increase the dispersion of reported rates of profit compared to the dispersion of true profit rates. Where firms show high profits or low profits relative to the rate of growth, the reported rates of profit disperse even wider. If it so happens that the rate of growth of the firm's capital is the same as its true profit rate, then there is no error in accounting profits, at least so far as they are affected by the practice of writing off R&D and advertising instead of capitalizing them.

Therefore, for most cases in the drug industry, a finding that a true rate of return (after capitalizing advertising and R&D spending) is less than the accounting rate of return is equivalent to a finding that the growth rate in their capital is less than their rate of return. Now, although P is the growth of the current investment in advertising and R&D, it equals, if it is a constant, the growth rate of accumulated advertising and R&D capital, correctly accounted.

Further, if the balance between physical capital and such intangible capital as advertising and R&D is undisturbed, that is, if both are growing at the same rate, then physical capital is also growing at the rate P. In that case, there is uniform growth such that each year the amount the firm is investing in all kinds of capital—tangible and intangible—equals its profits. It is plowing all its earnings back. That does not mean that it is retaining everything and paying no dividends, but rather that whatever it is paying out in dividends it is taking back from stockholders or other people in the form of new equity. Now, for industry as a whole, that is roughly true. It is investing, as reported by the Department of Commerce, an amount roughly equal to total industry profits. For drug companies, however, that seems not to be true. Their investment rate, that is, growth of capital, is less than their profit.

Does that mean that the drug industry is not doing well in terms of growth? Apparently right now it is not. There is something atypical in the finding that, for pharmaceuticals, the accounting rate of return is higher than the true rate. This could mean that the data we are looking at are unusual for that industry because it is going through a transition phase. Professor Schwartzman's paper emphasizes that there are new ground rules for the pharmaceutical industry that the law has set for FDA to administer. Under these rules the standards for the introduction of new drugs are much tougher than they used to be. Therefore, the industry's investment patterns are in transition, and the growth rate is changing while the industry adapts to the new rules.

That may or may not be the right way to interpret these results. However, we should expect that the pharmaceutical industry, if the ground rules ever stay constant for long enough, will look like other industries in the long run. That is, its accounting rates of return will not be much different from the true rates to the extent they are affected by intangible types of investment.

The conclusion I draw from Professor Schwartzman's analysis, similar to his but with a different emphasis, agrees with Sam Peltzman's recent article, which pointed out that the new ground rules reduce the rate of introduction of new drugs.[1] Professor Schwartzman, in some of his remarks, almost implied that the drug industry would quit. However, I do not think he meant that. The correct conclusion is that with tougher rules it will not be profitable to develop as many new drugs. There could be a reduction in the amount of spending, and assuredly there is a reduction in the rate of introduction of new drugs.

Now, whether that is a good or a bad thing depends on what we think about the benefits versus the cost of the drugs that are not introduced as a result of these rules.

That is a hard thing to appraise. On the one side, we might take Dr. Melmon's remarks (see Part One) at face value and say that the country would be better off if we had fewer drugs prescribed, new or old. The patient population would presumably be healthier if that were the case. Inasmuch as I am completely innocent of any knowledge of any data that may exist on this subject—he suggests there are some—I feel free to have any opinion I like. My opinion is very much in line with his. If we had an independent standard of tangible benefits and cost from the use of drugs, my guess is we would find the country is indeed on a drug

---

[1] "An evaluation of Consumer Protection Legislation: The 1962 Drug Amendments," *Journal of Political Economy*, vol. 81 (1973), p. 1049.

kick and would be better off, according to those tangible measures, with fewer drugs. By this reasoning it is a good thing that we are not introducing so many new drugs. Another reason that might lead to the same conclusion is that the drugs that are not developed will be the less promising ones. That is, they will come under some cutoff line at an early stage of their development and this decision will be based on some presumably valid information about how good the drugs are likely to be should the country go through the whole procedure of bringing them onto the market. A disproportionate share of those drugs held back as a result of the new regulations will be mediocre drugs, as the term was used. Hence, we should not use the average efficacy of drugs to decide how much harm is being done by the reduction in new drug development.

However, there is a problem about either one of these lines of thought. As a former Chicago economist, I have to agree with Professor Peltzman's remarks that a free market is better than a market entangled in regulation. Without these regulations, more drugs would be introduced, doctors would prescribe them, and people would use them. By the market test, whatever any objective evidence may say about tangible benefits, all we need to know is that people think the drugs are good for them. If they are deprived of drugs, they are, by the evidence of their own behavior, worse off. Now, how do I reconcile that line of thought with the earlier ones? My way of reconciling them is to say that the market is not free in some very important other respects that affect, to some degree, the usage of drugs.

The ideal reaction to all this is to go to a free market: abolish the FDA, allow all drugs to be sold freely without prescription, allow anyone to practice medicine without a license—abolish all state, local, and federal restrictions on the practice of medicine and use of drugs.

If we abandon that ideal as unattainable, what is a practical second best? The problem about the great tangle of interference in medical practice from state and federal law is that there is a considerable divergence of interest between the physician and his patient, of which the physician is well aware. The law has given local medical societies considerable power over the career of the doctor, through which they have enforced minimum fees for most medical services and, further, have prevented for thirty years the spread of prepaid medical practice. (Right now the issue of whether the federal government will succeed in making prepaid medical practice generally acceptable hangs in the balance.)

If we could have competition in the practice of medicine, with no interference, prepaid practice would become a major way for physicians to do business. In that case, anyone who went to a prepaid clinic that included drugs in the flat fee would find that the clinic would not be trying to give him drugs that he did not need. If he demanded a drug as a placebo, he would receive a sugar pill instead of some high-powered new thing that might hurt him. When the advantage of not using the drug is greater than the therapeutic value, it would be in the clinic's own interest to worry about side effects and to be sure no one had to be hospitalized because of them. In general, if drug-related medical services were priced competitively the doctor would have no financial interest in giving needless prescriptions.

So, my philosophical response to the information in these papers is that if the government could indeed succeed in encouraging prepaid medical practice and could generally increase the amount of competition in medicine, we would expect the amount of drugs prescribed to be reduced. If that happened, it would be best to have all the new drugs we could get, without restrictive regulations. Without increased competition, however, if doctors have a financial incentive to overprescribe due to fee-setting by local medical societies, the prospective demand for any drug is inflated. A larger than optimal number of drugs would therefore be introduced without regulation. The effect of regulation moves drug introduction in the socially better direction—namely, downward. However, there is no basis for saying whether it moves it too little or too much.

# HIGHLIGHTS OF
# THE DISCUSSION

After the prepared comments were presented by the panel, Professor Weidenbaum asked each of the three people who presented papers to reply to the discussants' remarks. What followed was a period of general debate among the six panelists. Most of the important points of this debate have been incorporated into these papers. This is not the case, however, with Professor Kitch's responses to Professor Bailey, which were the basis of much of the later comment from the floor on the effect of regulation on the supply of drug products "of limited commercial value."

It will be recalled that Professor Bailey argued that a disproportionate share of those drugs which were not developed as a result of tougher FDA rules would be mediocre drugs. This statement elicited two remarks by Professor Kitch. The first was that the term "mediocre drug" was misleading. If FDA regulation causes a reduction in the development of new drugs, the drugs which would be lost would be those which promise a low economic promise of return. In such a regulatory climate, the drug industry would develop more of those drugs for which they anticipate a large market. Kitch reasoned that the drugs which are not developed may be highly desirable drugs from a medical point of view but would tend to be those which are more condition-specific and patient-specific rather than those which would treat a large number of people.

Kitch's second point was that there was an important difference between the question Dr. Melmon was raising as to whether we have an overdrugged society that makes too great a use of the existing *stock* of drugs and the question of whether or not the rate of introduction of new pharmaceuticals is too high, too low, or optimal. To keep these two questions separate, Professor Kitch pointed out that if there is a built-in cultural bias toward excessive use of drugs, as Dr. Melmon suggests, then this over-consumption can be satisfied from the existing stock of drugs. However, if we could have an increase in drug research, it is quite possible that we could develop drugs which are therapeutically preferable, require shorter periods of administration, or have other characteristics which would reduce the use of drugs and thus ameliorate the problem of the excessive use of the present stock of drugs. To apply Kitch's analysis to a current controversy, if we could develop a virus-specific drug, doctors would prescribe this instead of using antibiotics for virus conditions.

Dr. John Curren noted that most cases of adverse drug reaction have been associated with the use of old drugs rather than newly developed ones. He concluded that regulatory policies that slow down the introduction of new drugs may increase our reliance on old drugs and thereby increase the risk of adverse reactions.

Dr. Rita Campbell brought up the ethical question of whether we should rely on foreign countries to gain experience with the human use of drugs. She said, "It bothers me to have my Mexican neighbors be the main testing ground for drugs that I may later take." Professor Bailey responded that the world population provides a very ample testing ground for gathering clinical experience on new drugs and that all possible worldwide information should be used to build up as soon as possible our systematic knowledge of the effects of drugs.

Dr. Kitch pointed out that "there is an old ethical standard that you should not apply rules to yourself that you are not willing to see everybody apply to themselves." Kitch concluded that we would probably become unhappy with our strict rules regarding human testing of drugs if other countries agreed with the American standards and decided to stop the use of human subjects for drug testing.

To summarize, most of the discussion in the second session related to the broad topic introduced in the first session—the risks and benefits of drug use. This developed naturally out of the subject of "incentives and performance" from Schwartzman's, Ayanian's, and Stauffer's analyses of the consequences of increasing the costs of drug research. As this discussion has pointed out, reasonable men will always disagree about the use of risky but potentially beneficial drugs and the degree to which government policy should affect the risk-benefit decision. Perhaps the only way out of this dilemma is to create a system that allows the individual drug user who stands to benefit from a drug more choice about its use.

# PART THREE

## EXTERNAL DETERMINANTS OF DRUG INNOVATION

# CHAIRMAN'S COMMENT

*Leon I. Goldberg*

The subject of this group of papers is the external determinants of drug innovation. It seems to me we should examine at least two important issues related to this topic. First, we have to determine if there is a problem in the United States—whether in fact we have a drug lag here and, if so, whether it has been a good or bad thing. Second, we have to think about whether there have been any changes in the system. Has anything happened to make it better, or is it still bad? If in fact there is a drug lag here, what could be done to improve the situation? How could it be done in the present climate, where ethical issues and legislation seem to predominate over everything else? These papers should provide stimulating material for later discussion of such questions.

# THE ECONOMIC AND REGULATORY CLIMATE: U.S. AND OVERSEAS TRENDS

*Harold A. Clymer*

## Introduction

My purpose today is to present the evidence that leads to the following hypothesis concerning the U.S. pharmaceutical industry: An adverse microeconomic environment, resulting principally from the regulatory climate, seriously threatens the leadership of the domestic R&D activities of the technology-intensive U.S. pharmaceutical industry. Their inability to grow in their home market through new product introductions and to obtain an adequate return on their R&D investment forces firms to give priority to foreign pharmaceutical markets, with eventual commensurate reallocation of their R&D resources, or to diversify into other business areas. In either case, the result is erosion of the extensive domestic technological resources of the U.S. pharmaceutical industry.

In support of this hypothesis, I would like to share with you some of the data that I believe to be leading indicators of trends in the pharmaceutical industry, with particular emphasis on the R&D impact. I shall compare changes in the United States with those taking place in major foreign countries, and discuss some of the economic factors that are behind these changes. In reviewing the trends, it will be apparent that their continuation would have public policy implications too important to be left for the pharmaceutical industry and the Food and Drug Administration to deal with as best they can.

You will note that the opening statement is labeled a hypothesis rather than a theory, since I am sure that today it will not be universally accepted. Were the facts so clear-cut, our deliberations here would be a waste of time, for it would probably be too late to influence public policy or alter the final course of events. Accordingly, the most important topic I want to cover in this paper is an outline of crucial new data that is obtainable and that would shed light on where and why the U.S. regulatory climate has had its greatest impact, thus leading to a less confused and more meaningful debate on issues of concern to all of us.

## History of the U.S. Pharmaceutical Industry

In order to gain a perspective on these current topics, it is useful to review briefly the evolution of the R&D-intensive industry we know today.

In the late thirties to mid-forties, the industry went through a metamorphosis. The major pharmaceutical companies of the 1930s were full-line houses. This meant they manufactured and sold a complete line of all medicaments the physican could prescribe. It would be more exact to say they supplied the pharmacist with all the needed ingredients to compound the doctor's prescriptions, for well into the 1930s prescriptions were multi-ingredient liquids, powders, and salves compounded in the pharmacy. Major firms manufactured mainly the tinctures, fluid extracts, syrups, elixirs, and ground crude drugs contained in the *United States Pharmacopoeia* (USP) and the *National Formulary* (NF). Until the 1940s, these official compendia changed little from one revision to the next and consisted mainly of products containing or derived from galenical drugs. The slow pace of advance in therapy can be seen from the tinctures and fluid extracts, for example, fluid extract of taraxacum (otherwise known as fluid extract of dandelion root), fluid extract of valerian, tincture of veratrum viride, and so forth, which were official in the pharmacopoeias of the 1800s, still official in the *National Formulary* of 1936, and still manufactured and used in the early forties. as evidenced by their listing in the 1943 catalog of Eli Lilly and Company. Although major companies had national or regional sales forces calling on physicians and pharmacists, the main thrust of their promotion was to stress the assured quality and purity of their firms' products and to get the physician to designate Lilly or Parke-Davis, or whatever the case might be, on every prescription he wrote.

If this description of the industry in the early part of the century sounds similar to current discussions concerning generic drugs, it is. Whether the term used is full-line house or generic house, it is still a commodity business with an economic profile entirely different from the research-based, innovative, speciality, pharmaceutical business. They are both important but they are different industries.

The economic profile of the industry in the 1930s was that of a commodity business. Cost of goods was in the range of 60 to 75 percent of sales, selling and administrative expenses, 20 to 25 percent, and pretax profit below 10 percent. Pretax profit is the only comparable profit figure, for prior to the excess-profits tax of World War II, the corporate tax rate was less than 20 percent. R&D as such was nonexistent in most firms; it certainly never appeared on income statements, nor was it mentioned in annual reports. Among my own firm's three-page annual reports for the 1930s, the first mention I could find of R&D was in a brief covering letter to the 1939 report by Mr. C. Mahlon Kline, the president of the company. Mr. Kline simply said, "We have increased our expenditures on research." It was in 1939 that I joined SmithKline; you can judge the magnitude of their R&D at that time by the fact that I was told I would have to consider the position temporary, since they had already hired two people within the previous year for their laboratory and were not sure that the business would warrant the continued expenditure.

What brought about the metamorphosis? It is a good deal easier to describe the pattern of investment behavior than it is to determine what set the changes in motion. The timing varied from firm to firm, and undoubtedly the impetus came from many factors: the advancement of scientific education in the United States and the transformation, starting in the 1920s, of our medical schools into more scientific and research-oriented institutions certainly were important. New ideas soon needed translation into practical therapy, and industry began to see a new role for itself.

In the case of my own firm, transformation was rather precipitous. In 1936 the younger managers, using the then relatively new management tool of cost accounting, convinced Mr. Kline that the firm was actually losing money on the hundreds of USP and NF items it made and that the profit was generated by three specialty products sold nationally. Why? Because each advertising and promotional dollar generated more sales and profits if the product had distinctive superiority and advantages for the physician. In what must have been one of the heroic business decisions of that era, SmithKline discontinued manufacture of hundreds of commodity USP and NF products, disposed of the inventory, and decided to concentrate its efforts on specialty products. Inherent in this major change in business strategy was the need for greater R&D effort to obtain the additional specialty products from which its growth was to come.

By the end of the 1950s, the pharmaceutical industry had transformed itself into an R&D-intensive business. It is interesting to observe the historical intensity of the reinvestment in R&D as a percentage of sales dollars, as shown in Table 1.

The creation and rapid expansion of a scientific and medical research capability within the drug industry has certainly played a role in the pace at which advances in therapy have been added to the physician's armament. It was a

## Table 1
### INTENSITY OF R&D INVESTMENT

| Year | R&D Investment as Percent of Sales |
|------|-----------------------------------|
| 1950 | 3.0 |
| 1955 | 5.5 |
| 1960 | 7.4 |
| 1965 | 8.3 |
| 1970 | 8.8 |
| 1971 | 9.0 |
| 1972 | 8.6 |

Source: PMA, *PMA Annual Survey Reports: Pharmaceutical Industry Operations and Research and Development Activity,* 1950 to 1973 editions (Washington, D.C.: Pharmaceutical Manufacturers Association).

consequence of vision on the part of management—a vision that recognized the plain economic facts of business life: profits and return on investment. It is often forgotten, overlooked, or misunderstood, but in the final analysis the incentive for risk investment in R&D is the prospect of future profits.

The pharmaceutical industry is part of a complex chain of institutions that play a role in the evolution of fundamental biological findings into utilizable new therapeutic agents. The other types of institutions involved are academic establishments and government research laboratories such as the National Institutes of Health (NIH). The pharmaceutical industry occupies a unique position in this chain, in that it encompasses the only workable system for doing the thousand and one things necessary to develop a drug product from a chemical compound— in other words, to carry out the innovative phase. I do not want to get involved in the semantic morass of fundamental versus applied research—which has greater social value or contributes more to the origin of new therapeutic agents, discovery or innovation?—for it is a sophomoric debate. However, since it is the innovative phase, or, as more commonly referred to within the industry, the developmental phase that is often pictured as routine and pedestrian, let me demonstrate just how critical and challenging a role it can play. Many past examples could be cited, but since most things after the fact have a tendency to appear easy, let me use an example in which the developmental problems are still unsolved. Interferon was discovered by Alick Isaacs at Mill Hill more than a decade ago. He demonstrated it to be a naturally occurring, intracellular antiviral material of great potential. The possibility of a much needed breakthrough in antiviral chemotherapy, akin to Sir Alexander Fleming's discovery of penicillin for the treatment and control of bacterial infections, was quickly perceived. The discovery was made; all that remained to be done was the developmental work of getting it into a bottle. In the intervening years, pharmaceutical firms around the world have spent millions of dollars and untold man-years trying to obtain sufficient material to evaluate fully interferon's activity in one human viral disease. It turns out that there are numerous types of interferon, each species-specific, and that human interferon is generated only by growing human cells. If the obstacles in the developmental phase are ever overcome, I predict the rules for the Nobel Prize will be changed to award it posthumously to Isaacs. If the difficulties are not overcome the discovery of interferon will be relegated to a minor mention in the history of medical science.

By the second half of the 1960s, it was obvious to those engaged in development of new therapeutic agents in the United States that the process of development had been radically altered, not principally through scientific advances, but by the new regulatory milieu created by the 1962 amendments to the Food, Drug and Cosmetic Act. Simply stated, the amendments brought about two basic changes. First, proof of efficacy was added to proof of safety as a requirement for marketing. Second, the investigational new drug (IND) process was instituted, by which the FDA would now regulate and monitor the developmental phase of

R&D. Few would argue with these basic requirements as concepts. Certainly there can be no turning back the clock, for in many ways the changes have had beneficial effects. They wrenched some of us out of old ways and headed us toward more thorough work and better science. They made R&D expenditures aimed at anything less than superior therapy a waste of stockholders' money. They have acted as an incentive for the development of keener methodology in many preclinical and clinical scientific disciplines. All of these changes were good and should have led to a giant step forward in therapeutics. However, after several years in practice, with a stream of interpretative regulations, quasi-official requirements, and regulatory minutiae, serious questions as to the basic system arose. In the late sixties leaders in the industry began to express concern about the future of drug research, since there was not only a marked and continuing increase in the time and expenditure required for developing compounds coming from research but also a continuing decline in products reaching the market. Unquestionably, the impact of these changes in drug development produced a perplexing set of economic constraints for the industry, combining a demand for increased investment with greatly increased uncertainty of return. The question asked more and more often was whether the new economic configuration would offer the profit potential to justify its inherently increasing costs and financial risks. Eventually, it must be the potential of tomorrow's profits, not the size of yesterday's or today's, that governs risk investment.

In a paper given in October 1971, I made some rather simple calculations of the total industry's return on its R&D investment under almost ten years of the new economics resulting from the 1962 amendments to the drug act.[1] Using minimal assumptions, I was able to get the closest prediction of return by using for input the Pharmaceutical Manufacturers Association (PMA) R&D expenditure for the total industry for the five-year period 1961–65 and for output the estimated peak sales of the products actually approved for marketing in the subsequent five-year period of 1966–70. The results of this exercise were disquieting to say the least. Without taking into consideration the time value of money (discounting the cash flow), at a 20 percent net profit or 40 percent pretax profit, the payback period was nineteen years after marketing! Since the 1971 paper, we have updated these calculations, using products approved through 1972, and the results show little if any improvement. The difficulty, if not impossibility, of industry earning a return on its R&D investment from the new products that have been approved in the current U.S. regulatory climate demonstrates the extent of the problem that is forcing the industry to give increased consideration to alternative resource allocation. Here the economist's concept of profit, rather than the accounting report of profit, is closer to the real world of management decision making. The

---

[1] H. A. Clymer, "The Economics of Drug Innovation" in M. Pernarowski and M. Darrach, eds., *The Development and Control of New Drug Products* (Vancouver, B. C.: Evergreen Press, 1971).

economist's concept includes only the profit made over and above what the investment would have earned elsewhere. This comparison then governs the rational choices among prospective alternatives. It is the future return potential of other alternatives for risk investment against which pharmaceutical R&D must eventually compete.

### Changes Taking Place in the Pharmaceutical Industry

The inability to grow in the home market through new product introductions and to obtain an adequate return on their R&D expenditures has presented U.S. pharmaceutical firms with the two major alternatives mentioned in my opening hypothesis: redeployment through diversification into other businesses and giving emphasis and priority to foreign markets. I do not intend to examine diversification in any depth in this paper. Certainly, this has taken place. In some cases, it has meant redeployment of R&D capabilities and investment into other high-technology areas. Some of this was originally the result of exploiting technology generated in pharmaceuticals; however, in the main, the purpose has been diversification per se. In other cases, diversification has taken the form of investment in less technology-intensive businesses such as consumer products, cosmetics and toiletries, and so forth. It is the second alternative that I want to examine in some detail—to describe the trends taking place and some of the economic factors that govern these trends.

**Priority to Foreign Markets.** The chairman of the Pharmaceutical Manufacturers Association (PMA) and president of Squibb Corporation, Richard M. Furlaud, in an address at the annual meeting of the PMA in April of this year, made the following statement regarding the importance of foreign markets:

> Indeed, when our profit structure is looked at from the point of view of the security analysts, who watch it with sharp and skeptical eyes, you get a picture very different from that created on Capitol Hill. For years, these analysts have been calling attention to the declining profit margins of our domestic operations, which they consider a negative factor in terms of our ability to finance future growth.
>
> Indeed, if the profitability of the industry is looked at closely, I think it will be concluded that pharmaceutical companies have been able to maintain their profit growth and largely to maintain their profit ratios primarily through their expansion in foreign markets, which has the effect of spreading their R&D and administrative costs over an increasingly large base.[2]

First, let us look at some of the figures that compare the growth of domestic and foreign markets. Table 2 is based on PMA sales figures and demonstrates

---

[2] R. M. Furlaud, "The Pharmaceutical Industry Faces the Future" (Paper presented at the Pharmaceutical Manufacturers Association meeting, Boca Raton, Florida, April 1974).

142

## Table 2
### PHARMACEUTICAL SALES OF PMA MEMBER FIRMS

| Year | Sales ($ millions) | | Total Sales (percent) | | Increase of Total Sales over Previous Year (percent) | |
|---|---|---|---|---|---|---|
| | U.S. | Foreign | U.S. | Foreign | U.S. | Foreign |
| 1965 | 2,779 | 930 | 75.0 | 25.0 | 12.1 | 15.4 |
| 1970 | 4,322 | 1,890 | 69.6 | 30.4 | 7.8 | 16.8 |
| 1971 | 4,667 | 2,113 | 68.8 | 31.2 | 8.0 | 11.8 |
| 1972 | 5,018 | 2,504 | 66.7 | 33.3 | 7.5 | 18.5 |

**Source:** PMA, *Prescription Drug Industry Fact Book,* rev. ed. (Washington, D. C., 1973).

a steady progression in recent years in the growth and importance of foreign markets. While these PMA figures are the best available as far as pure human ethical pharmaceutical sales are concerned, they understate the importance of foreign sales to the U.S.-owned industry, since they include the U.S. sales of subsidiaries of foreign-owned firms that are PMA members. The foreign sales of these foreign PMA members, of course, are not included in the PMA figures. Market surveys show that foreign subsidiary U.S. sales amount to approximately $1 billion; adjusting for this factor would bring the percentage of 1972 foreign sales for the U.S. firms up from 33 percent to approximately 38 percent and the domestic sales down to 62 percent rather than 67 percent. With foreign sales increasing significantly more rapidly than U.S. sales, within the next five years foreign markets will account for more than half of the U.S. pharmaceutical firms' total sales.

Another way to look at the relative importance to U.S. pharmaceutical firms of foreign versus domestic markets without the distortion produced by foreign firms' sales in the PMA figures is to use data given in annual reports. Table 3 shows the comparative foreign and domestic increases in 1973 sales over 1972 sales for fifteen major U.S.-owned pharmaceutical firms. The total foreign sales of all the firms increased 30 percent. On the other hand, their total domestic sales increase was only 10 percent. For these fifteen firms, the increase in foreign market growth was three times that of the U.S. growth. It is true that these figures are based on total corporate sales, since most of the firms in their annual reports do not segregate pharmaceutical sales within domestic and foreign categories. But from reports in which pharmaceutical figures are specifically given, and from general statements in most of the annual reports regarding the increase in foreign pharmaceutical sales, it is safe to assume that the differential between domestic and foreign increases in pharmaceutical sales is as great as, if not greater than, that reflected in total corporate sales figures. The same differential would apply to profits also.

## Table 3
### TOTAL CORPORATE SALES OF U.S.-OWNED PHARMACEUTICAL FIRMS, 1973

| Firm | Percentage Increase over 1972 | |
| --- | --- | --- |
| | U.S. | Foreign |
| Abbott | 15 | 26 |
| American Cyanamid | 2 | 23 |
| American Home | 8 | 23 |
| Bristol-Myers | 8 | 30 |
| Johnson & Johnson | 11 | 45 |
| Lilly | 13 | 31 |
| Merck | 10 | 25 |
| Pfizer | 11 | 24 |
| Robins | 11 | 21 |
| Schering-Plough | 11 | 40 |
| Searle | 16 | 22 |
| SmithKline | 9 | 15 |
| Squibb | 7 | 26 |
| Upjohn | 22 | 36 |
| Warner-Lambert | 6 | 22 |
| Percentage increase of all company sales | 10 | 30 |

**Source:** Annual reports of firms listed.

Table 4 shows the change in ratio between foreign and U.S. sales that took place from 1972 to 1973—a shift of 4 percent of total sales from U.S. to foreign. Again, the total sales figures understate the percentage of pharmaceutical sales made abroad. From the figures and comments in their annual reports, foreign

## Table 4
### FOREIGN AND DOMESTIC SALES OF FIFTEEN MAJOR U.S.-OWNED PHARMACEUTICAL FIRMS, 1972 AND 1973

| | Percent Distribution of Total Sales | | 1973 Sales Increase | |
| --- | --- | --- | --- | --- |
| | 1972 | 1973 | Millions of dollars | Percent of total increase |
| Domestic | 66 | 62 | 852 | 39.8 |
| Foreign | 34 | 38 | 1,286 | 60.2 |
| Total | | | 2,138 | 100.0 |

**Source:** Annual reports of firms in Table 3.

**Table 5**

SIZE OF MAJOR WORLD MARKETS

| Region | | Sales ($ billions) |
|---|---|---|
| United States | | 4.3 |
| Europe | | 6.5 |
|     United Kingdom | 0.6 | |
|     Germany | 1.9 | |
|     France | 1.9 | |
|     Italy | 1.6 | |
|     Other | 1.5 | |
| | 6.5 | |
| Japan | | 2.8 |
| Other developed markets | | 2.9 |

pharmaceutical sales for a number of firms are now over 50 percent. Table 4 also includes a breakdown of the absolute dollar growth in sales in 1973 for these fifteen firms and shows that 60 percent of the growth came from foreign markets. This is a pretty good indicator of why priority has to be given to these markets.

**Growth Factors in Foreign Markets**

**Market Size.** It is of interest to look deeper into the factors that have made these foreign markets conducive to growth. First, but not foremost, is size. The markets for pharmaceuticals in major European countries and Japan have had an average growth rate over the last decade about twice that of the U.S. Table 5 shows the size of these markets today compared with those of the U.S. From the standpoint of sheer size, the foreign markets no longer can be considered icing on the cake, or an opportunity to be exploited only after the U.S. market potential has been realized. Japan alone is over one-half the size of the U.S. market, Europe at $6.5 billion offers one and one-half times the potential of the U.S. market, and together the major developed international markets are approximately three times that of the U.S.

**Conducive Structure for New Product Introduction.** The industry is organized structurally and financially for growth from new product introductions. Market size in itself does not guarantee growth. During the last decade, the regulatory barriers to innovation have been considerably less formidable in the major foreign markets than in the U.S. I know I will hear the same argument I have heard for the last decade regarding this comparison, namely, that the development costs and times and delays in registration have been increasing in major foreign countries. Indeed they have. However, the United States somehow always manages to outpace them, with no indication that the gap is closing.[3] The FDA takes the rebuttal one step further and insists that our regulatory system is becoming the model for the world. If by this is meant that the world regulatory climate soon will approximate that existing in the United States for the last decade, it is hardly a reassuring argument for progress towards the relief of suffering and disease in the world. Fortunately, to date, the trends I am about to describe do not indicate that this is taking place.

The key critical factor that differentiates major foreign markets from the U.S. on an economic basis, and particularly that governing R&D investment, is the factor of uncertainty. This uncertainty is a result of the inability to perceive a dependable standard upon which to judge what degree of safety and efficacy will be required of a new compound and whether the chances of its ever being cleared for marketing in the U.S. justify continued investment. L. H. Sarett describes this uncertainty of regulatory approval as "extending at the far end into infinity." [4] The regulatory barriers to innovation in the pharmaceutical industry in the U.S. have not only been a moving target, but the upward trajectory at times has been extremely erratic. A case in point is the demand by the FDA in the 1970–71 period not merely for clinical studies to demonstrate the efficacy claimed, but for "clinically meaningful" effectiveness studies in certain therapeutic areas.[5] By this was meant long-term morbidity/mortality studies; for example, a drug sponsor was to provide evidence not only that a hypotensive agent lowers blood pressure safely and effectively but also that it will decrease long-term morbidity/mortality, or, in the case of an anti-appetite agent, that the resulting weight loss will result in increased life span for the patients.

To obtain some quantitative comparison of barriers to innovation and ability to obtain a return on R&D investment, it is interesting to look at new products introduced into the United Kingdom for the same five-year period, 1968–72, used earlier for the analysis of return on R&D investment in the United States. The United Kingdom has become the standard for comparison with the United States, principally because the quality of its science and medical practice are certainly on a par with that of the United States. In Table 6, the results of this comparison are shown. The number given in the first column is the number of products introduced that achieved a significant sales level of $1 million per year. In the second column are the estimated dollar sales to be achieved by these products in their peak years. There were forty-four such significant products introduced

---

[3] L. H. Sarett, "FDA Regulations and Their Influence on Future R&D," *Research Management*, vol. 27 (March 1974), pp. 18–20.

[4] Sarett, "FDA Regulations."

[5] K. H. Beyer, Jr., "What Pharmacology Is All About," *The Pharmacologist*, vol. 13 (Spring 1971), pp. 129–33; J. Freund and L. W. Preston, "FDA: Clinically Meaningful Data," *Science*, vol. 171 (29 January 1971), pp. 334–35.

## Table 6
## NEW PRODUCTS INTRODUCED, 1968–72

| Country | Number Reaching Sales of $1 Million per Year | Estimated Total Sales in Peak Year ($ millions) |
|---|---|---|
| United States | 26 | 240 |
| United Kingdom | 44 | 220 |

**Source:** NDA approval lists, *Monthly Index of Medical Specialities, Annual Compendium 1968 through 1972* (London), and market surveys for the United States and Britain performed by IMS America Ltd., Des Plaines, Illinois, and the British Pharmaceutical Index, Middlesex, England.

into the U.K. market during this five-year period versus twenty-six for the U.S. market. These figures indicate the relative difference between the two markets in receptivity to products of significant economic importance and ability to contribute to return on R&D investment. What is even more revealing is the fact that the total revenue from the new products introduced in the United Kingdom approaches the level of that for the United States. Even though the U.S. market is seven times as large, the U.K. market offers opportunities for growth and return on R&D investment approaching those offered in the United States.

### International Position of U.S. R&D Investment

What is the size of the U.S. pharmaceutical R&D investment as compared to that of other nations with major R&D activities? All of the comparisons I have seen stem from one source, which today is grossly outdated. This is the Organization for Economic Cooperation and Development (OECD) report, which contained comparative data for countries based on the 1964 level of R&D effort.[6] Given the changes that have taken place in the last decade in the pharmaceutical industry, the utility of this OECD report must be relegated to past comparisons.

From direct contact with foreign trade associations, as well as from international financial sources and annual reports of major pharmaceutical companies in foreign countries, we have compiled estimated annual R&D growth rates, which I believe is a more representative comparison of R&D intensity among the major countries today.

Table 7 gives the estimated growth rates for the two major indicators of R&D intensity, namely, level of financial expenditures and level of manpower. The growth rate of R&D in the major foreign countries is by any measure significantly greater than that of the United States and indicates that these countries

[6] *Gaps in Technology: Pharmaceuticals* (Paris: OECD Publications, 1969). As an example of how public policy can be influenced by lack of new data, the recently published report, *Chemicals and Health*, by the President's Science Advisory Committee, relied on this report.

## Table 7

### INTERNATIONAL COMPARISON OF PHARMACEUTICAL R&D INTENSITY

| | Estimated Annual Growth Rates | |
| --- | --- | --- |
| **Firms** | Expenditures (percent) | Manpower (percent) |
| United States | 4–8 | 0–1 |
| German | 15–20 | 8 |
| United Kingdom | 15–17 | n.a. |
| Swiss | 25 | n.a. |
| Swedish | 14 | 8 |
| Japanese | 22 | 15 |
| French | 15 | 8 |

**Source:** Estimates for United States derived from PMA *Annual Survey Report,* 1971–72, 1970–71, 1969–70; European, U.K., and Swedish estimates derived from European Trade Association data, financial publications such as *Financial Times,* or major company annual reports, whichever was most current for individual country; Japanese estimates derived from *Handbook of Japan Drug Industry, 1972,* and annual reports submitted to Ministry of Finance in accordance with "Japan Security Exchange Control."

are giving considerably greater emphasis to pharmaceutical R&D. Lest it be thought that the larger percentage increase abroad is principally a factor of a lower base, the 1972 dollar expenditure of the European Economic Community (EEC) on pharmaceutical R&D is, at a minimum, $900 million compared to the PMA figure for the U.S. industry of $667 million. In terms of R&D manpower, the employment in the Japanese pharmaceutical industry is currently 75 percent of that in the United States, that is, in the range of sixteen thousand for Japan versus twenty-one thousand for the United States.

## Table 8

### U.S. PHARMACEUTICAL R&D

| | Expenditures | | |
| --- | --- | --- | --- |
| **Location** | 1971 ($ millions) | 1972 ($ millions) | Increase (percent) |
| United States | 576.5 | 600.7 | 4.0 |
| Within firm | (510.1) | (526.6) | (3.2) |
| Outside firm | (66.4) | (74.1) | (11.7) |
| Other countries | 52.3 | 66.1 | 26.4 |
| Within firm | (45.8) | (58.3) | (27.2) |
| Outside firm | (6.5) | (7.8) | (20.0) |
| Total | 628.8 | 666.8 | 6.0 |

**Source:** Pharmaceutical Manufacturers Association, *Research and Development Expenditures 1972 Actual,* p. 2.

**Table 9**

DISTRIBUTION OF U.S. PHARMACEUTICAL R&D PERSONNEL

| | United States | | Foreign | |
|---|---|---|---|---|
| Year | Employees | Annual growth rate (percent) | Employees | Annual growth rate (percent) |
| 1965 | 16,375 | } 9 | | |
| 1966 | 17,555 | | | |
| 1967 | 19,400 | | | |
| 1968 | 20,480 | } 1 | | |
| 1969 | 20,230 | | | |
| 1970 | 20,605 | | | |
| 1971 | 21,725 | | 2,455 | |
| 1972 | 21,190 (−2.5%) | | 3,360 | 37 |

**Source:** PMA, *Annual Survey Reports.*

While the figures in Table 7 are indicators of loss of U.S. leadership in R&D intensity, let us also look at the U.S. R&D statistics in greater detail and examine the trends of domestic- and foreign-based R&D activities of U.S. firms. Table 8 compares the 1971 and 1972 expenditures for PMA member firms, broken down into amounts spent in the United States and abroad. While in absolute dollar terms foreign spending is still small, the percentage increase reflects the trend in priority for the use abroad of new or incremental funds for R&D. The PMA R&D figures present the same problem as previously noted regarding PMA sales figures, for they contain the U.S. spending of the foreign PMA member firms, while the figures for amount spent abroad are confined to U.S.-owned member firms. The average percentage increase for foreign-owned firms over the last four years has been three times the percentage increase for U.S. firms, so the figures in Table 8 for the amount spent in the United States by U.S. industry is actually overstated.

Table 9 is even more significant as a leading indicator of the changes actually taking place within R&D in the industry. It shows that, while in the early 1960s the level of personnel in R&D in the pharmaceutical industry in the United States was increasing at a rate of 9 percent per year, since 1968 the employment level has been essentially flat. Whether the drop in U.S. personnel in 1972 of 2.5 percent is actually the beginning of a downward trend in R&D employment remains to be seen. I am not at all sure that the PMA figures are sufficiently sensitive to make this drop significant. The PMA has published foreign R&D employment figures since 1971 only. This gives only a two-year comparison to indicate trends. However, the 37 percent increase, amounting to the addition of nearly one

**Table 10**

ORIGINS OF NEW CHEMICAL AGENTS MARKETED IN
THE UNITED STATES

| Year | Number of Compounds Introduced | Percentage Originated | |
|---|---|---|---|
| | | By U.S. firms | By foreign firms |
| 1940–70 | 809 | 70 | 30 |
| 1971–73 | 31 | 39 | 61 |

**Source:** Pharmaceutical Manufacturers Association, *Prescription Drug Industry Fact Book* for data 1940–70. Figures for 1971–73 derived from issued patents, annual reports, and personal communications.

thousand people, would appear to represent a real change. Together, the personnel and the dollar figures certainly indicate the trend toward emphasis on the spending of incremental R&D funds abroad.

### Origin of New Single Chemical Agents Marketed in the United States

Another indicator of concern is the origin of new single chemical agents approved for marketing in the United States. Table 10 compares the thirty-year record through 1970 of the origins of new products marketed in the United States with the recent record for 1971–73. While the number of compounds in this latter period is small, the percentage shift is too dramatic to be ignored. I suspect that the change started somewhere in the mid-sixties, for the prior three-year period of 1968–70 inaugurated a trend line, with figures of 48 percent for U.S. firms and 52 percent for foreign firms.

### New Information Obtainable

To begin to understand and judge the importance of the decrease that has taken place in the number of new therapeutic agents approved for marketing over the last decade, we first need new data on what parts of the process have been most involved. Let me outline only briefly the major questions that can and need to be answered, because I discussed this in great detail in a paper last year.[7]

**What Has Happened to the Rate of Discovery?** The first step is to recognize the need to separate the rate of discovery from the rate of innovation. To measure the rate of discovery, one must know what is entering the regulatory pipeline. By

[7] Presentation at the Second Seminar on Dynamics of Pharmaceutical Innovation and Economics, The American University, Washington, D. C., October 1973.

a myriad of preclinical research pathways originating years before, often with basic fundamental biological findings that evolved into applied research, synthesis, and animal testing, a new chemical agent reaches the critical decision-making stage. This is the point at which a compound has been identified with a unique pharmacological spectrum, sufficiently active and nontoxic to meet the criteria for potential new therapy. A decision is then made to take it into clinical trial. At this point it becomes a specific, identifiable product candidate, and the discovery phase has been completed.

The definitive sign of entry into the developmental phase is the filing of an application to undertake clinical trials, that is, the IND application. The rate of submission of such applications for product candidates and the number of INDs under active investigation provide a vital measure of research output. In total they represent the national portfolio of potential therapeutic assets bought at the cost of years and often decades of research and development. Each product candidate is a precious commodity the unnecessary loss of which results in incalculable loss in future new therapy.

Frankly, the FDA in its public disclosures and statements only adds confusion and obfuscates public assessment of the individual state of these different, though related, processes. The FDA, in trying to explain the drop in new drug application (NDA) approvals as a worldwide phenomenon, espouses the "we are on a plateau of discovery" or "the well has run dry—wait for the millenium" hypothesis. As an example, I quote the following from speeches given by Commissioner Schmidt earlier this year:

> But all of these are bits and pieces of a bigger problem. The bigger problem is the need for new knowledge of the basic mechanism of disease of aging, and even normal physiology. New drug development will follow advances in bio-medical science.[8]

> That reason begins with the fact that in many areas of biomedical knowledge, we are on a plateau. We have temporarily exhausted the exploitation of known concepts and tools. Truly dramatic new progress in medicine now waits on some basic innovation in molecular science, some breakthrough in our understanding of disease mechanisms, some new therapeutic concept or some new tool.[9]

But has the rate of discovery changed? The NDA approval rate and the number of new products introduced into the marketplace do not provide a measure of discovery. These are simply a measure of what has successfully completed the development phase. To know the rate of discovery, one must know what is entering that phase. How many IND applications for new chemical agents were

---

[8] Presentation at the Pharmaceutical Manufacturers Association meeting, Boca Raton, Florida, April 1974.

[9] Presentation at the American Cancer Society's Writers' Seminar, St. Augustine, Florida, March 1974.

filed last year? How did that number compare with the number filed in the previous year? Has the yearly rate significantly changed over the last decade?

The majority of people in industry, I believe, feel that the rate of discovery has not dropped and that the number of IND applications filed for new chemical agents has not decreased over the last decade.[10] I insert one caveat to the latter part of that statement—there may be some indication of a trend downward in such IND applications filed in the last two or three years, because the giving of priority to foreign markets has increased the tendency to carry out development and initial clinical investigations of new therapeutic agents in the market where product introduction is likely first to take place.

**What Is the IND Attrition Rate?**  What is happening to that vital new therapy represented by IND applications filed for new chemical agents? After these drugs enter the regulatory process, what has been the all-important attrition rate over the last ten years? Has it leveled, or is it still increasing? It was to be expected that the attrition rate would increase following the enactment of the 1962 amendments act, but has the rate of increase been that which Congress and the public expected? Prior to 1962, the dropout rate of the United States of new chemical agents during clinical investigation was approximately two out of three. Have the new regulations increased the rate two-fold, ten-fold, or a hundred-fold?

Again, information that the FDA makes public sheds little light on this all-important question. They do not separate applications for clinical investigation of new chemical agents from all the rest of the mishmash of IND applications that must be filed prior to undertaking many other types of clinical trials such as new uses of old drugs or formula changes with existing drugs, and the many duplicate IND applications filed by individual physicians for clinical use of such drugs as methadone, L-dopa, and so forth.

In testimony before the Senate Select Committee on Small Business on 5 February 1973, the FDA stated: "The FDA is currently monitoring several thousands of clinical drug investigations involving several thousand clinical investigators and tens of thousands of patients. The number of INDs received by FDA has been increasing over the past five years." [11] In their most recent annual report, the FDA states: "It has been alleged that the 1962 Drug Amendments have stifled progress in drug research and development. The facts appear to contradict this. . . . The number of INDs active during the year was the highest in the eleven years

---

[10] B. M. Bloom, "The Rate of Contemporary Drug Discovery," in R. F. Gould, ed., *Drug Discovery: Science and Development in a Changing Society*, Advances in Chemistry Ser. no. 108 (Washington, D. C.: American Chemical Society, 1971), pp. 176–84; M. Tishler, "What Information Does the Medicinal Chemist Really Need? Projections for the Future," *Journal of Chemical Documentation*, vol. 11 (1971), pp. 134–37; M. Tishler, "The Role of Industry in National Science Policy—The People's Welfare: Health and Medicine," *Perspectives in Biology and Medicine*, Summer 1970), pp. 528–36.

[11] U.S., Congress, Senate, Select Committee on Small Business, Subcommittee on Monopoly, Statement by H. E. Simmons, 5 February 1973, p. 35.

152

since the program started. New applications totaled 913." [12] The question of attrition rate of new chemical entity INDs is too important to be shaken off by generalized statements such as these. The facts regarding the fate of these all-important new chemical entities must be separated and made known in order to understand how, where, and why the development of new therapeutic agents has been altered. The dropout rate for new-chemical-entity INDs is the key to knowing whether the United States is suffering an economic and social loss beyond the benefit loss through delay described in the studies of W. M. Wardell [13] and the Dripps Committee [14] which call attention to the drug lag existing between the United States and the United Kingdom. There is a distinct possibility that we are experiencing a drug loss. The rate at which new chemical entities are entering and being lost in the course of the IND process would be a pretty fair indicator of whether the present regulatory process has increased the risk to the point that potentially useful compounds are being prematurely discarded and we are experiencing a loss of future new therapy. An article in the current *Chemical and Engineering News*, entitled Drug Regulations: Net Effect Is Not Good," contains the following striking sentence: "Although it is clear that far fewer drugs are now entering the market than before the Amendments, there is disagreement as to what the undeveloped drugs would have been like." [15] I believe that in addition to the straight figure-gathering I have just outlined, an examination of a representative sampling of case histories of IND applications for new chemical entities that have dropped by the wayside could give a pretty good indication of what the undeveloped drugs might have been like and whether Sam Peltzman was correct in his extrapolation of the loss to the public. [16]

Since the discussion began of the drug lag, a number of drugs of foreign origin, demonstrated to have medical and economic importance through five to ten years of marketing experience in major European countries, have been approved by the FDA. Whether this effort to close the gap in the case of these drugs of proven usefulness is a response based on recognition of past errors or simply a temporary effort based on vulnerability, remains to be seen. Enough of the history of three of these compounds in foreign markets and the United States can be pieced together from the public record to give the interesting comparison shown on Table 11.

---

[12] U.S., Department of Health, Education, and Welfare, Food and Drug Administration, *Annual Report 1973* (Washington, D. C.: Government Printing Office), p. 65.

[13] W. M. Wardell, "The Drug Lag: An International Comparison" (Paper delivered at the Fifth International Congress on Pharmacology, San Francisco, July 1972).

[14] See "American Scientists Charge U.S. Medicine Lags—Urge Major Change in Regulatory Policies," *Medical Tribune*, 5 April 1972.

[15] "Drug Regulations: Net Effect Is Not Good," *Chemical and Engineering News*, 8 July 1974, p. 7.

[16] S. Peltzman, *Regulation of Pharmaceutical Innovation: The 1962 Amendments*, Evaluative Studies (Washington, D. C.: American Enterprise Institute for Public Policy Research, 1974).

## Table 11
### COMPARATIVE CHRONOLOGY OF NEW DRUG MARKETING

| Foreign Marketing | | U.S. Chronology | |
|---|---|---|---|
| Alupent (metaproterenol) | | | |
| Germany | 1961 | NDA submitted | January 1964 |
| Japan | 1962 | NDA approved | July 1973 |
| United Kingdom | 1962 | • 12 years after marketing in Europe | |
| Italy | 1964 | • 9½ years after NDA submission | |
| France | 1966 | | |
| Approximately 25 countries by 1970 | | | |
| | | | |
| Pondimin (fenfluramine) | | | |
| France | 1963 | IND application filed | April 1964 |
| United Kingdom | 1964 | NDA submitted | March 1967 |
| Approximately 40 countries prior to U.S. approval | | NDA approved | May 1973 |
| | | • 10 years after marketing in Europe | |
| | | • 9 years after IND application filed | |
| | | • 6 years after NDA submission | |
| | | | |
| Intal (cromolyn) | | | |
| United Kingdom | 1967 | Clinical initiated | 1966 |
| Australia | 1969 | NDA submitted | December 1970 |
| Holland | 1969 | NDA approved | June 1973 |
| Canada | 1970 | • 5½ years after approval in United Kingdom | |
| Japan | 1971 | | |
| Approximately 60 countries prior to U.S. approval | | • 6 years after clinical initiated | |
| | | • 2½ years after NDA submission | |

A fuller description of the long and tortuous U.S. path from IND application to final NDA approval is available in other publications.[17] The confidence that led the sponsoring firms to persevere with these new drugs stems largely, I believe, from the fact that they were proven products, proven through medical acceptance and financial success achieved in their home and international markets. Should this not raise the even more important question of what happens to the unproven potential new therapeutic agent in this same regulatory climate?

At this point, I am not very sanguine that the information of the type I have just described ever will be made visible because, frankly, I do not see the right incentive in the right places to initiate such a study. The total data bank is available only at the FDA and, to be meaningful, the study should be carried out by a third party, with a blue-ribbon, independent, knowledgeable panel of experts. The object should be neither to laud nor to condemn FDA or industry but to gather without bias factual information on these and other important questions in order to evaluate dispassionately, and interpret for the future, the full impact of the regulatory climate on the health and vitality of U.S. research and development and the prognosis for new and improved therapy for the American public.

---

[17] J. S. G. Cox, "Intal and the USA," *Scrip* (30 March 1973), p. 10; R. B. Lee, "Three New Anorexigenics—From Chemist to Consumer," *Obesity/Bariatric Medicine*, vol. 2 (1973), pp. 120–23; Clymer, paper presented at the Second Seminar on Dynamics of Pharmaceutical Innovation and Economics.

# THE RATE OF
# NEW DRUG DISCOVERY

*Louis Lasagna and William M. Wardell*

Acrimonious debate has raged in recent years over the impact of the Kefauver-Harris amendments on the rate of introduction of new medicaments to the U.S. market. The many conflicting postures taken include the following: There has been a serious decline in this rate. The decline has been only in "me-too" drugs of little or no medical importance. The decline is a worldwide phenomenon. The decline has been seen most markedly (or primarily) in the United States. The decline is due to a failure of ideas. The decline is due to the currently excessive costs and risks of new drug development. The decline and delays are due to the unreasonable demands or ineptitude of the FDA. The decline and delays are due primarily to poor submissions by industrial sponsors. We are told from various sources that the situation is bad and getting worse, or good and getting better, or that it was bad but is now getting better. Finally, we hear variously that these matters have paramount medical implications or that they have no medical implications.

The debate might have been less acrimonious, and would certainly have been of higher quality, if definitions were clearer and postures supported by data. Instead, we have generally been treated to extravagant statements involving value judgments impossible to analyze, and to either no evidence or pseudo-evidence of the kind the late Senator Joseph McCarthy was so fond of: numbers whose origin and validity are forever hidden from the scrutiny of others. In the hope of elevating the level of debate, we deemed it worthwhile to obtain data about the process of drug development by U.S.-owned pharmaceutical firms.

## Methods

Our survey consisted of a questionnaire sent to the fifteen largest U.S.-owned firms, which we believe account for over 80 percent of all pharmaceutical research and development expenditure by the U.S.-owned pharmaceutical industry. The questionnaire sought numerical answers, for each year since 1962, to seven specific questions about new chemical entities that those firms had administered to man for the first time.

A new chemical entity (NCE) was defined as a compound of molecular structure not previously tested in man, excluding new salts, vaccines, and diag-

155

nostic agents. The seven items of information we requested for each year were these: total number of NCEs administered to man worldwide, number of these administered to man in the United States first (as against those administered abroad first), number of NCE IND applications filed in the United States, disposition of these applications as of 30 April 1974—namely, number still active, number discontinued or terminated prior to NDA approval—and number of successful NDAs (with years of approval).

Anonymity was promised to individual firms.

## Results

All fifteen firms responded to the questionnaire, and (after followup where necessary) there were no missing data. The data for 1974, where given, are to 30 April only. All data in this study have been corrected to eliminate drugs that had been

### Figure 1

### NUMBER OF NCEs ADMINISTERED TO MAN WORLDWIDE BY FIFTEEN MAJOR U.S.-OWNED COMPANIES, 1963–73

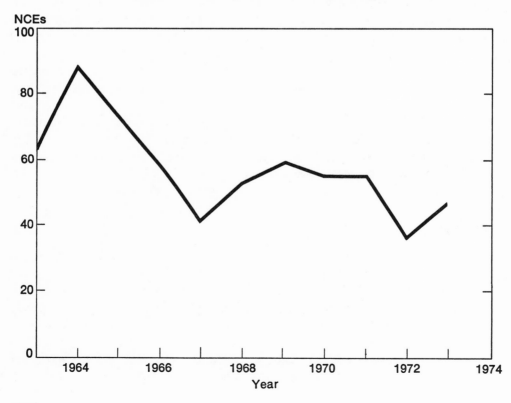

administered to man before 1963 but for which IND forms were filed in that year or later to fulfill the requirement of the new regulations.

The results, summed over the fifteen firms, are depicted in Figures 1 through 7, which deal with the following questions:

(1) Has there been a decline in the number of NCEs administered to man? The answer to this question appears to be "yes." See Figure 1, which plots NCEs administered to man worldwide by these companies. Each of the three years following the Kefauver-Harris amendments shows a substantially higher number of such NCEs than the period following; the average rate for the initial three-year period was 75 per year. A plateau seems to have been reached by 1966. For the latest three complete years, 1971–73, the average rate was 46 per year, which is 40 percent less than the earlier period.

(2) Where are American companies first studying new chemical entities in man? The drop in NCEs studied first in the United States has been disproportionately greater than the drop in NCEs studied worldwide. That is, U.S. firms now tend increasingly to conduct their first human studies abroad. This trend, shown

**Figure 2**

LOCATION OF FIRST HUMAN STUDIES OF NCEs, 1963–74

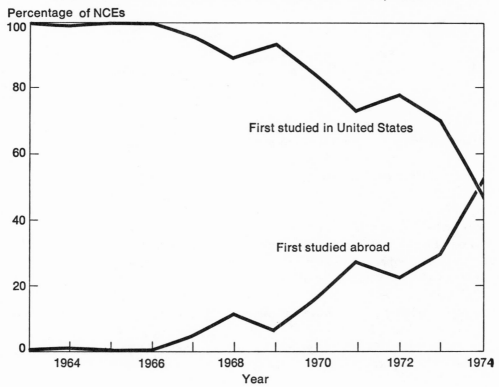

157

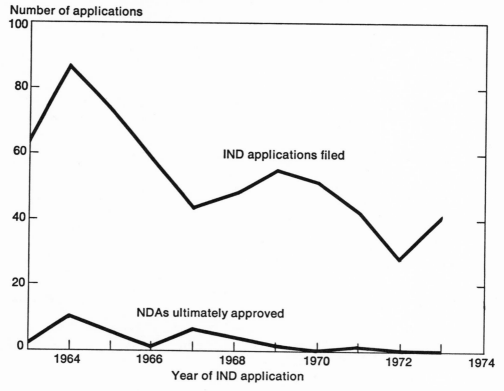

**Figure 3**

NUMBER OF NCE IND APPLICATIONS FILED AND APPROVED
AS NEW DRUGS IN THE UNITED STATES

in Figure 2, has accelerated rapidly over the last five years. Before that time, American companies rarely studied a drug in man first abroad; in the first third of 1974, half such studies began there.

(3) What has been the fate of the NCEs for which IND applications were filed? This question requires several answers. To begin with, the number of NCE IND applications filed per year has decreased; in the three years 1963–65, they were filed at the rate of 74 per year, while in the most recent three-year period (1971–73), this rate had fallen to exactly half—37 per year (see Figure 3). Second, the number and percent approved for marketing is small (Figures 3 and 4); by April 1974, 7.1 percent of all NCE IND applications filed from 1963 through 1967 had resulted in approved NDAs, while 3.1 percent of those filed from 1968 through 1971 had been approved by that date. The year 1966 seems to have been a particularly bad one to file an IND application; none of the 58 NCEs for which applications were filed in that year have yet been marketed. Third, the mean time (Figure 5) required for clinical study and approval has risen steadily from

158

## Figure 4

### PERCENTAGE OF NCE IND APPLICATIONS RESULTING IN APPROVED NDAs[a]

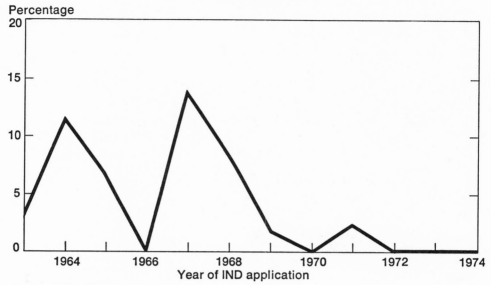

a As of 30 April 1974.

## Figure 5

### MEAN TIME TO NDA APPROVAL, BY YEAR OF APPROVAL

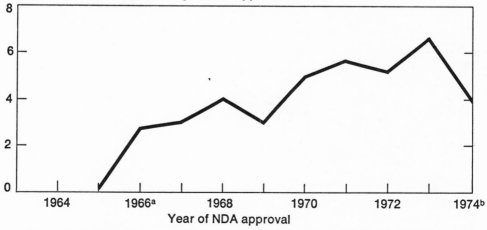

a Earliest year of NDA approval of an NCE for which IND application was filed after 1962.
b Based on two drugs approved by 30 April 1974.

159

2.7 years for those NDAs approved in 1966 to 6.6 years in 1973. An apparent fall to four years occurred in the first four months of 1974, but this is based on only 2 NCE approvals. Data for the whole year will be needed to determine whether a real change is occurring.

Some lengthening of the mean time to approval is to be expected, since we are dealing only with compounds administered to man since 1962, and the maximum time available is thus steadily increasing. However, it is worth noting that so far only 2 of the 232 NCE INDs that have entered human study in the United States since 1968 have been approved for marketing here. Further, despite the slowdown in filing of IND applications, the number of active INDs has accumulated (Figure 6).[1] At the time of the survey, 170 of the 604 total NCE INDs were still

**Figure 6**

ACCUMULATION OF NCE INDs

Cumulative total active as of 30 April 1974[a]

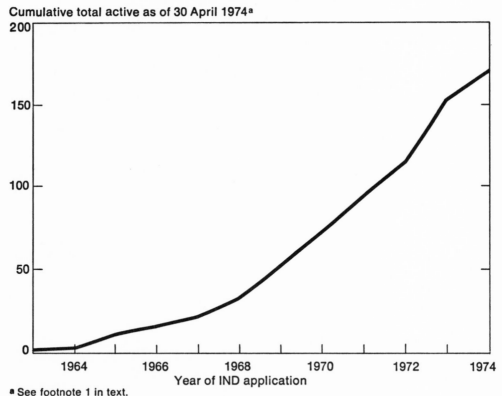

Year of IND application

[a] See footnote 1 in text.

---

[1] The "still active" category has to be interpreted with caution, since some INDs are kept active after NDA approval, to allow, for example, exploration of new uses. In the responses received, this caused some duplication, but the size of this error was very small.

160

active; Figure 6 shows that applications for 72 of these had been filed in 1970 or earlier.

Finally, in Figure 7 is plotted, by year of filing, the percentage of NCE IND files closed prior to obtaining NDA approval. The process appears to be a function of time, and from this figure it can be seen that about half of the unsuccessful INDs are dropped within three or four years of filing.

**Figure 7**

ATTRITION OF NCE INDs

Percentage of IND files closed prior to obtaining NDA approval

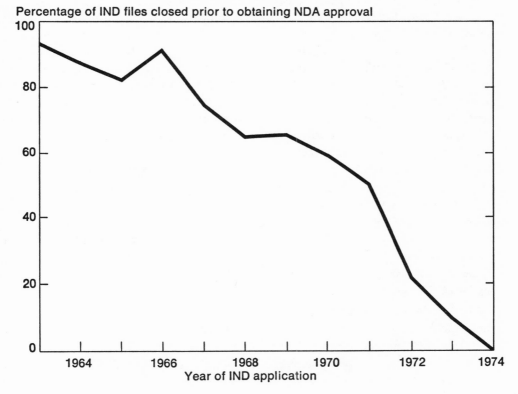

Year of IND application

**Discussion and Conclusions**

What can one conclude from the foregoing? First, it is obvious that the percentage of approvals of all NCEs administered to man is low: 29 out of 649 applications, or 4.5 percent overall. This is, to be sure, an underestimate, since presumably some of the NCEs still pending will ultimately be approved. Nevertheless, the number approved out of those INDs filed since 1968, is, as we have shown, vanishingly small (less than 1 percent). When one recalls that the drugs administered to man constitute only a small percentage of drugs studied in indus-

161

trial laboratories, we are reminded forcefully of how inefficient the process of drug development really is.

Do we know any more, after this study, about why the flow of new drugs has slowed down? A little, perhaps. We know that the number of NCEs administered to man has dropped, but we do not know why. Is it because the easy nuts have been cracked and we are suffering from a lack of new knowledge? Has industrial creativity slowed down? Was it always low, with the old higher rate merely reflecting approval of drugs of dubious merit or of data of dubious quality? Or is there now increased timidity in industry due to the greater current cost, complexity, and frustrations of drug research?

We surely have data showing that the process of human drug study and approval takes longer than it used to, but we do not know in absolute terms whether this is good or bad. If bad, whose fault is it—the FDA's, the sponsors', or both? Whatever the reason, the time required seems (at least through 1973) to be still increasing, and our data provide no evidence that a reduction in approval time is occurring. If the trend through 1973 continues, by 1979 it will require ten years for a drug to be evaluated in man and approved in the United States. The implications of this for the duration of patent protection are obvious. Perhaps, on the other hand, the data for recent years simply reflect the expiation of past sins on the part of either FDA in the form of more reasonable regulatory postures or of industry in the form of the submission of better data. In this case the time to approval should show a downward trenJ in the next few years, and these gloomy extrapolations will not hold.

Finally, it is clear that U.S.-owned companies are shifting their initial studies abroad. Is this good or bad from the standpoint of the U.S. economy, U.S. patients, or the standard of clinical pharmacology in this country? We know that while R&D expenditures of U.S. firms abroad are still only about 10 percent of their total R&D expenditures, these foreign expenditures have increased at a much more rapid rate than domestic outlays over the last decade.

It should be emphasized that the present study deals with the research performance of the U.S.-owned pharmaceutical industry only. We also need data on the performance in the United States of foreign-owned companies, who have been studying drugs abroad at an earlier date for some time; have they, paradoxically, had more NCEs introduced here in recent years because of this practice?

We would make the following recommendations:

(1) Data of the sort presented above need to be accumulated and analyzed in many areas of drug development. Case histories of NCEs and INDs might prove invaluable in trying to analyze the reasons for the time taken for drug investigation and approval. Drug firms need to be scrutinized to evaluate the ways in which they are contributing, directly or indirectly, to the slowdown. Also we should not ignore the fate of drugs scrapped prior to the IND stage, before the FDA becomes

involved. That is an area of great importance about which little is known outside the pharmaceutical industry.

(2) A corollary to the foregoing is that these studies should be done by parties whose impartiality and credibility are as great as possible. In our opinion, this rules out both the FDA and the drug industry.

(3) The role of the FDA needs redefinition. Former FDA commissioner Dr. Charles Edwards has defined this role as one of "consumer protection." Unfortunately, the usual definition of "protection" is hopelessly myopic, since the patient is only being protected from drug hazards and not from disease and discomfort.

We prefer the attitude of the President's Advisory Committee on Chemicals and Health: "Each regulatory agency concerned with agents that can affect health as well as threaten it should recognize its twin responsibilities: to make available without undue delay agents that improve health, and to protect health by restricting the availability of agents that may threaten health."

# DEVELOPMENTS IN THE INTRODUCTION OF NEW DRUGS IN THE UNITED STATES AND BRITAIN, 1971-74

*William M. Wardell*

## Introduction

In 1972, I examined the pattern of introduction of new therapeutic drugs to the United States over the decade since the Kefauver-Harris amendments of 1962 and compared this pattern with that of Britain for the same period.[1] That study documented a situation that is widely known in medical circles abroad but has met with slow recognition inside the United States, namely, that the delayed availability of new drugs in the United States had led to the development in this country of conservative therapeutic patterns, some of which could be seen to have adverse medical consequences.

The notion that this difference exists and is of some medical consequence has been only grudgingly accepted in this country. This is surprising, because it is so well known outside the United States that these earlier papers are simply a statement of the obvious. It is obvious to every English-speaking medical student outside the United States who buys an American textbook of pharmacology or medicine, only to find that the sections on current drugs and therapeutics are so out of date that he has to buy a British textbook as well. This is well documented in book review columns.

This drug lag and its effects are also obvious to those of us who are teachers of pharmacology and therapeutics abroad (as I have been in two countries outside the United States), who depend, for maintaining the credibility of the subject and the interest of the students, on having books and materials that describe what is being used in one's own hospital today. The fact is that while all textbooks are out of date, American textbooks are so hopelessly out of date when used abroad as to be often irrelevant. That explains how I came to be interested in this phenomenon.

---

[1] W. M. Wardell, "The Drug Lag: An International Comparison," *Proceedings of the Fifth International Pharmacological Congress* (July 1972); Wardell, "Introduction of New Therapeutic Drugs in the United States and Great Britain: An International Comparison," *Clinical Pharmacology and Therapeutics*, vol. 14, no. 5 (September-October 1973), pp. 773–90; Wardell, "British Usage and American Awareness of Some New Therapeutic Drugs," *Clinical Pharmacology and Therapeutics*, vol. 14, no. 6 (November-December 1973), pp. 1022–34; and Wardell, "Therapeutic Implications of the Drug Lag," *Clinical Pharmacology and Therapeutics*, vol. 15, no. 1 (January 1974), pp. 73–96.

The results of the original study were as follows. In nine therapeutic categories during the decade 1962–71, nearly four times as many new drugs (single chemical entities) became exclusively available in Britain as became exclusively available in the United States.[2] In addition, where differences occurred in the dates of introduction of drugs introduced in both countries, twice as many drugs were introduced first in Britain as in the United States. When examined by therapeutic category, this drug lag was found to be most marked in the areas of cardiovascular, gastrointestinal and respiratory medicine, and diuretic and anti-bacterial therapy.

British usage and American awareness of some new therapeutic drugs were then surveyed in five therapeutic areas (angina, hypertension, asthma, pyelo-nephritis and gastric ulcer).[3] It was found that certain drugs then unavailable in the United States had made a great impact on the prescribing habits of British experts, whose therapy was likely to be substantially different from that which could be prescribed by Americans. By contrast, most of the American specialists surveyed had a very low level of knowledge about those and other new drugs not yet available to them, despite the fact that some of those drugs had been in wide-spread use abroad in their own specialities for as long as a decade. Those Americans who were aware of a drug's properties, however, usually wished to have that drug available to them. The lack of American awareness of new (and even not-so-new) drugs was unexpected and surprising.

The implications of these substantial international differences in the avail-ability, use, and knowledge of new therapies were analyzed to determine whether, in therapeutic terms, Britain had gained or lost from adopting the less restrictive policy.[4] The therapeutic impact of a new drug on the whole community was found to be difficult to assess, mainly because there are few methods or data available for measuring the benefits drugs confer. On the evidence currently available, Britain probably did not lose appreciably from the introduction of a greater number of new drugs, nor from the possibility that a few of these may have been of questionable value. The main deleterious effect was that Britain suffered more toxicity from new drugs than did the United States, as could be anticipated from the fact that more new drugs were marketed in Britain. However, in com-parison with the size of the *total* burden of drug toxicity, that portion attributable to new drugs was found to be extremely small, and would in any case be at least partially offset by the adverse effects of older alternative drugs had the latter been employed instead. Conversely, Britain experienced clearly discernible gains by introducing useful new drugs either earlier than the United States or exclusively. On balance, Britain appeared to have gained in comparison with the United States

[2] Wardell, "Introduction of New Therapeutic Drugs."

[3] Wardell, "British Usage and American Awareness."

[4] Wardell, "Therapeutic Implications."

from its less restrictive policy toward the marketing of new drugs coupled with a more rigorous program of postmarketing surveillance.[5]

The present paper brings the original study up to date, extending the analysis from the beginning of 1972 to the middle of 1974. The object is to determine whether any changes have occurred in the past two and one-half years in the pattern of each country, and in the relationship between them. Such changes would be of interest, because over the past two and one-half years, regulatory approaches in both the United States and Britain have altered. In Britain, the Medicines Act (1968) became law in 1971. As a result, the review process for new drugs has become more institutionalized in nature, resembling in some respects that of the U.S. (including, according to some observers, the involvement of a slow-moving bureaucracy). In the United States, on the other hand, there have been considerable regulatory efforts over the past few years to enlighten the review process for new drugs to bring it into line with modern standards of medical practice and scientific thought. One way to determine the relative positions of the regulatory systems in the two countries is to examine their effects on current patterns of new drug introduction.

**Methods**

These were similar to those of the previous study. For the United Kingdom, the identity and marketing dates of new compounds were obtained from the month of publication in the periodical *MIMS*.[6] For the United States, the marketing date was obtained from the month of first citation in the marketing survey *IMS*,[7] or from the de Haen *New Product Survey*.[8] For those drugs introduced since 1970, we have the date of marketing to the nearest month. (For those introduced prior to 1970 this was not always available, and in those cases it is assumed, in the tables and graphs that follow, that marketing occurred in the middle of the year concerned.) It should be noted that *MIMS* covers only those drugs introduced into general practice in Britain. Thus, the following results understate the priority of marketing in Britain for those drugs that were introduced there earlier or exclusively in hospitals rather than in general practice.

**Results**

The results are shown in tabular form (Tables 1–9, pages 173–77) using the same headings as were used in the previous papers already cited. (Table 1 is an overall summary.) In addition, a graphical display is given (Figures 1–4, pages 178–81) to

---

[5] Ibid.

[6] *Monthly Index of Medical Specialities (MIMS)* (London: Haymarket Publishing Ltd., Medical Division).

[7] Intercontinental Medical Statistics, Ltd. (London: York House, Queen Square).

[8] *de Haen New Product Survey* (New York: Paul de Haen, Inc.).

show when, and for how long, drugs were exclusively available in either country. For each therapeutic topic, time is represented horizontally, and a horizontal line bisects the field. Those drugs that were exclusively available in the United Kingdom are plotted above this line, those exclusively available in the United States below the line. The bar representing each drug extends from the time the drug was marketed until its exclusive availability ceased (usually because the drug was marketed in the other country).

Thus, a preponderance of drug bars above the line would indicate a British lead, while a preponderance of bars below the line would indicate an American lead. The length of the bar shows how long the disparity persisted. What is important is not so much the number of drugs available, but their identity; this arrangement allows us to see that clearly. One of the main points of these graphs is that a vertical line at any point on the time scale allows us to see at a glance the differences between the range of drugs available in each country at that time.

**Cardiovascular Drugs and Antihypertensive Therapy (Table 2 and Figure 1).** The main drugs used in the treatment of hypertension are, apart from diuretics, those shown in Figure 1. Here I have divided the drugs into a mixed group largely composed of adrenergic-neurone blocking drugs, and the β-blockers.

In the first group (nondiuretic antihypertensives) there has since 1963 been a steady accumulation of exclusively available drugs in Britain, beginning with bethanidine and debrisoquin (which are useful alternatives to guanethidine), and in 1971, clonidine, which is a useful alternative to reserpine or methyldopa.

The β-blockers are one of the major developments of the past decade in the treatment of both angina and hypertension; it is now just ten years since the first papers demonstrating the efficacy of propranolol in hypertension were published. The pattern with β-blockers resembles that of the other antihypertensive agents. There is an accumulation of agents exclusively available in Britain, and none exclusively available in the United States. Propranolol was first marketed in Britain nine years ago. It was available there exclusively for three years before becoming available in the United States. When propranolol did become available in the United States, it was only approved for relatively minor uses; it was not approved for the treatment of angina for a further five years, and it has still not been approved for the therapy of hypertension. This is markedly out of line with expert medical opinion even in the United States. Then there are other β-blockers that are exclusively available in Britain, some of which offer advantages over propranolol in some patients. Thus, the pattern for the hypertension category is a steady and continuing British lead in the agents available, and the pattern for angina is similar with respect to the β-blockers.

**Diuretics (Table 3 and Figure 2).** In the group of thiazide and related diuretics, there have been no major developments in the last few years, although there are a number of new arrivals that deserve closer comparison with established drugs. The main advances of the past decade are still furosemide and ethacrynic acid, both of which were introduced two years earlier in Britain.

Looking at potassium-sparing diuretics, we again find the pattern present— triamterene was marketed first in Britain, and amiloride is still marketed there exclusively (Figure 2).

In view of this, it is hard to understand why slow-release potassium supplements have not been more vigorously sought by industry, government and the profession. The *Medical Letter* continues to criticize the outmoded and dangerous enteric-coated K+ supplements available in the United States, and the correspondence columns of American journals continue to report disasters due to this dosage form. Meanwhile the number of types of the safer slow-release potassium supplements continues to grow abroad both alone and in combination with diuretics. This hazardous anachronism in the U.S. market has now existed for eleven years.

**Respiratory Drugs (Table 4 and Figure 3).** The antiallergic drug cromolyn sodium became available in the United States some five and one-half years after its introduction in the United Kingdom. This closed one obvious gap, although cromolyn is still available in Britain in dose forms and for indications that have not been approved in the United States—for example, for nasal insufflation in the treatment of allergic rhinitis, for which it offers some unique advantages.

An interesting recent development in Britain is the renewed attention being given to corticosteroids administerable by inhalation for the treatment of asthma, as seen in the introduction there of inhaler versions of beclomethasone and betamethasone. This idea is not entirely new. People have for a long time been fascinated by the idea that local application of steroids to the bronchioles would permit local control of allergic bronchospasm by a dose of steroid that was too small to exert much systemic effect, thus eliminating the worst objections to steroid therapy for asthma. Indeed, an inhalable form of dexamethasone has been available for many years on the U.S. market, although it is not at all widely used at present.

What is new is that the concept has now been fairly well vindicated. Relief of bronchospasm occurs with very small doses of steroid. It has been found possible to maintain patients on inhaled, rather than systemic steroids, at very small doses that have much fewer—and in some cases, no—systemic effects such as adrenal suppression. This is the main advance represented by those newer preparations in use in Britain. Whether the improvements are due to the nature of the steroids, or to refinement of the metered delivery system, or simply to increasing sophistication in the evaluation of these drugs, does not seem to have been conclusively established. The main side effect reported so far is candidiasis, and it is not yet certain how serious this side effect will prove in long-term therapy.

This development represents a modest advance overall, but one that is of very definite importance to some patients in reducing the systemic side effects of steroids.

The other main area of interest in the respiratory field is that of orally active, longer-acting bronchoselective bronchodilators (see Figure 3). Here the gap between the United States and Britain was to some extent reduced by the marketing of metaproterenol (orciprenaline) in the United States in 1973, some eleven years after its introduction in Britain, where it had already been largely superseded by more bronchoselective agents such as albuterol and terbutaline. Note that there is still no oral or inhaled highly bronchoselective agent available in the United States, since terbutaline has so far been marketed here only in a dose form for injection. The developments subsequent to metaproterenol have been of less incremental medical importance, but they are all in the direction of increasing bronchoselectivity, with an attendant reduction in acute cardiac side effects.

In summary, the main gaps in the respiratory field have been substantially reduced by the introduction of moderately bronchoselective bronchodilators and cromolyn. There are, however, signs of continued innovation in Britain, particularly with inhaled steroids and more bronchoselective bronchodilators such as rimiterol. Bromhexine continues to be exclusively available in Britain, showing modest utility as a sputum liquifier in chronic bronchitis.

**Antibacterial Drugs (Table 5).** While there have been delays in the admission to the U.S. market of several useful antibacterial drugs, the recent marketing of co-trimoxazole in the United States, five years after its marketing in Britain substantially clears the backlog of significant drugs in this category that were unavailable in the United States. Furthermore, at least two newer antibiotics (spectinomycin and minocycline) have been introduced earlier in the United States.

In the field of penicillins and cephalosporins, there have been some minor advances in which both countries have shared equally. Thus, in the antibacterial field the gap between the two countries has been virtually eliminated.

**Anti-inflammatory Analgesics (Table 9 and Figure 4).** With the marketing in Britain of six more anti-inflammatory analgesics, there are now eight of these agents exclusively available there.

The medical impact of this is obscure. As far as one can tell, these drugs are all similar in terms of efficacy. The main claim that might be made for them is a diminished incidence, or at least a different spectrum, of side effects compared with such classical alternatives as aspirin or phenylbutazone. In the case of some of these drugs, side effects do seem to be less, but the type of proof available is not yet of high standard. There are few rigorous demonstrations of an enhanced therapeutic ratio.

One medical effect of this international difference appears to be that there is more use of this class of drug in Britain than in the United States; it has been estimated that the per capita utilization rate of anti-inflammatory analgesics in Britain is double that found in the United States. Whether this is on balance good or bad is at present unknown.

**Gastrointestinal Drugs.** No new drugs in this category have been marketed in either country since 1971. The British lead in this field remains unchallenged.

## Summary and Conclusions

In the original papers, which covered the decade through 1971, I found obvious differences between the United States and the United Kingdom in the therapeutic fields represented by cardiovascular, diuretic, respiratory, antibacterial and gastrointestinal drugs. This preliminary examination of developments over the past two and one-half years shows that this relationship has changed perceptibly in most areas.

In the antibacterial area, the British lead has disappeared, and there is now little difference between the two countries. Some useful new antibiotics have recently been approved earlier in the United States than in Britain. In the respiratory field, the previous differences have been substantially reduced, but not completely eliminated, while some interesting new advances have appeared in Britain. Fields in which the United States is still noticeably behind Britain include the treatment of hypertension and the problem of potassium balance in diuretic therapy. The obvious shortcomings that currently exist in these two areas have both been present for ten years. A major new development is the large number of anti-inflammatory analgesics that have appeared in Britain, the medical impact of which is unknown and deserving of careful scrutiny.

What can be learned from studies like this? First, it is clear that changes have occurred, particularly in the United States, where the pattern of available drugs and approved uses has, in the past two and one-half years, come to be more in line with current world standards of professional and scientific thought. Some of the major discrepancies between the United States and the United Kingdom have been reduced, although anachronisms remain, particularly in the cardiovascular area. This progress is at least partly due to a more enlightened regulatory approach in the United States.[9] It is conceivable that the narrowing of the dif-

[9] Whether such enlightened progress will be allowed to continue may depend on the outcome of some extraordinary Congressional reaction to the approval of the $\beta$-blockers for angina. This reaction is destined to become a classic in the history of political pharmacology, with very wide implications for legislation and regulation of drugs. In recent hearings of the Subcommittee on Intergovernmental Relations, Senate Committee on Government Operations, on this topic, the FDA—Dr. Crout in particular—was criticized for approving propranolol for angina on the grounds that this action went against the supposed recommendation of an

ferences between the two countries could be caused by a more conservative trend in Britain. The data available do not suggest this yet, but in any case this type of comparison would not be sensitive enough to pick up small changes at an early stage.

A second suggestion arises from the ease with which gross disparities can be detected between countries. Some organization ought to be continuously monitoring such therapeutic differences. This would be a relatively simple task, but one that does not at present seem to be receiving attention. We do not even know much about what is going on in the other English-speaking countries—Canada, Australia, New Zealand, and South Africa—let alone what is happening in non-English-speaking countries.

Third, as discussed previously,[10] these simple and obvious comparisons between countries, although necessary, should be only the beginning of our attempts to chart therapeutic progress and to measure the impact of drugs in absolute therapeutic terms. We need to know in addition how to measure the therapeutic impact, for better or worse, that a new drug has on the community; and (perhaps further in the future) how to assess the potential therapeutic impact of drugs that are prospective candidates for approval.

---

advisory committee, and that the exact requirements of the law for proving efficacy were not strictly fulfilled in the technical sense.

The fact is that there is no doubt in the highest professional circles about the efficacy of propranolol in this situation. Its efficacy is proven thousands of times a day the world over. Beta-blockers are by far the most important development in the therapy of angina since the nitrites were discovered one hundred years ago. They have long been used in the United States and abroad as the treatment of choice for some patients.

After reading the voluminous testimony of these hearings, I came to the conclusion that the criticisms of the FDA in this matter were so out of touch with medical reality that in any other country they could scarcely have seen the light of day in 1964, let alone 1974. For such criticisms to be seriously entertained, there has to be profound ignorance within the medical profession about what is going on in the regulation of drugs.

The FDA in this case has made a long overdue move to bring American regulatory practice into line with the best standards of American medicine. I would like to support the FDA and Dr. Crout very strongly, because I believe that criticism of his action poses a real threat to the very desirable efficacy requirements of the law. If these requirements were ever to be implemented in such a manner that they made medical nonsense, then this would obviously impair the credibility of the law in the eyes of physicians and patients to such an extent that the law could be destroyed. Therefore, I believe that this criticism undermining FDA's attempts to adopt a medically sound approach is not only misguided and unwarranted, but it is a severe disservice to patients. Whatever the outcome, this episode is already a landmark in the development of regulatory philosophy in this country.

[10] Wardell, "Therapeutic Implication."

## Table 1

### SUMMARY OF NEW DRUG INTRODUCTIONS IN BRITAIN AND THE UNITED STATES, JANUARY 1972–JUNE 1974

| Category | Total Drugs | Mutual | | Exclusive | |
|---|---|---|---|---|---|
| | | U.K. first | U.S. first | U.K. | U.S. |
| Cardiovascular | 7 | 1 | 0 | 5 | 1 |
| Diuretic | 2 | 1 | 0 | 1 | 0 |
| Respiratory | 4 | 3 | 0 | 1 | 0 |
| Antibacterial and chemotherapeutic | 17 | 2 | 4 | 6 | 5 |
| CNS | 15 | 3 | 3 | 6 | 3 |
| Anesthetic | 3 | 2 | 0 | 0 | 1 |
| Analgesics, etc. | 7 | 0 | 0 | 7 | 0 |
| Gastrointestinal | 0 | 0 | 0 | 0 | 0 |
| Total | 55 | 12 | 7 | 26 | 10 |

## Table 2

### INTRODUCTION OF CARDIOVASCULAR DRUGS

| Drug | Date of Introduction | | Lead in Years (Months) | |
|---|---|---|---|---|
| | U.K. | U.S. | U.K. | U.S. |
| Antihypertensive Diazoxide (Hyperstat) | Oct. 1969 | Feb. 1973 | 3(4) | |
| β-adrenoreceptor antagonist Timolol (Blocadren) | June 1974 | — | | |
| Sotalol (Beta-Cardone) | June 1974 | — | | |
| Antiarrhythmic Di-isopyramide (Rythomodan) | Sept. 1972 | — | | |
| Bretylium tosylate (Bretylate) | Nov. 1972 | — | | |
| Antianginal β-blockers, q.v. | | | | |
| Vasodilators and other Nattidrofuryl (Praxilene) | May 1972 | — | | |
| Dopamine HCl (Intropin) | — | May 1974 | | |
| Hypolipidemic Cholestyramine (Questran) | 1970 | Aug. 1973[a] | 3 | |
| Polidexide (Secholex) | May 1974 | — | | |

[a] New indication.

## Table 3
### INTRODUCTION OF DIURETICS, SLOW-RELEASE K+ SUPPLEMENTS, AND RELATED DRUGS

| Drug | Date of Introduction U.K. | Date of Introduction U.S. | Lead in Years (Months) U.K. | Lead in Years (Months) U.S. |
|---|---|---|---|---|
| **Diuretic** | | | | |
| Metolazone (Zaroxolyn) | June 1973 | Nov. 1973 | (5) | |
| Bumetanide (Burinex) | Sept. 1973 | — | | |
| **Potassium supplement** | | | | |
| K-Contin | May 1973 | — | | |
| **Sodium supplement** | | | | |
| Slow sodium | Aug. 1972 | — | | |

## Table 4
### INTRODUCTION OF RESPIRATORY DRUGS

| Drug | Date of Introduction U.K. | Date of Introduction U.S. | Lead in Years (Months) U.K. | Lead in Years (Months) U.S. |
|---|---|---|---|---|
| **Bronchodilators** | | | | |
| Metaproterenol/orciprenaline (Alupent) | 1962 | Dec. 1973 | 11(6) | |
| Terbutaline (Bricanyl) | June 1971 | May 1974 | 2(11) | |
| Rimiterol (Pulmadil) | June 1974 | — | | |
| **Antiallergic** | | | | |
| Cromolyn sodium (Intal, Aarane) | 1968 | June 1973 | 5(0) | |
| Beclomethasone (Becotide inhaler) | Nov. 1972 | — | | |
| Betamethasone (Bextasol inhaler) | Sept. 1973 | — | | |

174

## Table 5
### INTRODUCTION OF ANTIBACTERIAL AND CHEMOTHERAPEUTIC DRUGS

| Drug | Date of Introduction U.K. | Date of Introduction U.S. | Lead in Years (Months) U.K. | Lead in Years (Months) U.S. |
|---|---|---|---|---|
| Pencillins, cephalosporins, etc. | | | | |
| Amoxicillin (Amoxil) | April 1972 | March 1974 | 2 | |
| Cephradine (Eskacef, Velosef) | Oct. 1972 | Aug. 1974 | 1(10) | |
| Carbenicillin indanyl sodium (Geocillin Tabs) | — | Nov. 1972 | | |
| Cephazolin sodium (Ancef) | June 1974 | Oct. 1973 | | (8) |
| Cephapirin (Cefadyl) | — | March 1974 | | |
| Other | | | | |
| Co-trimoxazole (Septra, Bactrim) | 1968 | Sept. 1973 | 5(3) | |
| Spectinomycin (Trobocin) | June 1973 | Sept. 1971 | | 1(9) |
| Minocycline (Minocin) | Sept. 1973 | 1971 | | 2 |
| Antifungal | | | | |
| Flucytosine (Ancobon) | — | Nov. 1971 | | |
| Haloprogin (Halotex Cream) | — | March 1972 | | |
| Clotrimazole (Canesten) | Feb. 1973 | — | | |
| Miconazole nitrate (Monistat cream) | June 1974 | March 1974 | | (3) |
| Antiparasitic | | | | |
| Nitrimidazine (Nulogyl) | Feb. 1971 | — | | |
| Pyrantel pamoate (Antiminth Oral) | — | Jan. 1972 | | |

## Table 6
### INTRODUCTION OF ANTICANCER AND IMMUNOSUPPRESSIVE DRUGS

| Drug | Date of Introduction U.K. | Date of Introduction U.S. |
|---|---|---|
| Thioguanine (Lanvis) | Nov. 1972 | — |
| Bleomycin sulfate (Blenoxane) | — | Aug. 1973 |
| Tamoxifen (Novaldex) | Oct. 1973 | — |

## Table 7
### INTRODUCTION OF CENTRALLY ACTING DRUGS

| Drug | Date of Introduction U.K. | Date of Introduction U.S. | Lead in Years (Months) U.K. | Lead in Years (Months) U.S. |
|---|---|---|---|---|
| **Psychotropic** | | | | |
| Flupenthixol (Depixol) | May 1972 | — | | |
| Lorazepam (Ativan) | Feb. 1973 | — | | |
| Fluphenazine decanoate (Prolixin Deconoate) | — | April 1973 | | |
| Chlorazepate (Tranxene) | Sept. 1973 | Sept. 1972 | | 1 |
| Benperidol (Anquil) | Oct. 1973 | — | | |
| Molidone (Moban) | — | March 1974 | | |
| **Hypnotic** | | | | |
| Flurazepam (Dalmane) | Jan. 1974 | Jan. 1971 | | 3 |
| Triclofos (Triclos) | Before 1962 | June 1972 | 10 | |
| **CNS stimulant** | | | | |
| Fencamfamin (Reactivan) | June 1971 | — | | |
| **Muscle Relaxant** | | | | |
| Baclofen (Lioresal) | June 1972 | — | | |
| Dantrolene (Dantrium) | — | Feb. 1974 | | |
| **Anorectic** | | | | |
| Fenfluramine (Pondimin) | 1964 | July 1973 | 9 | |
| Mazindol (Sanorex) | Jan. 1974 | June 1973 | | (7) |
| Clortermine (Voranil) | — | June 1973 | | |
| **Antiparkinsonism, tremor, etc.** | | | | |
| Benapryzine (Brizin) | Sept. 1973 | — | | |
| Carbidopa (Sinemet) | Nov. 1973 | — | | |

## Table 8
### INTRODUCTION OF ANESTHETIC DRUGS

| Drug | Date of Introduction | | Lead in Years (Months) | |
|---|---|---|---|---|
| | U.K. | U.S. | U.K. | U.S. |
| General anesthetic | | | | |
| Trifluoroethyl difluoromethyl ether (Ethrane) | — | Jan. 1973 | | |
| Alphaloxone + Alphadolone (Althesin) | July 1972 | — | | |
| Local anesthetic | | | | |
| Bupvivacaine (Marcaine) | 1968 | March 1973 | 4(9) | |
| Neuromuscular blocking | | | | |
| Pancuronium (Pavulon) | 1968 | Nov. 1972 | 4(5) | |

## Table 9
### ANALGESIC AND RELATED DRUGS

| Drug | Date of Introduction | |
|---|---|---|
| | U.K. | U.S. |
| Anti-inflammatory analgesic | | |
| Benorylate (Benoral) | Aug. 1971 | — |
| Alclofenac (Prinalgin) | March 1972 | — |
| Naproxen (Naprosyn) | Sept. 1973 | — |
| Ketoprofen (Orudis) | Oct. 1973 | — |
| Fenoprofen (Fenopron) | Feb. 1974 | — |
| Narcotic and narcotic antagonist | | |
| Piritramide (Dipidolor) | June 1972 | — |
| Miscellaneous | | |
| Bufexamac (Feximac)-Topical | Sept. 1973 | — |

**Figure 1**

EXCLUSIVE AVAILABILITY OF CARDIOVASCULAR DRUGS

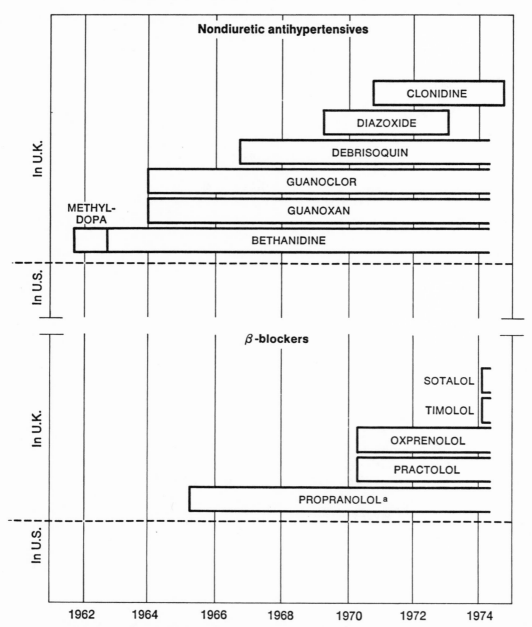

a Not available for angina and hypertension from 1968 to 1973, when it was approved for angina only.

**Figure 2**

## EXCLUSIVE AVAILABILITY OF DIURETICS AND POTASSIUM SUPPLEMENTS

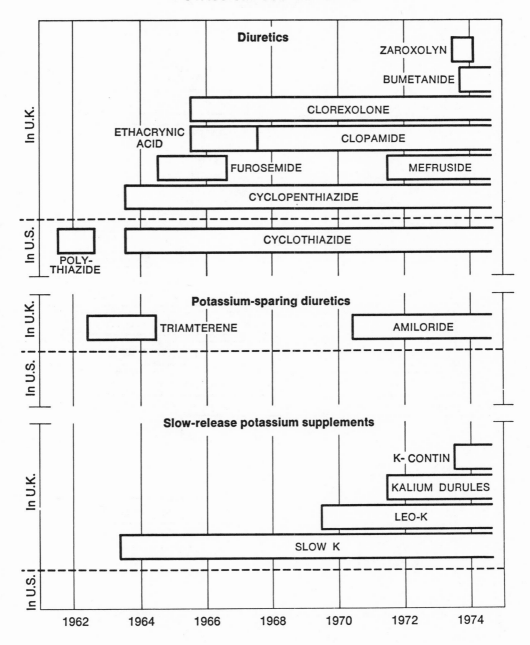

## Figure 3
### EXCLUSIVE AVAILABILITY OF RESPIRATORY DRUGS

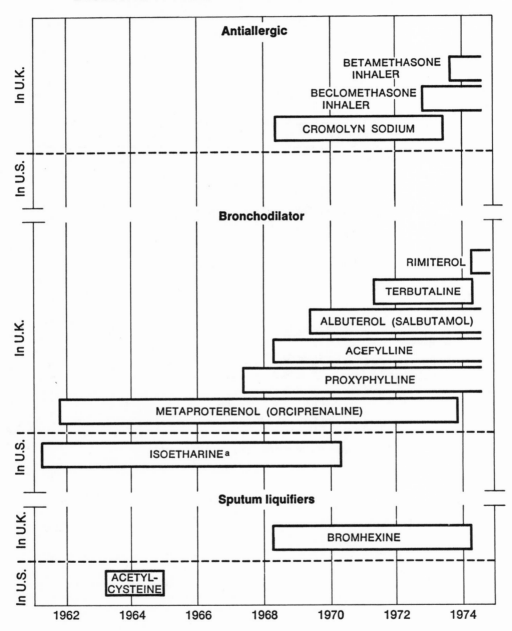

[a] Not available as single entity. For details, see W. Wardell, "Introduction of New Therapeutic Drugs in the United States and Great Britain: An International Comparison," *Clinical Pharmacology and Therapeutics*, vol. 14, no. 5 (Sept.-Oct. 1973), p. 781.

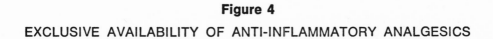

**Figure 4**

EXCLUSIVE AVAILABILITY OF ANTI-INFLAMMATORY ANALGESICS

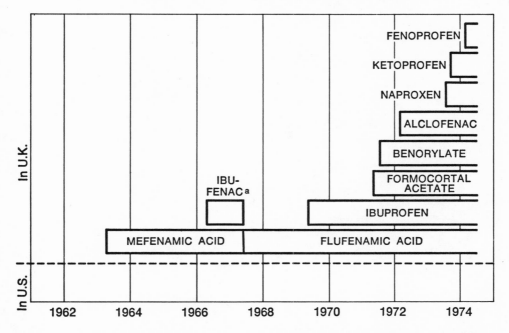

a Ibufenac was withdrawn in Great Britain for toxicity reasons. For details see Wardell, "New Therapeutic Drugs in the United States and Great Britain," p. 785.

## J. F. Dunne

I am in a somewhat invidious position as an outsider. First, I must explain that I present my views in a personal capacity, and they are not necessarily representative of the Committee on Safety of Medicines in the United Kingdom. Second, as an interested party, it would be improper for me to offer any judgment on the relative merits of drug regulatory systems in our two countries. Several differences are obvious.

In the United Kingdom all product licenses and clinical trial certificates are issued on the recommendation of a single standing committee that meets monthly and is representative of a wide variety of clinical and preclinical opinion. In some respects our procedures are more restrictive than yours. For instance, no clinical investigation of a new compound can be undertaken in the United Kingdom without definitive approval from the committee. But in other ways we adopt a more flexible approach. For example, presentation of clinical evidence to the committee is accepted in the form of reasoned papers suitable for publication and large numbers of individual case reports are not usually required.

Since 1971 the committee has operated under statute. Administrative procedures have changed, but the Medicines Act has had no effect on technical assessments, nor, now that initial teething problems are over, on the time required for decision making.

None of this, of course, accounts for the apparent systematic difference in the marketing dates of the same compound on the two sides of the Atlantic described by Dr. Wardell, and it may well be that hitherto the FDA has demanded a greater weight of evidence than its British counterpart, particularly in relation to efficacy. Clearly, the two regulatory agencies operate with laudable independence of judgment.

Dr. Wardell implies that the trend toward introducing new compounds into routine clinical use somewhat earlier in the United Kingdom is advantageous to medicine and states that the total burden of toxicity attributed to drugs recently introduced there is small. One can sympathize with the frustrations evoked among clinicians and within sponsor companies when the introduction of an interesting new compound to an important market is delayed by a failure to meet registration requirements; but I know of no standard by which the attendant benefits and risks

183

of earlier introduction could be measured without having much more precise information of the circumstances determining each case.

Mr. Clymer's thesis that the pharmaceutical industry relies for growth potential on continuous introduction of new products raises issues outside the purely commercial ambit. Innovation is beyond criticism when it offers tangible advantage to the patient as well as to industry. Otherwise, all that is achieved is a superfluous extension of the spectrum of choice for the prescriber. In a free economy this is inevitable, but in many instances we have reached the stage where a confusing number of drugs is available for the same indication. This can operate against the interest of the patient, for each time a new preparation is placed on the market a calculated risk is taken both by the sponsor and the drug regulatory authority: the safety of a drug is unequivocally established only after its use has become established in routine practice. On occasion, disillusionment follows initial enthusiasm.

Professor Lasagna questions whether the tendency for drugs to undergo increasingly prolonged clinical investigation prior to marketing reflects a remorseless increase in the demands of drug regulatory authorities. Despite the reservation I have just made, there is no conscious move in this direction in the United Kingdom. In part his data may reflect a change in the nature of the clinical problems that are now engaging attention. An increasing number of new drugs such as nonsteroidal anti-inflammatory agents and lipid-lowering agents are developed for uses that demand prolonged clinical investigation. No one can seriously dispute that these drugs should be marketed only when they have been shown to produce tangible clinical benefit and not merely on short-term evidence showing that they produce biochemical changes of questionable clinical significance.

Drug regulatory authorities appreciate the commercial implications of their decisions, but their only concern and consideration in determining a marketing application is to see that reasonable criteria of quality, efficacy, and safety are met. Inevitably these decisions are taken in default of much evidence that, ideally, should be available, and they are the more onerous because of the shortcomings of any practicable system for monitoring adverse reactions so far devised.

In conclusion, I suggest that the data presented by these papers underscore two basic problems.

First, inadequate information about the performance of drugs subsequent to marketing puts pressure on drug regulatory authorities to adopt a conservative approach to marketing applications. To some extent we have overcome this problem in the United Kingdom by allowing monitored release of selected preparations—a procedure committing the sponsor to the provision of a report on all clinical usage of the preparation for, say, the first year after its introduction.

Second, Dr. Wardell's comments about the number of nonsteroidal anti-inflammatory drugs on the United Kingdom market suggests there is much parallelism of research within the industry at the present time. But how, or if, this problem should be tackled is a matter outside my competence to judge.


## John A. Oates

I would like to focus initially on the process of drug discovery, because the failure to discover a drug is an absolute loss. By contrast, a delay in the approval of a drug is simply a rate phenomenon, which from the standpoint of the future is not so great a loss. While Drs. Lasagna and Wardell have been able to measure the lag between the introduction of a compound into man and the approval of a new drug application (NDA) and to compare this in different countries, it is much more difficult to quantify the number of discoveries that have not been made. This is essentially a unmeasurable loss.

How then do we approach the question of whether we are doing things at the present time that prevent discovery? The only method is to look at the history of drug discovery and to examine Dr. Lasagna's current data on the introduction of new chemical entities and their attrition rate in the light of drug discovery in the past. A look at this history is important because there are many misconceptions about how current drugs have been discovered. Even Mr. Clymer, in his definition, treated discovery as a process that took place only prior to the introduction of a drug into man. This misconception is further emphasized in Commissioner Schmidt's remarks quoted by Mr. Clymer: "We have temporarily exhausted the exploitation of known concepts and tools," and "New drug development will follow advances in bio-medical science." It is certainly true that science must provide a basis for new drug discovery, but the statement is only partially true if biomedical science does not include research on chemical compounds in man.

There are different points in the research process at which new drugs are discovered. Figure 1 depicts a discovery pathway that is classical for antibiotic and cancer research. In this mode of discovery, research in laboratory systems and experimental models leads to a disease-specific potential drug. If it is not too toxic, you then evaluate it in man and, if again it is not too full of ill effects, it will become a therapeutic agent. However, I believe this model from the antibiotic field is too broadly generalized in terms of drug discovery.

Figure 2 shows a drug discovery pathway in which an agent with biochemical or pharmacologic activity is a basis for an experimental hypothesis. I emphasize *experimental* hypothesis, because this is a far broader basis for introduction of new chemicals into clinical research than is a disease-specific hypothesis. These compounds may be investigational tools. It is important to note in the light of what has been said today, that they also may be agents that are being tested in man as possible "me-too" drugs. They further include some compounds introduced for a disease-specific hypothesis that is quite different from the therapeutic effect actually discovered during investigation in man. One reason for the greater possibility of discovering certain drugs in man is that he has diseases such as essential hypertension and depression for which drug therapy has antedated the

**Figure 1**

DISCOVERY PATHWAY I

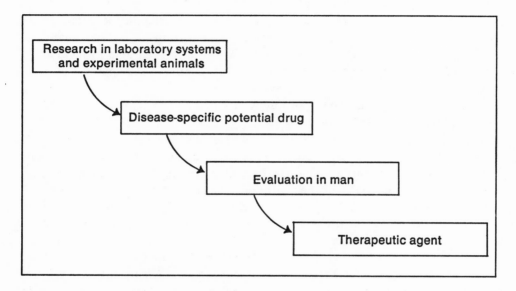

**Figure 2**

DISCOVERY PATHWAY II

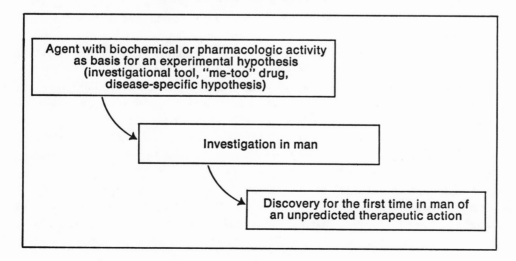

development of adequate animal models. Thus, the therapeutic actions of many of the valuable drugs currently in use have been recognized initially in clinical studies. Much of the discussion about drug discovery has ignored the fact that, in order to make these discoveries, compounds must first be studied in man, frequently with only a research hypothesis. I would like to illustrate just a few of the drugs that have come through this pathway to show that it is not an imaginary phenomenon.

The discovery of the use of propranolol for the treatment of essential hypertension is particularly important in terms of the number of people affected. This is probably the most important advance in this therapy in the last ten years. Propranolol was found to be effective in hypertension while Pritchard was studying it in patients with angina. This alert investigator then began to study it systematically in hypertensive patients. It is important to realize that at that time pharmacologists in academia, people in other drug companies, and those within the regulatory agency were referring to propranolol as "a drug in search of a disease" in a pejorative way, with the idea that this novel pharmacologic compound with the capacity to inhibit the $\beta$-adrenergic receptors really should not be out there looking around for a disease. It is now quite clear that the addition of this drug to the treatment of hypertension offers many patients a therapy with fewer side effects and increases, therefore, the possibility of their compliance with drug therapy. They do not become ill as a result of the drug quite as often.

Methyldopa is another drug that is widely used for hypertension. Prior to its introduction into clinical investigation, this drug had not been found to be hypotensive in experimental animals. It was being studied in man as part of a biochemical research project to evaluate its effect on decarboxylase enzymes in the human.

In regard to the increasing difficulty of studying drugs in the United States as compared to other countries, hydralazine offers an interesting case. This compound did enter human studies initially with a disease-specific hypothesis for hypertension. It was studied outside the United States by a very competent investigator, who promptly reported to the company that "this drug will never be of any value in the human as it produces tremendous tachycardia and palpitations which were quite unpleasant to the patient. You might as well forget it." Fortunately, it took his interlocutors some time to assimilate this information and communicate it to their American counterparts; by that time, a group in St. Louis had found that hydralazine could be used for the treatment of hypertension if the sympathetic nervous system was first interrupted so as to prevent the tachycardia.

Hydralazine was introduced because an American investigator made this observation after a very competent investigator elsewhere had indicated it was not of value. Recent studies using this drug in conjunction with propranolol make it quite obvious that hydralazine—and perhaps new vasodilators that have followed hydralazine—will be increasingly useful in the treatment of patients with hypertension. This example shows the value of studying drugs in multiple places with investigators having different viewpoints, rather than relying on single clinical trials in a foreign country followed by a decision based on a limited input of data and imagination.

The psychopharmacology area is another that has been built almost entirely on investigations in man with hypotheses that had little to do with the final outcome: Chlorpromazine was not investigated initially as an antipsychotic. The first antidepressant, iproniazid, was discovered while being studied as an anti-tuberculous drug. The tricyclic antidepressants were really "me-too" drugs in the line of phenothiazines that were being investigated as major tranquilizers. Only then were they found to have antidepressant activities. This is one of many examples of how chemical congeners when studied in man may be found to have useful properties that were not predicted by preclinical evaluation.

As a by-product of cancer chemotherapy, allopurinol was introduced and was found in man to lower uric acid. As a consequence, it has become a leading drug for the treatment of gout. The treatment of Parkinson's disease with L-dopa occurred as a result of studies in humans with neurologic disease; it was developed, not directly by industry, but as an investigational tool sponsored by an investigator. Similarly, the decarboxylase inhibitors, which are being used to enhance the value of L-dopa in Parkinsonism, were initially introduced as part of structure-activity relationship studies of the decarboxylase inhibitors. After these studies demon-strated a potent biochemical effect in man, these drugs lay dormant for some time until it was found that they might readily be used in Parkinson's disease together with L-dopa. Without this initial human experience, it might have been difficult to persuade someone to put these compounds through the necessary studies to get them into man for the first time. Pharmacologic properties of dopamine first observed during studies in man led to further investigations on this drug and its subsequent application in the treatment of shock. These, then, are a few examples of chemical entities that were introduced into man on the basis of an experimental hypothesis that led to the discovery of valuable therapy.

When we consider on the basis of past history the data that Dr. Lasagna has presented regarding the introduction of new chemical entities into the innova-tive new drug (IND) process and the rate of their removal from clinical research, we have to extrapolate that not only does the reduction of new chemical entity entrance decrease disease-specific drug discovery, but also it decreases the possi-bility of discoveries that may be made only when investigative compounds are introduced into clinical research.

What can be done about this? It is too narrow a view to say that this is simply a problem of the regulatory agency. I think that part of the problem of new chemical entity introduction into man depends on the objective, attitude, and research philosophy of the pharmaceutical industry. There still is a possibility, albeit limited, of their being creative and innovative if they do not indulge in a defeatist attitude toward the regulatory agency. An ever-present risk in industry is that dealing with Washington may excessively intimidate one to the point of stifling the creativity that leads to drug discovery in man.

The decisions of some pharmaceutical firms to take their early research abroad may be a response to the regulatory situation in this country, but it is a clearly voluntary decision. Since some of our considerations are economic, it may be worth considering the probable economic impact on the U.S. market of starting the initial investigations of a drug abroad. A model drug from this standpoint might be bethanidine, which was studied very late in this country. Could that be one reason why it has not reached the market here? It had already been studied so extensively abroad that there was very little investigator interest here by the time it was finally available as an IND in the United States.

In addition to the influence of industry's actions on research, one must logically ask if the regulatory agency can relate to pure research on new chemical entities in man without impeding investigation. This very difficult question must be divided into considerations of both administration and the law that controls the FDA. Certainly, under Dr. Crout, the Bureau of Drugs is taking steps to improve the administrative processes that deal with the initial work on new chemical entities. Whether or not the law needs to be clarified in regard to how FDA regulates research on all chemical compounds at their earliest stages needs real consideration, particularly because the Congress has heretofore not been very interested in the process of drug discovery.

Dr. Goldberg has emphasized the changes that are taking place in present attitudes toward drug research. This is very important, because one problem in encouraging research in man is that the real consumer—the patient with disease—does not have a valid advocate. The self-styled consumer advocates currently are proposing that long-term toxicity studies of questionable justification precede even short-term studies of any foreign chemical compound, drug, or other product in man. This is not the present—or even the past—problem of the consumer. First-phase testing in man and the introduction of foreign chemicals for the first time in man historically has been a remarkably safe process considering its inherent uncertainties. What problems there have been frequently can be related to the competence of the investigators, or to the failure of the sponsors to use those short-term toxicity studies currently recognized as necessary. Thus, the present attention of the self-styled consumer advocates is not justified on the basis of history or of consumer need. As Dr. Lasagna pointed out, the need of the patient with arthritis is to have a drug that will relieve his pain and increase the range of motion of his limbs. The need of a patient with hypertension is to have a drug that does not produce so many side effects that he refuses to take it and ends up with a crippling stroke.

In addition, there is a need for the patient to avoid the danger of reactions to current drugs. From a statistical standpoint, that is the consumer's largest risk. Four to six percent of hospitalized patients have drug reactions that range in seriousness from those that delay recovery or prolong hospitalization to those that are fatal. One solution to this problem is the development of newer drugs that are safer. A second solution is to facilitate clinical research that will expand our understanding of how currently available drugs can be employed more safely.

Certainly, the introduction of chemical compounds into man in first-phase studies will always carry potential risk, even when conducted with precautions meeting current standards. There is reason to believe, however, that these risks are minimized by present procedures to the greatest extent possible with current technology. Further limitations on the introduction of new compounds into the clinical research process are not in the best interest of the patient-consumer who is subject to real risk with current drugs and needs new and safer therapeutic agents.

An additional risk, not only in phase-one testing but all the way through therapeutic research, lies in the marginally qualified investigator. The past history of clinical research shows that an important assurance of patients' safety is the care with which studies are conducted. There is no question at the moment but that, with the regulatory climate and the industry's response to it, we are progressively expelling clinical research from the United States, a trend certain to lead to an atrophy of our national competence in this area. To patients and to subjects of investigation this trend is a matter of considerable concern. The patient who needs new and safer therapy could be served well by an advocate who recognized that his needs include more careful research with compounds of pharmacologic interest and qualified investigators to conduct this research.


## Aaron J. Gellman

I would like to do three things in this commentary. The first is to make some specific comments on the three papers. The second is to mention some issues that were either not addressed or, in my opinion, not adequately discussed in the papers. Finally, I will consider the possibility of generalizing from what we can learn from the recent history of the drug industry in the United States and the comparisons that have been made in these papers between the U.S. experience and the histories of other countries.

Each of the papers at hand suffers in some measure from data problems, usually not of the author's making. This is not a problem unique to the study of the innovation process or to research designed to shed light on the relationship between regulation and technological change, and it is not unique to this particular industry. It is a problem we face in virtually every industry we try to study.

In the drug field I think it is imperative that resources be devoted to providing more extensive and more relevant data than some that have appeared in these papers. Great problems arise from drawing general conclusions from the data presented in several cases; in many of them, I am sure, the author faced a resource limitation problem. No criticism of the authors is implied in any respect, since there clearly are problems in using data derived, for example, from "fifteen major firms" in the industry being studied. I shall return to this subject in another context in a moment.

Again, there are problems associated with deriving or using data comparing sales overseas with those in the United States without some explanation of the reasons for the change being greater in the overseas sales than it has been in the United States in the dozen years or so that were analyzed.

My second general comment relates to the foreign activities of U.S. firms and the difference between foreign practices and markets and our own. It seems to me that there is insufficient discussion of the difference in nature between foreign and U.S. markets and what this means for the process of innovation in each case. There is no field our firm has ever studied in which the process of innovation, when efficiently carried out, was not determined by the nature of the market. I think that this nexus between the market and the process of technological innovation has been essentially ignored in most of these papers.

In connection with the foreign activities of U.S. firms, it is important to ask just how bad it is that U.S. firms are emphasizing overseas growth. It is not so bad, I suggest, from a business standpoint—if that is what interests you. Indeed, it is possible that the United States would have even less drug innovation without these apparently vigorous foreign markets which enable industry to combine the foreign with the U.S. demand for certain drugs and get a better result than would be obtained without dynamic foreign markets to stimulate research and innovation. But the effect may be undesirable too. These papers do not present the data needed to determine whether the effect is good or bad, nor do I know of any other place they can be found.

One of the unfortunate results of the overseas emphasis flows from the fact that innovation is a *people* process. Whatever else may be said about innovation, those who have been studying the field intensively recognize this fact. This idea has cropped up repeatedly—most recently from the gentleman here who said that young investigators, and their recruitment and development, are handicapped by certain constraints found in the United States. This statement reflects an understanding that innovation is a people process. To the extent that people in the United States are not able to engage in innovation in the drug field, innovation will ultimately be less ubiquitous in our economy, probably to our great and collective detriment.

No data have been presented here to indicate whether there is less innovation activity in the drug field in the United States than there would have been without the 1962 legislative changes. It has been suggested that there is less, but there is precious little evidence to support that hypothesis. I think convincing evidence can be developed. There surely appear to be raw materials from which useful data could be derived.

I would like to raise a question in another vein: What does the growth of overseas markets for U.S. drugs owe to the existence of a strong FDA? It seems to me that the FDA may actually have increased the desirability of U.S. drugs. We know, for example, that the foreign demand for U.S. transport aircraft owes a great deal to the very strict Federal Aviation Administration certification requirement; and I submit that some similar process may be at work in the case of drugs. If so, it is beneficial from the balance-of-payments standpoint, if from no other. I am not suggesting that the net effect of a strong FDA is good for promoting innovation in pharmaceutics; I am simply suggesting that there are some things on the asset as well as on the liability side of the balance sheet.

My third general comment relates to research and development. There is little understanding, not only in the drug field but in other fields as well, that research and development is part of that continuum leading to successful market introduction which we call innovation. There are real data problems here, too. They are significant in some of these papers if only because the R&D data have been derived from a very limited sample which appears to be somewhat biased in favor of large enterprises.

Still, with drug R&D expenditures in the United States growing both in absolute terms and as percentages of revenue, as shown in one paper, why does it also seem that research and development output (as defined by the physical scientist) is down? Although I am admittedly from outside your field, I still cannot quite accept the reason given, which is that it is increasingly difficult and expensive to achieve R&D results. Frankly, that is an evasion that is employed in every field when fortunes turn down. You have to supply a great deal more data than has been presented in this forum or elsewhere to support the hypothesis that we have reached the point of diminishing returns in research and development in the drug field. This is especially true given some of the claims made for drug R&D overseas.

I think that, in fact, it is probably a case of increasing or constant returns on true R&D dollars and that we apply the label R&D to many things that are actually subsequent to R&D in the process of innovation which, if successful, gets you to the market. Accounting is part of the problem; so is the fact that the FDA has lengthened the proof-of-efficacy portion of the process and thus has caused investment in what, in the accounting sense, is lumped in with R&D to make R&D very much greater than it used to be. I believe we ought to understand clearly that some of the dollars that go into the R&D category for accounting purposes do so because of FDA action and because of the tax treatment often accorded R&D. Furthermore, we ought to distinguish what really constitutes

R&D investment from investment in the technology delivery system, which begins where R&D ends in the process of innovation. I suggest that virtually all the FDA requirements impinge on the latter and not on R&D itself.

Doctor Wardell makes a specific contribution by showing that there are significant differences between the United States and the United Kingdom where drug innovation is concerned; but it seems to me that he fails to explain the difference adequately, perhaps because of a lack of data beyond his control. For example, I would like to know the role socialized medicine in Britain played in generating this difference. I am certain there is ample material in Britain to develop and support a hypothesis on this point.

Let me turn now to the diversification of U.S. drug firms through entry into other fields. This issue was raised, but unfortunately there was no real discussion of it. I would suggest that somebody find out to what extent U.S. drug firms are, in fact, diversified outside the drug field—with the latter precisely defined.

Several of these papers contain assertions concerning the international mobility of R&D results but do not convincingly support them. Those of us interested in the process of innovation are always sensitive to data that will tell us something about such mobility. For example, our firm is now doing a National Science Foundation study that includes an analysis of five hundred innovations transferred internationally in the course of their development. Some are drug innovations; this is a very important dimension of the problem and there should be much more done on this type of transfer.

I have said that R&D is only part of a much larger process called innovation, a process that is only partially understood even by those who consider themselves experts in the field. But it is very clear that the authors of the papers entertain at times the notion that R&D is synonymous with innovation. It is not. Of the total resources required to carry through the process of innovation from idea or creation or invention to market introduction, typically only about 10 percent goes into R&D. Ninety percent of the resources are typically applied after R&D—in what we call the technology delivery system.

I think it is important to recognize that regulatory agencies, without exception, clearly do not understand this fact. Certainly the FDA has demonstrated very little understanding of what the process of innovation is about or how it does or should work. There is ample evidence in these papers to demonstrate this fact. Innovation is a continuum. It is not to be looked at strictly through comparative-statics analytical methods. You must use dynamic economic analysis because innovation is a dynamic process. Consider how long it takes to go from conception or creation to market. Furthermore, the greatest resources need to be employed beyond the R&D phase, in technology delivery. This is the basis for my suggestion that the FDA type of regulation is so pernicious for the drug industry. It directly influences not the R&D but the route that the R&D output must take to get to the market where, for the first time, the output of R&D becomes economically significant.

There are four issues that were either not addressed or inadequately dealt with in these papers. First, we need to know more than any of these papers tells us about the differences between large firms and small firms in this field. I have read some very interesting data on what happened to the small firm as a result of the Kefauver-Harris amendment. These seemed to support the conclusion that small firms were squeezed out or acquired by larger firms and that the formation of new enterprises in the drug field has been very much less than it was before and would have continued to be in the absence of this legislation. This is crucial to judging whether current FDA regulation is good, bad, or indifferent. Yet the case has not been made in these papers, nor is it often made elsewhere. What happened to small firms is important, of course, because there is good reason to believe that in fields of this nature the small firms are more the hotbed of innovation than are the large firms.

A second point that needed coverage was barely touched upon. It relates to the education of researchers and entrepreneurs in the process of innovation in the drug field. This was discussed in the context of the young investigator, but there also needs to be education for innovation incorporated into the curricula of medical schools, physical science education and, certainly, general public education.

I am absolutely convinced that if we continue long enough without introducing the concept of how important innovation is and what the process is about in fields like medicine, we absolutely guarantee there will be little or no innovation in such fields. Not only should the medical curriculum be laced with medical economics, which I understand is often the case these days, but also medical economics ought to include something explicit about the process of innovation.

A third question concerns the reversibility of the phenomenon of innovation in the drug field. If we were to repeal the Kefauver-Harris amendment, would the original nature of the innovation process in the drug industry be restored? Would we return to the kind of innovation activity we had in this field prior to the passage of such legislation? I do not know that we can produce a conclusive answer, but the issue ought to be considered.

Fourth, something needs to be said about the exportation of U.S. drug standards overseas. This was touched upon, not in the written papers, but in the authors' remarks. This is an extremely important point. What are we doing to ourselves, to the exportability of our drugs, and to the rest of the world if we export our drug regulatory standards? We have surely done grievous harm to a number of countries by exporting our environmental standards. I am not sure what the effect is if we are, in fact, exporting standards like the FDA's as well, but somebody ought to determine what the net effect is—for us and for other countries. Are we so sure we are right?

Finally, I would like to talk about a very important aspect of the conference itself. This concerns the possibility of generalizing from what we can learn through the history of the drug industry, especially its recent history. First, a historical analysis would delineate the responsibilities of various sorts of professionals in the face of regulation. The professionals in the field, scientists and businessmen, should react. They should come forward with the proper kinds of discussions and arguments about what such regulation does and will do to the process of innovation in their industry. They should come forward when rules are being considered. They should do so continually as they are being applied and when the regulatory framework is being revised.

This conference is one form of discharging this responsibility, but it is not enough. The drug field can be useful here because it actually or potentially touches everybody, including congressmen. Its situation offers a graphic way to demonstrate the benefits and the detriments of regulation to the process of innovation. Moreover, I believe there are many facets of drug industry history which can be applied to other fields of endeavor where regulation touches technology.

Certainly there is a need for a broader and deeper analytical framework in which to consider prospective regulations and to judge the performance and impact of such regulations in terms of technological change and innovation. I can think of no more effective context for this framework than the drug field.

Some oars ought soon to be bent to accomplish this. There is under discussion at the Bureau of Standards, as part of its Experimental Technology Incentives Program (ETIP), the creation of something that is often called the Center for Regulatory Analysis. This center would be devoted principally to taking a look at the technology impact of regulation in conjunction with other kinds of impacts. We are required to forecast environmental impacts on everything these days, but no one has yet formalized or even suggested that we require a technology impact statement which would address the question of the probable impact of each regulation or policy on innovation and technology.

It is time we did something along these lines. There would seem to be no better area in which to start than the drug industry, broadly defined. These papers, compared with papers that come out of other industries, persuade one that you are asking many of the right questions in this field. This indicates that you are likely to be able to forecast the effect of regulation on innovation and technology, although you have not yet done so. While there has been some forecasting of this sort, most of it has been of a highly private, firm-oriented, profit-maximizing type. For example, there is evidence that some of the larger drug firms were not too unhappy about Kefauver-Harris; they recognized the possibility of its eliminating some competitors and making the survivors cheaper to acquire because of the increased investment necessary to get into the market.

In conclusion, it seems to me that there is a need for teams to be formed to look at the process of innovation in general and in regulated industry in particular. The sort of people represented by these papers, working with economists, can demonstrate the interrelationships between innovation and regulation quite graphically in terms that the public and, in particular, Congress can understand.

We need to develop something that I often refer to as foregone-benefits analysis. The drug field seems to be the very best place for such analyses because many benefits were lost through the kind of regulation applied to it. This type of loss ought to be pointed out.

The economics of consumer protection also ought to be thoroughly discussed in the context of drugs. Further, it is very clear that such economic analysis ought to be taken directly into consideration in the regulatory agencies' calculations.

The FDA, among other agencies, absolutely and clearly does not understand what the discount rate is all about and what regulation does to the economics of those businesses they directly or indirectly affect. It is wise to remember that a riskless existence means little or no growth or improvement. Then one begins to understand what can happen as a result of regulation that is single-valued and fails to look at the overall picture in dynamic terms.

## J. Richard Crout

There are three important points that should be brought out. One is the very unfortunate fact that the modern organization and management of the Food and Drug Administration really began only about 1969. The agency was plagued with management instability for too many of the first seven years after the 1962 amendments. It had an enormous mission but received relatively little support. So in predicting what the future will be like, we should pay closest attention to the principles that have been laid down since 1969.

The second point is that some of those principles are paying off in terms of more rapid decision making at the Food and Drug Administration, and this will continue to improve as time goes on. We have had, for example, seventeen new molecular entities approved in the last year. That is higher than any year since 1967. This did not come about from any change in scientific standards. What it reflects is simply management procedures and practices designed to force more rapid decision making. If you do that in the presence of a backlog and a steady input, you will have a better output for a while. This is an important thing, but in the great scheme of things it is a ripple on the water. It is not a major wave because, as the panel has brought out, the larger issue involves societal standards, not just technical management.

Therefore, a third thing I would emphasize very strongly is that the Food and Drug Administration regulates health policy, not economic matters. That is terribly important to understand. We do not pay any attention to the economic consequences of our decisions and the law does not ask us to. That does not mean that FDA people are necessarily lacking in breadth as people or that we are blind to costs, but the point I emphasize strongly is that our decisions deal solely with the safety and effectiveness of chemicals intended for use as drugs. Because its primary mission is the regulation of health matters, the FDA is a different kind of regulatory agency from many others in the government. Also, as Dr. Gellman and Mr. Clymer have pointed out, it is the only regulatory agency that regulates the innovative process.

I would like to comment on three societal questions concerning health policy that from my perspective greatly influence decision making at the Food and Drug Administration. The first one is this: How much attention should we pay to animal toxicity, especially that which is untestable in man except by the test of the marketplace? For example, the scientific community does not have a universal solution to the problem of a drug that is carcinogenic in animals and yet may be of some health benefit in man. Should we approve such a drug? How much health benefit is needed to outweigh the risk? These are judgmental issues, not really data issues in science.

A second societal question is, what is the quality of evidence required for decision making on a health problem? Do we always need the raw data? Is our role mainly to weed out the marginal or deviant performer? Or is our role to require an increasing standard of excellence from everyone? Those are societal questions that all free men can debate, but there are no final answers. They are matters of policy, not of law.

The third societal question has not been touched on at all at this conference and is a very important one: To what extent are the data derived from a clinical trial to be considered the proprietary property of a drug firm rather than a societal asset? The drug industry cannot simultaneously say that data submitted to the Food and Drug Administration are proprietary information which cannot be viewed in public and also complain about FDA decisions made in private. We will either have the review of scientific data in this country conducted in the usual public arena of science or we will continue to have industry-FDA arguments going on and on. Proprietary data keep the regulatory approval process out of the open environment in which scientific decisions are usually made.

I think I have revealed my prejudice that nothing improves anything like the light of day.

# HIGHLIGHTS OF
# THE DISCUSSION

The relatively short floor discussion in the third session revolved primarily around two topics: the causes of the movement abroad of drug testing, and the pros and cons of selective approval or monitored release of drugs for marketing.

Mr. Paul de Haen started the discussion about the comparative drug lag by pointing out that his own studies of new drugs in several European countries show that quite commonly a large percentage of the drugs developed in any one country are introduced only in that country. To explain why this occurs would help explain the reduced introduction of new drugs in the United States and the apparent decision of U.S. drug firms to locate more of their development and testing work outside of the United States.

Professor Joseph Cooper pointed out that there is some evidence that the rate of new drug submissions in Germany was greatly reduced when that country adopted a tighter system of regulation. The German companies reduced their submissions while orienting themselves to the new requirements.

Dr. Lasagna added that in addition to differences in regulatory posture, other causes of international differences in drug innovation and development might be the availability of clinical investigators and differences in the cost of doing research. What is needed is more systematic research to explain differences between countries.

Dr. John Bunker responded that the shift in research outside the United States was not due to a lack of clinical investigators in the United States compared with other countries. He related that until about three years ago he received frequent calls from drug companies asking him to recommend U.S. investigators. But now he is asked to recommend British, Swedish, or other European investigators who can do the requisite studies. Dr. Bunker concluded that there has been a decision made by the drug companies to have the studies done abroad and that this decision is not based on the unavailability of domestic research personnel.

The second major topic of floor discussion was initiated by Dr. Arthur Carol who asked if we have to have a yes-or-no decision every time we introduce a new drug. As an example, Dr. Carol pointed out that we might want to approve a drug for use with the aged if it provided beneficial short-run effects even though it might be highly toxic if used for an extended period. He asked if we could not have a system of regulation that would recognize "degrees of marketability."

199

Dr. Leon Goldberg, the chairman of the session, responded that, while it has been extremely difficult to approve a drug for limited use, the FDA has recently suggested approval of the drug chymotrypsin for disc disease with the restriction that it be injected by an orthopedic surgeon.

Dr. Richard Crout of the FDA responded that the FDA had tried to avoid restricting drugs according to a man's specialty by saying instead that a particular drug released for limited use should be administered by "a physician experienced in back surgery" or a doctor "experienced in dermatological consultation," and so forth. He pointed out that there has long been resistance in the United States to approval of drugs for limited use. This posture has been based on the premise that "every doctor is a doctor" and therefore standards should be such that every doctor could use an approved drug. Dr. Crout pointed out, however, that the FDA was making some progress in approving drugs for limited use but was moving "gingerly" and without the enthusiastic support of the medical profession.

Dr. J. F. Dunne of the United Kingdom Committee on Safety of Medicines pointed out that British doctors have also resisted monitored release of drugs, insisting that they be given complete freedom to use the tools of their collective trade. Dr. Dunne said that it had only been in the last five or six years that the committee has introduced the system of monitored release. He pointed out that this is done with drugs, such as those for leukemia or disc disease, which obviously have use only to a specialist. Instead of restricting use to a named specialist, he said the British system is to restrict use of the drug to people with the "facilities" to treat and monitor patients with a particular severe disease.

Dr. Dunne added that a requirement for each clinician's use of a restricted drug is that he return to the committee a report on all such uses for a stated period, perhaps a year. This system of monitored release thus allows the committee to make a more informed decision about the safety of a drug than was possible at the time the drug was approved for marketing.

Dr. Louis Lasagna commented that one effect of the 1962 Kefauver amendments has been to squeeze out small drug firms. Two of the things Senator Kefauver was most concerned about in the hearings that led to the amendments were competition and costs. "[Kefauver] certainly did not want to squeeze out the small firm, and he certainly did not want to increase the cost of drugs," said Dr. Lasagna. However, the effects of the amendments have been just the opposite of the intent. Costs of R&D have increased, and small firms have declined relative to larger firms. Dr. Lasagna's point was that in drafting legislation, Congressmen, staff personnel, and witnesses have a responsibility to think through the implications of legislation and regulation and do the best job possible to predict "what this Pandora's box will let out when the lid is taken off."

The papers and discussion of the next session provide some interesting evidence on the effects of drug legislation.

# PART
# FOUR

## FACTORS AFFECTING
## DRUG INDUSTRY STRUCTURE
## AND COSTS

# CHAIRMAN'S COMMENT

*Rita Ricardo Campbell*

As an economist, I would like to remark briefly on the subject matter of this session. I think that all economists are in agreement that there is a need to develop and use better data and more precise definitions. These should be used in a consistent fashion in discussions about the supply and utilization of drugs and about various drug prices, such as *Red Book* list prices, discount prices to hospitals or chain drugstores, retail pharmacy prices, and so forth. Further, the economist—and here I am indebted to one of my very early preceptors, Professor Joseph Schumpeter of Harvard—makes a clear distinction between innovation, the creative act of discovery, and the entrepreneur's function, the marketing of the discovery. This distinction has not always been observed in our earlier discussions.

It is possible to invent a new way of doing things, to discover a new drug, and yet not see that new process marketed because it is not economic to do so. That is, the cost of producing the invention is not equal to the price for which it can be sold. Although to state this concept precisely would involve a discussion of marginal or incremental price and cost, I think that this simple statement is clear enough to help those who are not economists to follow these papers.

Furthermore, drugs can be viewed as part of a joint product, medical care. It is well-known that third parties pay a large percentage of the medical care bill in this as well as other countries. It is true that, although third-party medical payments in the United States do not usually cover costs of prescription drugs, the prescription drug is conjoined with a physician's services as part of medical care. This means that drugs also have a demand curve shifting to the right, that is, demand increasing at all prices, as the third-party share of payment increases. This, of course, helps to account for the increasing profits of some pharmaceutical companies.

The following papers will examine the supply response to the level of profits in the industry by existing companies and by the entry of new companies. However, the authors do not explicitly relate such management decisions to the increasing demand derived from third-party payments, but rather implicitly assume increasing demand and then ask how supply has responded.

It was noted earlier that initial research and development of new drugs by American international companies is increasingly being shifted from the United States to foreign countries. This shift is usually explained by cost differentials, by foreign exchange rates and, in the case of the drug industry, by differences in government regulations among countries. An additional reason in the drug industry may be that earlier marketing abroad is more feasible if the initial research has been done abroad, and that markets there are more fully underwritten by third-party payments, thus assuring some level of demand. Third-party payments in some countries take care of all or most of the total drug bill for the patient, which is not usual in the United States except under Medicaid and some private, comprehensive plans and health maintenance organizations. In other words, the size of the market abroad for drugs may be larger and more steady than in the United States. The recent limitations by the British National Health Service on the prices it will pay for prescription drugs such as Valium and Librium may, however, weaken the tendency to move research abroad.

In the group of papers on incentives and performance, it was noted that the pharmaceutical industry is often attacked because it appears to have, compared to other industries, a high level of profits. Economic theory assumes that, when profits are high in an industry with relatively few large firms, these firms, or oligopolies, set prices that, although competitive with each other, are higher than would be the case if there were more firms producing an identical product and competing only by price. Thus they obtain larger profits than might otherwise be possible. In the pharmaceutical industry, one drug product can often be substituted for another, very similar drug; companies tend to compete not on the basis of price for a given standard product, but rather, as the third paper of this group points out, primarily on the basis of product differentiation. This analysis is in line with the traditional economic theory of monopolistic competition, where relatively high profits depend in part on how close the substitutes are and how free is entry to the industry.

The first paper notes that, although the apparently large profits in the pharmaceutical industry should attract entry of new firms, this has not been the general rule. Here, however, I might make a personal observation. I live in an area of the country where several new pharmaceutical firms have developed recently, notably Syntex and Alza. In both cases, these firms have developed a very innovative idea that has been translated into a marketable product or products.

The first paper also points out that in an industry dominated by large firms, collusion is not necessary for prices to be above the free-market competitive level, but firms individually may tend to hold their prices only slightly above the competitive level to avoid attracting new firms into the industry. The second paper supports the contention that introduction of new products by existing firms encourages price competition among these firms.

One may infer from the first paper that existing firms have relatively protected markets because government regulation makes entry of new firms more difficult. The question is raised of how a new firm can get a start in an industry that requires large amounts of capital to be spent over several years, without any revenue coming in from sales, for initial and developmental research to substantiate claims to meet the new drug approval requirements. Persons lending capital for such an operation are called entrepreneurs. Much of the expansion of supply and the development of new products is by firms already in the industry.

Comparison of the first two papers is difficult because each author uses a different set of therapeutic categories, and it is not clear whether their somewhat different estimates of how innovative the industry is are due to this, or to the slight difference in the time period they use, or to some other factor.

# THE SUPPLY RESPONSE TO SHIFTING DEMAND IN THE ETHICAL PHARMACEUTICAL INDUSTRY

*Lester G. Telser*

## Introduction

The research described in this paper has two main purposes: to sketch a theory of entry, and to test it empirically using data for the ethical pharmaceutical industry. Success in these endeavors will increase our confidence in the validity of some economic theories of entry and decrease confidence in some rival theories, thereby contributing to an understanding of how entry works in all industries. Since the data refer to the ethical pharmaceutical industry, the findings have special relevance for this industry.

In stating the goals of this research, I am careful to exclude certain issues that are prominent in many discussions of the economics of industries. This work makes no attempt to discover whether an industry is competitive, nor does it determine the goodness of the behavior of the firms in the industry. This means that we do not ask whether the industry is monopolistic or bad. Nevertheless, some may find the results relevant to the debate about whether the pharmaceutical industry is competitive or monopolistic.

Because the world is much too complicated to describe in words, theories are devised to furnish compact mental images useful for understanding some portions of complex reality. Such mental images should not only advance our understanding of reality but should also be correct; both considerations are important. For instance, we may believe that the stars and the planets affect the lives of men. This belief may satisfy some, but I doubt its usefulness in revealing hitherto unknown aspects of the real world. By the same token, economic theory should not only provide satisfaction, but also give insights. Therefore, it should be tested by whether it correctly predicts previously unknown relations among real phenomena. The empirical results I shall report serve this purpose.

Of particular interest are the empirical results bearing on whether high levels of promotional outlays constitute a barrier to entry. If they do, we should find that when entry is lower, promotional outlays are higher. The reverse is true!

A more technical version of this material will appear in an article to be published in the *Journal of Law and Economics*, vol. 18 (1975). I wish to thank Yoram Barzel, Harry Johnson, Sam Peltzman, and George Stigler for their comments. I assume responsibility for all errors.

207

There is a positive relation between entry and promotional outlays divided by sales.

This study shatters another widely held belief that entry is less likely in those industries where firms must be large. This belief rests partly on the assumption of imperfect capital markets. Hence the existence of large firms in itself constitutes a barrier to entry. This is so, according to this argument, because it is more difficult for the entrant to secure the large capital necessary for success. In fact the empirical results for the therapeutic categories in this study show that, in markets of a given initial size, the smaller the number of firms initially in a category, the more entry occurs. Also, for a given initial number of firms, there is more entry in the markets of larger initial size. Both results mean that the larger the size of the firms initially in the category, the more entry occurs. There is virtually no relation between entry and the oligopoly as measured by the four-firm concentration ratio.

## A Theory of Entry

The theory of entry that guides this work postulates an optimal supply response to given demand conditions. Assume that the quantity demanded is a stable function of certain variables including the price of the good concerned, prices of competing and complementary goods, the wealth of the buyers, and so forth— in short, a normal demand function. The optimal supply response to a given quantity demanded is to produce that quantity at the least total cost. Doing so requires appropriate combinations and amounts of the inputs, which include the various factors of production such as raw materials, machinery, factories, labor, and management. Some of these inputs are combined into packages that economists call a plant and the *Census of Manufacture* calls an establishment. A firm is a collection of one or more plants under the general control of one person, the entrepreneur. A firm constitutes a single entrepreneurial input. It does not produce a single rate of output, but rather a range of outputs at different costs. The entrepreneur exercises control over this range of firm outputs, and the number of entrepreneurs constitutes one of the inputs to the industry. Therefore, to postulate that a total industry rate of output is made at the least total cost by the industry is equivalent to saying that to a given rate of output there corresponds an optimal size distribution of firms.

To understand and develop this argument a diagram is helpful. Figure 1 shows a demand schedule, the negatively sloped curve $DD$ relating the price on the vertical axis to the quantity demanded on the horizontal axis. Letting $N$ denote the number of firms in the industry, if $N$ is constant, the minimum total cost of producing at the rate $Oq$ is given by the area of the figure $OqAB$ in Figure 1. The locus of these points is shown by the upward sloping $S(D,N_0)$.

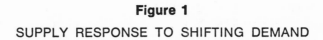

# Figure 1

## SUPPLY RESPONSE TO SHIFTING DEMAND

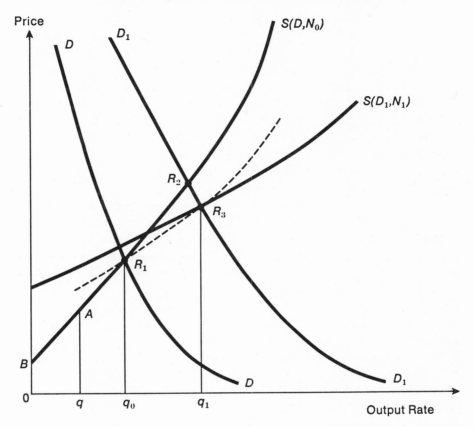

This is the supply schedule for a given number of firms in the industry. The intersection of $DD$ and $S(D,N_0)$ gives the industry rate of output $Oq_0$ at which the industry total cost is a minimum. Therefore, given the demand schedule $DD$, the optimal supply response is the rate of output $Oq_0$. Supply response depends on demand conditions, and for each demand schedule there is an optimal response in supply. Therefore, the supply function depends on the whole demand schedule. Movements along any schedule $S(D,N)$ hold constant the number of entrepreneurs in the industry. That is, the response to a shift in demand along the schedule $S(D,N_0)$ assumes an increase in all of the inputs other than the entrepreneurial input. But this does not give the optimal supply response. The curve $S(D_1,N_1)$ shows a supply schedule when there is a larger number of firms in the industry. In general, it is less costly to satisfy an increase in demand (a shift of the demand schedule to the right) by increasing the entrepreneurial input together with all of the other inputs than by simply having each firm produce more. Thus, a shift

209

in the demand schedule from $DD$ to $D_1D_1$ calls forth a change in the supply schedule from $S(D,N_0)$ to $S(D_1,N_1)$ and an equilibrium output rate such as $Oq_1$, which is the optimum response to the new demand schedule.

The analysis so far ignores the costs of entry. The optimal supply response does reckon with the cost of movement from one optimal rate of production to another. The more rapid the rate of change, the higher is the cost. Just as there is an optimal rate of output, so too there is an optimal path leading from one optimal rate of output to another. When a new firm enters the industry, it incurs certain costs that do not apply to the established firms. These costs of entry arise from establishing trade connections, making the new firm known to the buyers of the product, and learning how to operate efficiently under new conditions. Existing firms in the industry also have costs associated with changing output rates, but these are probably smaller than those of entry. There are also costs of finding new products and new methods of production.

This theory postulates an efficient supply response in the sense that all inputs in the industry adjust at appropriate rates to a level that can satisfy new demand conditions at the least total cost. The incentive for setting these changes in motion is the expected rate of return. If the current rate of return to firms presently in the industry rises and remains high, this gives evidence to potential entrants of better prospects in the industry and induces entry. In terms of Figure 1, the initial response to a rise in demand is an expansion of output by the firms presently in the industry accompanied by a rise in price. This gives incentives for entry and shifts the supply schedule to the right to $S(D_1,N_1)$. Therefore, the factors increasing demand encourage entry, and those decreasing demand discourage entry. Entry, by shifting the short-run supply schedule to the right, results in a further expansion of output and a decrease in the price. The locus of long-run output-price combinations will be given by the positively sloped curve $R_1R_3$ in Figure 1.

The empirical work uses this formal model. An algebraic formulation is helpful. Let $x$ denote entry and $q$ the quantity demanded at a given price. The first relation then postulates that

$$x = F(q) \text{ and } \frac{\delta F}{\delta q} > 0. \tag{1}$$

Let $p'$ denote the rate of change of prices; the second function postulates an inverse relation between $p'$ and $x$ as follows:

$$p' = G(x) \text{ and } \frac{\delta G(x)}{\delta x} < 0. \tag{2}$$

The first relation represents the shift in supply due to a change in the level of demand. The second relation shows how the shift in supply [$S(D_1,N_1)$ in Figure 1] resulting from entry affects the rate of change of prices. Let $y$ denote a variable that tends to raise the rate of demand at a given price so that $\delta q/\delta y > 0$. According to this theory, $x$ should increase with $y$ and $p'$ should decrease with $y$. The empirical relations furnish estimates of the two functions given in equations (1) and (2). The movement from $R_1$ to $R_2$ in Figure 1 is represented by equation (1); that from $R_2$ to $R_3$ is represented by (2).

## Description of the Sample [1]

The ethical pharmaceutical industry makes and sells those drugs that require a physician's prescription. Products are classified by therapeutic category. The rationale for a category depends on both supply and demand conditions. Categories based solely on demand conditions would include all drugs designed to treat a single illness. Were supply conditions the sole criterion, a category would include all those drugs with a high cross elasticity of supply regardless of the final uses of the drugs. The emphasis would then lie on similarity of methods of manufacture, distribution and promotion. It is probably accurate to say that demand conditions are more important than supply conditions in defining the ethical therapeutic categories. Almost all categories are in the sample. Table 1 lists the seventeen used, together with brief descriptions of them.

There are two submarkets for each category, the hospital market and the drugstore or, simply, drug market. For some purposes it is better to study these as distinct markets; for other purposes it is wiser to combine them.

Certain additional facts about the industry are pertinent. Almost all new drugs have patent protection. In addition, Food and Drug Administration (FDA) approval is required before drug companies may release them on the market. Drug companies spend large sums on research and development. New drugs are constantly sought and few, if any, old drugs have an assured market. This is apparent not only within therapeutic categories but also in the appearance of new categories and the declining importance of some old ones. The sample includes two categories that sprang into existence in the late 1950s: diuretics and oral contraceptives. The changes that constantly occur in the drug industry remind one of book publishing. Some close analogies between these two industries, illuminating the economic factors common to both, will be developed later.

There is finally the fact that the ultimate consumer of drugs does not completely control his drug purchase decisions. These decisions are made by physicians. Although this situation is more obvious in the drug industry, similar phenomena

---

[1] The data and the empirical analysis described in this section and the following one are incorporated in a study of entry in the ethical pharmaceutical industry by A. T. Kearney, management consultants, for the Pharmaceutical Manufacturers Association (PMA). I am grateful to my associates at Kearney, William Best, John Egan, and Tom Higbee for their helpful collaboration. The views herein are those of the author and do not represent those of the organizations cited.

## Table 1
### ETHICAL THERAPEUTIC CATEGORIES IN THE SAMPLE

| Category | Description |
|---|---|
| Anorexics | for treatment of obesity. |
| Anthelmintics | for treatment of intestinal worm conditions. |
| Antibiotics, excluding penicillin | choramphenicals, erythromicins, and tetracyclines, and their derivatives. These are broad-spectrum antibiotics. |
| Anticonvulsants | for the treatment of disorders of cerebral functions including epilepsy. |
| Antihypertensives | for the treatment of high blood pressure. This category includes rauwolfias and some combination drugs with diuretics. |
| Ataractics | tranquilizers or antianxiety agents. |
| Bronchial dilators | for asthma, bronchitis, pulmonary emphysema. |
| Coronary vasodilators | antianginal agents for relaxing spasms of the smooth muscles of the coronary vessels in the treatment of angina pectoris to prevent myocardial infarction. |
| Diuretics | for the reduction of the volume of extracellular fluid to eliminate or prevent edema, which is a state of excess volume of extracellular fluid. |
| Oral contraceptives | to prevent conception and to treat certain hormonal disorders. |
| Oxytocics | for the prevention and treatment of postpartum and postabortal hemorrhage. |
| Penicillin | |
| Psychostimulants | antidepressants. |
| Sedatives and hypnotics | |
| Sulfanomides | bacteriostatic drugs popularly known as sulfa drugs for the treatment of certain bacterial infections resistant to the antibiotics. |
| Thyroid preparations | for the treatment of a number of thyroid diseases including goiter, hyperthyroidism, and so forth. |
| Trichomonacides | for the treatment of trichomonas vaginalis, a bacterial infection of the vagina. |

pervade consumer markets. The purchaser of an automobile does not decide which piston rings should be used in the manufacture of the engine. The buyer of bread does not determine for the baker which flour he should use. The buyer of furniture does not decide on the glue and nails to use. The lady who buys a dress does not stipulate which thread to use. Most consumer products are such joint products. Consumers choose ingredients by deciding which of competing final products to buy. Similarly, drugs are an input to the consumer product we may call medical care. The physician's services are also an input. In choosing among physicians, the consumer selects a very complicated joint product which includes the drugs prescribed, the stethoscope used, the x-ray machine, the nurses, and so forth. The fact that the physician determines the drug to be administered creates little fundamental difference between the economics of consumer choice of drugs and, say, furniture. Indeed the patient may still search among drugstores for the one that will offer the prescribed drug at the lowest price. The obstacles to doing so are those that inhibit competition among drugstores, such as the common state prohibition of drug price advertising by pharmacists.

There is one other aspect of this industry deserving attention: the methods of promotion. Much of the advertising and promotion of ethical drugs is aimed at physicians and may include direct mail, advertising in medical journals, and the promotion of drugs by detail men, who call on physicians and describe the drugs made by their companies. In this respect, the drug and textbook-publishing industries are similar. In the latter, salesmen call on instructors and describe textbooks in the hope that the instructors will adopt them. The students who take a course must use the textbook assigned by the instructor just as the patient must use the drug prescribed by the physician. In both industries, salesmen promote a product to those who dictate the customer's choice. Publishers stress new textbooks and drug companies stress new drugs. In both industries the costs of promotion constitute one of the main elements in the cost of entry.

The larger drug companies operate in almost all of the therapeutic categories, while the small ones tend to specialize in a few. It is fair to say that any company in the drug industry is a potential entrant in any given category. Furthermore, many chemical companies are also potential entrants into this industry. By studying a cross-section of therapeutic categories we can observe a group of firms with very similar skills and cost conditions and at the same time obtain enough replication to apply statistical methods.

The sample period begins in 1963 and ends in 1972.. The measure of entry is the proportion of sales (in dollars) in 1972 in a therapeutic category by companies who were absent from the category in 1963 or some other specified initial date. This measure of entry is more closely related to successful or net entry than it is to gross entry. That is, if a company entered a category in 1963 and left it before 1972, its action has no effect on the calculation of entry for the period 1963 to 1972. The use of measures with shorter time periods would reduce the difference between gross entry and net entry but would have the disadvantage of making the measure of entry more erratic. That is, the choice of shorter periods for the measure of entry would lead to differences among the categories that would be difficult to explain without uncovering considerably more detail about the category than time would allow. This measure of entry also makes no explicit allowance for the number of entrants. There can be large entry in a category due to a single entrant. The statistical analysis does take into account the number of firms in the category in the initial period as an explanatory variable for entry. There are separate measures of entry for the drug and hospital markets, and it is important to note that the average size of entry is larger in the hospital than in the drug market. The correlation between entry in the two markets is 0.955.

This measure of entry is compatible with either high or low concentration ratios. The analogy between the drug industry and book publishing is again useful to understand the reasons for this. Suppose the book publishing industry were divided into categories by type of book: mystery novels, science fiction, love stories, cookbooks, dictionaries, financial investment advice, and so forth. For each category calculate the market share of the four leading books. Can anyone doubt that the observed four-book concentration ratios will be high? Even so, entry will probably also be high, because few books in any category will maintain their leading position for any considerable period. Therefore, a large measure of success coupled with a high rate of entry is normal in book publishing. Some therapeutic categories show similar patterns. Successful new drugs appear and seize a commanding position only to falter after five or more years and to be replaced by presumably better rivals. A high concentration ratio will persist under these conditions at the same time as a high rate of entry. Different market conditions prevail where a high level of concentration accompanies a low rate of entry. This can occur if firms cannot or will not enter highly concentrated categories. Those who argue that rates of return rise with concentration ratios would argue that high concentration by itself stimulates entry because it signals a high rate of return. They infer the presence of barriers to entry from lack of entry in highly concentrated categories. Consequently, it is of some interest to compute the correlation between rates of entry and such variables as the concentration ratio or the number of firms within therapeutic categories.

With barriers to entry, the correlation between the concentration ratio and entry should be negative. In fact, it is virtually zero (0.0028) between the four-firm concentration ratio in 1963 and entry from 1963 to 1972. This bears on the effect of concentration on entry since it measures concentration at the beginning of the period for which entry is calculated. The correlation between entry and concentration at the end of the period (in 1972) is 0.0921. For the purpose of making simple tests of the barrier-to-entry hypothesis, the number of firms in specific therapeutic categories is better than the four-firm concentration ratio. For 1972 the correlation between the four-firm concentration ratio and the number of firms in specific therapeutic categories is −0.763. Using the 1963 data, this correlation is −0.675. The correlation between entry from 1963 to 1972 and the number of firms in 1963 is −0.504. Hence entry was more likely in those therapeutic categories with fewer firms initially and less likely in the categories with many firms initially. This is direct evidence against the barrier-to-entry hypothesis. The next section gives more refined tests of this theory and of the presence of barriers to entry.[2]

---

[2] The simple correlation between the 1972 four-firm concentration ratio and the 1963 number of firms by therapeutic category is lower, −0.646, compared with the simple corre-

## Tests of the Basic Theory

The basic theory employs two equations. Entry is the dependent variable in the first, and the price change is the dependent variable in the second. The first equation postulates that entry is an increasing function of those variables that raise the level of demand at given prices and of certain other variables. The second equation postulates that the rate of change of prices is a decreasing function of entry. Therefore, the variables that enhance entry tend to lower prices, and those that retard or inhibit entry tend to raise prices.

Consider the nature of the sample to determine the number of degrees of freedom. There are two sets of observations for each of the seventeen therapeutic categories, one for the drugstore market and one for the hospital market. Do the thirty-four observations constitute thirty-four degrees of freedom? Classical statistics would answer that the number of degrees of freedom equals the number of independent random drawings from the population. In fact most of the ethical therapeutic categories for which data are available, and all of the important ones, appear in the sample. The correlation between entry in the drug and hospital markets is high (0.955). Nevertheless, the variables used to predict entry are not so highly correlated, and even though there is a high correlation between entry in the two markets, it does not follow by arithmetic or by logical necessity that the explanatory variables should work equally well in the submarkets. The question of whether the theory works as well in the drug as in the hospital market is empirical. Moreover, despite the high correlation between entry in the two markets, the mean entry rates differ: 12.2 percent for the seventeen hospital submarkets and 10.7 percent for the seventeen drugstore submarkets. Therefore, there is no spurious increase in sample size resulting from the study of both markets. On the contrary the theory is more easily tested with the replication provided by two markets. A single regression is calculated for the two sets of submarkets including a dummy variable that equals 1 for the drugstore market and 0 for the hospital market. In this way we can test for differences in the levels of the two markets while holding the explanatory variables constant. Put differently, we wish to see whether the differences in entry levels between the two markets can be accounted for by the explanatory variables. The main advantage of combining the two markets is to allow the use of more explanatory variables in the regression equation. High correlations among the explanatory variables make their presence known by raising the estimated standard errors of the regression coefficients. Therefore, if the estimation of a single regression equation for both the hospital and the drugstore markets were invalid, then the t-values of

---

lation of $-0.763$ between the 1972 number of firms and the 1972 concentration ratio. Also, the simple correlation between entry from 1963 to 1972 and the 1963 number of firms is $-0.504$. Therefore, there is more entry in those categories where there is a smaller number of firms initially. These figures are consistent with the finding of no negative correlation between the 1963 concentration ratio and entry from 1963 to 1972. As reported in the text, this correlation is virtually zero.

the regression coefficients would be low. The procedure, therefore, is subject to empirical test.

The regression equation with entry as the dependent variable has several obvious explanatory variables including growth in dollar sales, market size as measured by the log of total dollar sales in 1963, the log of the number of firms in the category in 1963, and promotional intensity. One variable, market stability, requires some explanation. This is a variable derived from certain regression equations fitted to each market as subdivided by therapeutic category across companies and years. This variable is designed to measure the stability of all companies' sales from one year to the next in such a submarket.

The greater the market's acceptance of the existing drugs in a given therapeutic category, the higher is this measure of market stability. A precise description is as follows: Let $s_{ijt}$ denote the sales of company $j$ in therapeutic category $i$ in year $t$. Let $d_t$ denote a dummy variable that is 1 in year $t$ and is 0 otherwise. The measure of stability for therapeutic category $i$ is the regression coefficient $b_i$ in the following regression:

$$s_{ijt} = \Sigma_t \, c_{it} \, d_t + b_i \, s_{ij,t-1} + u_{ij,t}, \tag{3}$$

where $c_{it}$ is the coefficient of the year dummy $d_t$ and $u_{ij,t}$ denotes the regression residual.

There is another way of writing this equation that illuminates the interpretation of $b_i$. For year $t$ equation (3) becomes

$$s_{ij,t} = c_{it} + b_i \, s_{ij,t-1} + u_{ij,t}. \tag{4}$$

Let $n_{it}$ denote the number of companies in therapeutic category $i$ in year $t$. Summing over $j$ in equation (4) and dividing by $n_{it}$, we obtain

$$\bar{s}_{i.t} = c_{it} + b_i \, \bar{s}_{i.t-1} + \bar{u}_{i.t}, \tag{5}$$

where

$$\bar{s}_{i.t} = \left(\frac{1}{n_{i.}}\right) \sum_{j}^{n_{i.t.}} s_{ijt},$$

$$\bar{s}_{i.t-1} = \left(\frac{1}{n_{i.}}\right) \sum_{j}^{n_{it-1}} s_{ijt-1}, \text{ and}$$

$$\bar{u}_{i.t} = \left(\frac{1}{n_{i.}}\right) \sum_{j}^{n_{it}} u_{ijt}.$$

Replacing $c_{it}$ in equation (3) according to the expression (5), we obtain

$$s_{ij,t} - \bar{s}_{i.t} = b_i \, (s_{ij,t-1} - \bar{s}_{i.t-1}) + u_{ij,t} - \bar{u}_{i.t}. \tag{6}$$

Thus, equation (6) is equivalent to equation (3). In equation (6) the measure of market stability $b_i$ gives the degree to which the deviation of a company's sales from the mean sales of all companies tends to change from one year to the next. In this way the year dummy removes common-year effects from company sales.

Equation (3) gives very good fits; the lowest $R^2$ is 0.89. The stability measure ranges from 0.962 to 1.150 in the drugstore market and from 0.954 to 1.248 in the hospital market. The simple correlation between entry and this measure of market stability is quite low, only 0.0742. Only in the limiting case where the multiple $R^2$ for equation (3) were 1 for *all* therapeutic categories would the correlation between the entry measure and market stability be zero. However, as we shall see, this variable plays an important role in all of the subsequent empirical analysis. It is worth noting that the stability measure is most closely correlated with the growth of sales for the period 1968 to 1972, the correlation being 0.883. The correlation of stability with sales growth from 1957 to 1963 is $-0.0785$ and with sales growth from 1963 to 1968 it is 0.2633.

One explanatory variable, promotional intensity, is the same for both the drug and hospital markets. This results from a lack of separate data for the two markets. The regression equations use as promotional intensity the total outlays on promotion divided by total sales.

Table 2 gives the pertinent statistics for the regression analysis. Entry is an increasing function of growth in sales, a decreasing function of stability, an increasing function of market size, an increasing function of promotional intensity, and a decreasing function of the number of firms. Therefore, holding the number of firms constant, there was more entry in the markets in which existing firms were of larger size. Holding market size constant, there was more entry in the markets with a smaller number of firms initially. Both of these results furnish more refined evidence against the hypothesis that there are barriers to entry. Nor is this all. The regression shows that entry rises with promotional intensity. If promotional outlays were a barrier to entry, the coefficients of promotional intensity would be negative; in fact they are positive. A more refined test would separate the promotional outlays into those of the entrants and those of the established firms. The barrier theory implies that entrants would allocate larger sums to promotion than do the established firms. Their outlays would decrease as their products gained acceptance.

The coefficients for growth in sales show an erratic pattern. Experiments with some other regression equations, where sales growth is calculated for different periods, show that the sum of the elasticities giving the effect of growth on entry tends to remain constant. Thus, in the Table 2 regression the sum is 0.666. In a regression that drops the 1957 to 1963 sales growth variable, the sum of the elasticities is about the same (0.638). It seems that estimates of the effect of long-term growth on entry are more reliable than are those for the subperiods. That is, the sum of the elasticities shows the effect of a 1 percent rise in growth from 1957 to 1972.

Price change has little effect on entry. However, as we shall see, the factors determining entry have much effect on price change. As expected from a comparison of the sample means, other things being equal, entry is larger in the hospital

## Table 2
### SELECTED STATISTICS FOR REGRESSION EQUATIONS EXPLAINING ENTRY (1963–72) AND PRICE RATIOS (1972/1964) FOR 17 ETHICAL THERAPEUTIC CATEGORIES IN HOSPITAL AND DRUGSTORE SUBMARKETS

| Explanatory Variables | Dependent Variables | | | |
|---|---|---|---|---|
| | Entry 1963–72 | | Price 1972/Price 1964 | |
| | Elasticity[a] | t-ratio | Elasticity[a] | t-ratio |
| Growth in sales (dollars) | | | | |
| 1957–1963 | 0.158 | 1.83 | — | — |
| 1963–1968 | −0.308 | −1.76 | −0.030 | −0.85 |
| 1968–1972 | 0.816 | 2.65 | −0.195 | −2.57 |
| Market stability | −8.802 | −1.75 | 3.586 | 3.19 |
| Log of dollar sales, 1963 | 0.307 | 2.10 | −0.115 | −4.04 |
| Price ratio | | | | |
| 1968/1964 | 0.737 | 0.45 | — | — |
| 1972/1968 | −0.206 | −0.13 | — | — |
| Entry 1963–72 | — | — | 0.089 | 1.97 |
| Promotional intensity | | | | |
| 1964–68 | 1.278 | 2.09 | −0.206 | −1.35 |
| 1968–72 | 0.550 | 1.00 | 0.084 | 0.66 |
| Log of number of firms, 1963 | −0.701 | −2.49 | 0.108 | 1.75 |
| Dummy variable = 1 in drugstore market, = 0 in hospital market | −2.906 | −0.69 | 0.224 | 2.92 |
| Constant term | 72.61 | 1.63 | −1.814 | −1.62 |
| $R^2$ | 0.817 | | 0.548 | |

[a] Calculated at sample mean.

market. This is shown by the negative value of the coefficient of the dummy variable. The t-value is low.

A more powerful test of the theory underlying this regression is to see whether the variables enhancing entry tend to lower price change while those decreasing entry tend to raise the price change. Equation (2) says that

$$p' = G(x) \text{ and } \frac{\delta G(x)}{\delta x} < 0.$$

Let $z$ denote a variable that affects entry. It follows that

$$\frac{\delta p'}{\delta z} = \left( \frac{\delta G(x)}{\delta x} \right) \left( \frac{\delta x}{\delta z} \right). \tag{7}$$

Therefore, the sign of the coefficient of $p'$ with respect to $z$ is determined by (2) and (7). Hence if $\delta x/\delta z > 0$ so that $z$ tends to increase entry, then $\delta p'/\delta z < 0$. If $\delta x/\delta z < 0$ so that $z$ tends to reduce entry, then $\delta p'/\delta z > 0$.

Consider the second regression in Table 2, which gives the price ratio from 1972 to 1964 as the dependent variable.[3] According to the preceding argument, sales growth should have a negative coefficient, market stability a positive coefficient, market size a negative coefficient, promotional intensity a negative coefficient, and number of firms a positive coefficient. In addition, since there is more entry in the hospital markets, prices should have risen more rapidly in the drugstore markets. These predictions are confirmed by the regression coefficients in Table 2 in seven cases out of eight. If a positive or a negative coefficient were equally likely, so that the probability of a coefficient's having a positive sign was .5, agreement between the hypothesis and the observed results could occur by chance with a probability given as follows:

$$8(.5)^7 + (.5)^8 = 0.0664.$$

Even this calculation understates the odds, since the t-value for the one exception, promotional intensity for 1968–72, is only 0.66.

One important fact remains about the regression equation with the price change as the dependent variable: it includes entry from 1963 to 1972 as one of the explanatory variables. The elasticity of entry is 0.089, and the t-value is 1.97. By hypothesis, holding entry constant is equivalent to holding the supply schedule constant and observing the effect of a shift in demand. Also, the theory implies that holding constant the remaining variables in the regression equation is equivalent to fixing the level of the demand schedule. Indeed, it is by the latter hypothesis that we predict the signs of the coefficients in equation (7). It follows, if this view is correct, that the coefficient of entry with the price change as the dependent variable should be positive, and it is.[4] Therefore, the theory correctly predicts the signs of eight out of nine coefficients. This or a better result would occur by chance with a probability as follows:

$$9(.5)^8 + (.5)^9 = 0.037.$$

## Promotional Outlays: Avenue of Entry

It is a widely held view that large promotional outlays by firms are designed to cement the loyalties of their customers, and therefore the established firms in an industry occupy a secure place. According to this view, the high promotional outlays constitute a barrier to entry. If this is true, we should observe an inverse

[3] Prices come from invoices and not from price lists. Details are given in the A. T. Kearney report.

[4] Although the regression coefficient of entry is positive, the simple correlation between the price ratio and entry is negative and small, −0.0348.

relation between entry and promotional intensity. The purpose of this section is to furnish some empirical evidence relevant to this debate. Since the promotional outlays refer to the combined hospital and drug markets, we shall use the data for the combined markets, that is, seventeen observations.

The sample is split into two subperiods, 1963–68 and 1968–72. We can then see the nature of the relation between changes in entry and changes in promotional intensity between the two subperiods. There are only three categories for which the change in promotional intensity is of an opposite sign to the change in entry, and one case where there is no change in promotional intensity while entry decreased. In the remaining thirteen cases the change in promotional intensity is of the same sign as the change in entry. This gives a crude indication that promotional intensity and entry tend to move in the same direction.

Examination of a scatter diagram relating promotional intensity to entry reveals a nonlinear relation as shown in Figure 2. Promotional intensity has an upper boundary independent of the level of entry. As entry increases, promotional intensity increases at a decreasing rate. This raises the question of what nonlinear relation between promotional intensity, $y$, and entry, $x$, can furnish a good fit. Consider

$$y = \alpha_0 - \alpha_1 e^{-\beta x}, \ \alpha_0, \ \alpha_1 \ \beta > 0. \tag{8}$$

**Figure 2**

POSITIVE RELATIONSHIP OF ENTRY AND PROMOTIONAL INTENSITY

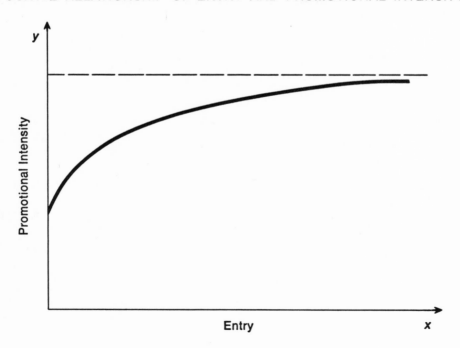

This form does have the properties shown by the curve in Figure 2. It has the disadvantage of being nonlinear in the parameter $\beta$ and consequently difficult to estimate. Equation (8) implies that $dy/dx = \alpha_1 \beta e^{-\beta x}$. Hence

$$\log \left( \frac{dy}{dx} \right) = \log (\alpha_1 \beta) - \beta x. \tag{9}$$

The transformation to this form gives an equation linear in the parameter $\beta$. We can estimate (9) using an approximation to the slope $dy/dx \simeq \Delta y/\Delta x$ where $\Delta y$ is the change in promotional intensity from the subperiod 1963–68 to the subperiod 1968–72. Similarly, we can calculate the change in entry for the same subperiods. However, since only logarithms of positive numbers are defined, this procedure works only for the thirteen therapeutic categories for which $\Delta y/\Delta x > 0$. The results are as follows:

$$\log \left( \frac{\Delta y}{\Delta x} \right) = \log (\alpha_1 \beta) - 7.492\, x,$$

$$R^2 = 0.480, \text{t-ratio} = -3.186. \tag{10}$$

Entry in this equation, $x$, is measured for the whole period from 1963 to 1972.

The results in (10) are encouraging and show that the hypothesis of a positive relation between entry and promotional intensity passes a second, more rigorous, test. However, four observations are excluded from this sample; three because $\Delta y/\Delta x < 0$ and one for which $\Delta y = 0$ because the logarithm is undefined in these cases. A more demanding test is to see how well equation (8) fits all of the data for the combined markets and all seventeen therapeutic categories. The correlation between $y$ and $e^{-7.49x}$ is $-0.496$. Hence the hypothesis of a positive relation between promotional intensity and entry passes a third test. A better procedure for showing how entry affects promotional intensity takes account of how other factors affect promotional intensity. We now consider some of these.

It is a well established fact that the effects of promotion endure for a time after the actual outlays. This is analogous to a form of capital which gradually wears out and disappears unless it is sustained by maintenance outlays. Therefore, the current outlays on promotion may serve two purposes: to maintain the existing stock of promotional capital and to increase this stock. Let $A$ denote the current stock of promotional capital, and let $a$ denote the current outlays on promotion. This argument implies that

$$a = \delta A + \left( \frac{dA}{dt} \right), \tag{11}$$

where the depreciation of promotional capital $\delta A$ is proportional to the stock of promotional capital, and $(dA/dt)$ denotes the net change in the stock. Equation (11), therefore, says that the current outlay on promotion has a component that maintains the existing stock and a component that represents additional investment in promotional capital. Assume that sales are proportional to the stock of promotional capital. Thus, $s = k A$, where $s$ denotes sales. The factor of proportionality, $k$, may itself depend on numerous variables so that it is neither constant nor beyond the control of the companies. Promotional intensity as measured herein is $a/s$. Therefore,

$$\frac{a}{s} = \left(\frac{\delta}{k}\right) + \left(\frac{1}{k}\right) \underbrace{\left(\frac{dA}{dt}\right)}_{A}. \tag{12}$$

This equation gives a relation between promotional intensity and some of its determinants, of which one is $\delta$, the rate of depreciation of the promotional capital. One of the empirical variables, namely, the stability of sales by therapeutic category, is an inverse function of the rate of depreciation of promotional capital. The more stable are the sales, the lower is the rate of depreciation of the promotional capital. Therefore, we expect that if the investment in promotional capital is held constant, promotional intensity should be lower, the more stable the sales. Also, entry is positively correlated with investment in promotional capital. Therefore, the higher the rate of entry, the higher promotional intensity should be.

The regression results are as follows:

$$y = 0.4677 - 0.0661\ e^{-7.49x} - 0.2744\ \text{stab.}$$
$$\text{t-ratio} \qquad -2.35 \qquad\qquad -1.59 \tag{13}$$
$$R^2 = 0.361,\ n = 17\quad \text{S.E.} = 0.0338.$$

These results confirm the hypothesis.

Finally, consider that version of the hypothesis that asserts promotional outlays constitute a barrier to entry so that the higher the four-firm concentration ratio, the higher the promotional intensity. The result of introducing the 1963 four-firm concentration ratio as a third explanatory variable in the regression equation is as follows:

$$y = 0.5439 - 0.0736\ e^{-7.49x} - 0.2321\ \text{stab.} - 0.1473\ \text{conc. (1963)}$$
$$\text{t-ratio} \qquad -2.95 \qquad\qquad -1.52 \qquad\qquad -2.26 \tag{14}$$
$$R^2 = 0.541,\ n = 17,\ \text{S.E.} = 0.0297.$$

In fact, promotional intensity varies inversely with the four-firm concentration ratio.[5] Even the simple correlation between promotional intensity and the 1963

---

[5] It is also of interest to calculate the regression corresponding to (14) using the 1972 four-firm concentration ratio. The results are as follows:

$$y = 0.5095 - 0.0658 e^{-7.49x} - 0.2434\ \text{stab.} - 0.0947\ \text{conc. (1972)}$$
$$\text{t-ratio} \qquad -2.47 \qquad\qquad -1.52 \qquad\qquad -2.26 \tag{15}$$
$$R^2 = 0.467,\ n = 17,\ \text{S.E.} = 0.03202.$$

We see that the results are better for the concentration ratios at the beginning of the period for which the promotional intensity is calculated than it is for the end-of-period concentration ratios. This is to say that equation (14) gives a much better fit than does equation (15).

four-firm concentration ratio is negative, $-0.392$. There is less, not more, promotional intensity in the more concentrated therapeutic categories. This suggests the explanation that firms in the more concentrated categories have less need to convey information than the many relatively smaller firms in the less concentrated categories. The general problem of explaining differences in promotional intensities among the categories deserves a more searching and detailed examination. It is plain from these results that promotional outlays do not constitute a barrier to entry. On the contrary, they are a means of competition. The view that such outlays are a form of capital receives strong confirmation from these results. Finally, the empirical results in this section and especially equations (13) and (14) are the first successful explanations of the different promotional intensities among products.

## Conclusions

One of the main empirical results of this study shows that prices tend to fall in response to entry. It is, therefore, of interest to compare the change in prices for the period prior to 1963 with that following, since there was more entry before 1963 than afterwards. From 1949 to 1961, the wholesale price index rose by 20.1 percent, while the Pharmaceutical Manufacturers Association (PMA) index of drug prices fell 12.1 percent. The real price of drugs consequently fell 32.2 percent. From 1961 to 1971 the wholesale price index rose by 17.5 percent, while the PMA index of drug prices fell 2.2 percent. Thus, in the decade 1961–71 the real price of drugs fell 19.7 percent. Even after adjustment for the slightly longer period, twelve years as against ten years, it is plain that the real price of drugs fell more during the time when there was more entry, thereby giving additional confirmation to the theory presented here.

More work needs to be done on this subject. We need data for other industries to provide additional means of testing this theory. We also need to see how much the patent laws and the FDA regulations tend to retard entry. I believe that despite these factors the rate of return on patents remains at a competitive level, that is, at levels comparable to those prevailing in other industries. Hard empirical work is necessary to see whether this theoretical prediction can be verified.

# PRODUCT INNOVATION AND THE DYNAMIC ELEMENTS OF COMPETITION IN THE ETHICAL PHARMACEUTICAL INDUSTRY

*Douglas L. Cocks*

## Introduction

Since the late 1950s, the economics of the ethical pharmaceutical industry have been scrutinized in congressional debate and by industrial organization economists. For the most part, economic studies of the industry have looked at its structure, conduct, and performance characteristics.[1] These studies have generally concluded that the industry's nature results in a substantial misallocation of resources. In addition, evidence has been gathered recently that reflects the fact that the 1962 Kefauver-Harris amendments (the 1962 drug amendments) to the 1938 Food, Drug, and Cosmetic Act represent a major institutional change in the ethical drug industry, and that this change has had a significant structural impact.[2] It is generally concluded that one of the primary results of this structural change has been a greatly increased cost for research and development and a significant lessening

---

[1] William S. Comanor, "The Drug Industry and Medical Research: The Economics of the Kefauver Committee Investigations," *Journal of Business,* vol. 39 (January 1966), pp. 12–18; idem, "Research and Competitive Product Differentiation in the Pharmaceutical Industry in the United States," *Economica,* vol. 31 (November 1964), pp. 372–84; idem, "Research and Technical Change in the Pharmaceutical Industry," *Review of Economics and Statistics,* vol. 47 (May 1965), pp. 181–89; P. M. Costello, "Economics of the Ethical Drug Industry: A Reply to Whitney," *Antitrust Bulletin,* vol. 14 (Summer 1969), pp. 397–409; idem, "The Tetracycline Conspiracy: Structure Conduct and Performance in the Drug Industry," *Antitrust Law and Economics Review,* vol. 1 (Summer 1968), pp. 13–44; Estes Kefauver, *In a Few Hands: Monopoly Power in America* (New York: Pantheon, 1965); Jesse W. Markham, "Economic Incentives in the Drug Industry," in Paul Talalay, ed., *Drugs in Our Society* (Baltimore: Johns Hopkins University Press, 1964), pp. 163–73; Leonard Schifrin, "The Ethical Drug Industry: The Case for Compulsory Patent Licensing," *Antitrust Bulletin,* vol. 12 (Fall 1967), pp. 893–915; Henry Steele, "Monopoly and Competition in the Ethical Drugs Market," *Journal of Law and Economics,* vol. 5 (October 1962), pp. 131–63; idem, "Patent Restrictions and Price Competition in the Ethical Drugs Industry," *Journal of Law and Economics* (July 1964), pp. 198–223; Hugh D. Walker, *Market Power and Price Levels in the Ethical Drug Industry* (Bloomington: Indiana University Press, 1971).

[2] Martin Neil Baily, "Research and Development Costs and Returns: The U.S. Pharmaceutical Industry," *Journal of Political Economy,* vol. 80 (January–February, 1972), pp. 70–85; Douglas L. Cocks, "The Impact of the 1962 Drug Amendments on R and D Productivity in the Ethical Pharmaceutical Industry" (Ph.D. diss., Oklahoma State University, 1973); Joseph M. Jadlow, "The Economic Effects of the 1962 Drug Amendments" (Ph.D. diss., University of Virginia, 1970); and Sam Peltzman, *Regulation of Pharmaceutical Innovation: The 1962 Amendments* (Washington, D. C.: The American Enterprise Institute, 1974), pp. 46–48.

of competition in the industry.[3] This conclusion seems to have given a greater urgency to recommendations of direct economic regulation of the industry, manifested in such things as the industrial reorganization bill introduced by Senator Hart [4] and the policy recommendations of the Task Force on Prescription Drugs.[5]

The present paper investigates the possibility that the previous analyses did not fully allow for the dynamic nature of the drug industry. A model is applied to the industry that takes into account certain of the dynamic elements flowing from the research and development activity of drug firms.[6] The model depicts the competitive nature of these firms. In addition, preliminary empirical evidence that tests the predictive power of the model is presented. Finally, through the application of this model, it is concluded that further research is necessary before appropriate public policy can be devised applicable to the ethical drug industry.


**A Comparative Static Model of the Drug Industry** [7]

Prior analyses of the ethical drug industry have generally adhered to the standard industrial organization framework, stressing concentration, entry barriers, pricing behavior, and profit performance. Several writers have recognized that product competition through research and development activity is an important characteristic of the industry, but they have generally regarded this as an element barring entry to drug markets.[8] It is one of the purposes of this paper to investigate the possibility that product competition through R&D provides the institutional basis for substantial price competition. This R&D product competition is primarily a supply-side characteristic, and only recently have its price competitive effects been considered.[9]

If a firm directs a great deal of effort toward the development of new products, and if in fact such development is a primary objective of its R&D effort, then a

---

[3] Jadlow, "Economic Effects of the 1962 Drug Amendments," pp. 197–98 and Peltzman, *Regulation of Pharmaceutical Innovation*, p. 82.

[4] U.S., Congress, Senate, *Congressional Record* (12 March 1973), pp. S4631–S4636.

[5] U.S., Department of Health, Education, and Welfare, Task Force on Prescription Drugs, *Final Report* (Washington, D. C.: Government Printing Office, 1969), p. xvii.

[6] The need for utilizing dynamic models of the firm when research and development is an important firm characteristic has been recognized by several economists. For example, see Jacob Schmookler, "Technological Change in the Law of Industrial Growth" in Zvi Grilliches and Leonid Hurwicz, eds., *Patents, Invention, and Economic Change* (Cambridge, Mass.: Harvard University Press, 1972), pp. 70–84; and Werner Z. Hirsch, "Technological Progress and Microeconomic Theory," *American Economic Review*, vol. 59 (May 1969), pp. 36–43.

[7] The author is grateful to Janice Jadlow who, while we were graduate students at Oklahoma State University, first suggested that the model outlined in this paper might be applicable to the drug industry.

[8] Comanor, "Research and Competitive Product Differentiation," p. 380; and Schifrin, "The Ethical Drug Industry," pp. 911–12.

[9] Peltzman, *Regulation of Pharmaceutical Innovation*, pp. 46–48.

possible method of analyzing the dynamics of this situation is suggested in a model introduced by Clemens.[10] In applying this model to the ethical drug industry, it is assumed that development of new drug products through the R&D process is the primary objective of a substantial number of firms. The main incentive is that a firm can obtain a preferred market position by developing new products significantly different from existing drug therapy.

Clemens's model deals with multi-product production where new products are an important element of a firm's strategy and are devised with the intent of using a firm's idle capacity.[11] In the drug industry it is assumed that, while this new product introduction may be intended to employ idle capacity, it also seeks to meet unfulfilled demand in various areas of drug therapy.

The essence of Clemens's analysis is that the existence of a market where the price of a product is greater than its marginal cost encourages firms to enter that market. Firms will expand output to the point where the least profitable unit of output will be produced at a marginal cost equal to its price. Specifically, drug firms will attempt to enter particular areas of therapeutic activity in which their R&D effort develops new entries significantly different from existing medical therapy. At the same time, they are encouraged to introduce new products that may have only slight advantages over, or even duplicate, existing therapy. It is assumed, however, that their primary interest lies in introducing new products that are significant improvements in therapy.

The Clemens model is used here to illustrate how technological innovations in the form of new products are translated into the production activity of the ethical drug firm. Several assumptions are made:

(1) Products are not considered to be homogeneous, but there is a relatively homogeneous unit of output. "Units of output are defined as blocks of output, without distinction as to products, which have equal direct costs under standard conditions." [12] In essence this implies that the output of heterogeneous products can be measured in terms of the inputs required. This allows the measurement of output in commensurate units (in input units required) that can be summed to give the aggregate demand curve for these heterogeneous products. This means that the firm can produce several different products utilizing the same production processes (input units). The demand being considered is really the demand for these production processes and for R&D effort (R&D inputs). R&D inputs can be diversified across a wide range of potential therapies and are also considered to be homogeneous.

---

[10] Eli W. Clemens, "Price Discrimination and the Multiple Product Firm," in Richard Hefelbower and George W. Stocking, eds., *Readings in Industrial Organization and Public Policy* (Homewood, Ill.: Irwin, 1958), pp. 262–76.

[11] Ibid., p. 263.

[12] Ibid., p. 265.

(2) Closely allied with the first assumption is the assumption that resources are easily transferable within the firm, a condition allowing the production of several products. Clemens cited the chemical industry as an example of the relative ease of transfer of resources among products. This high cross elasticity of supply is evident in both production and R&D activities.[13]

(3) The market positions of the firm's various products range from strong "market power" to pure competition. This appears to be a realistic assumption for the drug industry. Newly patented drugs may have "market power" positions dependent on their therapeutic uniqueness. As drugs mature commercially and substitutes become available, markets move closer to pure competition.

(4) Clemens assumes that the demand curves faced by the firm are not related—the new product areas are relatively diversified. Previous analyses of the industry have drawn conclusions that would contradict this assumption.[14] However, the present study suggests that this assumption does apply to the ethical drug industry. As shown in the empirical section, there is the possibility of a large number of firms introducing new products in many therapeutic areas, a situation that indicates fairly extensive new product diversification among these firms and unrelated demand for many of their products.

(5) It is assumed that the firm has a certain amount of excess capacity or can apply its technological knowledge to its production processes to increase productivity when demand is growing. This allows the firm to increase production without a great increase in marginal cost. The first part of this assumption follows from the tendency of the demand for a firm's individual drug products to deteriorate. Also, the largest portion of the drug firm's total costs are fixed, so that marginal costs are low for added outputs.[15]

(6) New markets are invaded in the order of their profitability. This clearly applies to the ethical pharmaceutical industry, because firms enter those markets to which R&D activity has been directed and has resulted in a patentable product. R&D activity yields significant new drug products that may be profitable if the demand for them is large enough.

(7) Finally, it is assumed that the firm maximizes profits.[16] It strives to develop products of unique therapeutic effect that can establish a substantial

[13] Several economists have recognized the importance of the cross elasticity of supply when considering competition. For example, refer to Robert L. Bishop, "Elasticities, Cross Elasticities, and Market Relationships," *American Economic Review*, vol. 42 (December 1952), pp. 779–803; A. G. Papandreau, "Market Structure and Monopoly Power," *American Economic Review*, vol. 39 (September 1949), pp. 883–97; and Robert Triffin, *Monopolistic Competition and General Equilibrium Theory* (Cambridge, Mass.: Harvard University Press, 1940).

[14] Schifrin, "The Ethical Drug Industry," pp. 897–98.

[15] Comanor, "Research and Competitive Product Differentiation," p. 375.

[16] An analysis of the relevance of profit maximizing behavior on the part of drug firms to their R&D activity is presented in Jadlow, "Economic Effects of the 1962 Drug Amendments," pp. 16–23, and in Clemens, "Price Discrimination," pp. 266–67.

## Figure 1
### MULTI-PRODUCT PRODUCTION

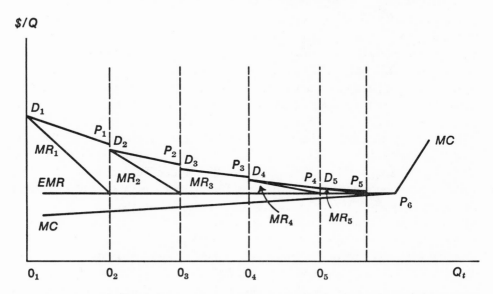

market preference and for which the demand will be large. R&D projects are selected which are expected to yield the most profitable products among those that might be developed.

To illustrate his model, Clemens presented an analysis of five markets in which profits are maximized when production is distributed among them in such a manner that marginal revenue in each market is equal to marginal cost. In Figure 1, *EMR* is the horizontal line depicting equal marginal revenue. This is established by the intersection of the firm's marginal cost curve and the marginal revenue curve for the last market that can be secured profitably. The limit to this is a market with a perfectly elastic demand curve. In Figure 1 each market has its own 0 output axis with a corresponding demand curve. From these demand curves it is possible to derive the marginal revenue curves for each market. The steepness of these demand curves, when applied to areas of drug therapy, could reflect the uniqueness and therapeutic value of the product in treating disease. These demand curves are shown in Figure 1 as $D_1$ through $D_5$ with their respective marginal revenue curves, $MR_1$ through $MR_5$. In these five markets, five product prices are established as $P_1$ through $P_5$.[17]

For a drug firm, $D_1$ could be the demand curve for the most recently patented, therapeutically unique of five drugs. The demand for it would be relatively less elastic. The other demand curves could represent maturing brand name products,

---

[17] Clemens, "Price Discrimination," p. 267.

229

or the relatively more elastic demand curves could represent generic products that the firm produces to fill out excess capacity.

Thus, a drug firm may devise new drug products to gain a profitable market position and then fill out the rest of its productive capacity, or increase its capacity, in the manner shown. As long as a profitable market exists, a drug firm is encouraged to enter it.[18] Because of the low marginal cost, it may enter markets which increase its profits but which would provide insufficient returns to a new firm with no existing plant or organization. Thus, drugs are made available that would not be placed on the market if no firm had excess capacity or if there were not economies of scale or of learning.

On the surface the above analysis is basically a static framework. However, if we use the model on a comparative static basis, it highlights the dynamic characteristics of drug R&D and its effects on the productive processes of the firm. Price competition among drug firms would be reflected by a shift of the demand curves $D_1$ through $D_5$ downward and towards greater elasticity.

This price competition can be illustrated in two ways. In both examples, the demand for each of the firm's products is made more elastic by the competitive products introduced by other firms; the demands facing other firms are made more elastic by the products introduced by the firm depicted in Figure 1.

Figure 2 depicts the drug firm shown in Figure 1 in a subsequent period when it has successfully introduced a new drug significantly better than existing drug therapy. Demand curve $D_6$ represents this new drug. While the firm was developing this product, competitors could readily see the profit potential of the product associated with, say, $D_5$. They had an incentive to enter with products of their own, and such entry would cause the elasticity of $D_5$ to become greater. The introduction of the new product, $D_6$, alerts competitors to the profit potential of the new therapy also. At the same time the firm in Figure 2 is introducing its significant new product, it could also be entering product areas of competitive firms $(D_7)$ with demand curves like $D_5$ in Figure 1, or any other product area in which price is greater than marginal cost. This increases the elasticity of the demand curves faced by these competitors.

An important aspect of the model outlined above is the depicting of several different demand curves associated with a single marginal cost curve. This indicates that the drug firm's production function is singular in that it can utilize common production processes to serve several demand-side markets. Thus, the firm, in making its profit maximizing decisions, considers all of the demand curves it is confronted with and allocates its productive capacity accordingly.

Innovation in the form of new drug products is the key element in both of the cases shown in Figures 2 and 3. However, the uniqueness of the products coming out of the R&D process is crucial in determining the relative magnitude

---

[18] This discussion of the application of Clemens's model to the ethical drug industry was first presented in Cocks, "Impact of the 1962 Drug Amendments," pp. 32–36.

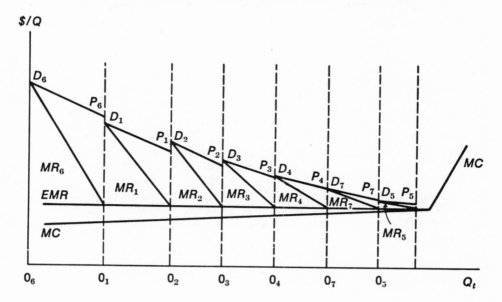

**Figure 2**

MULTI-PRODUCT PRODUCTION IN PERIOD
WHEN SIGNIFICANT NEW DRUG IS INTRODUCED

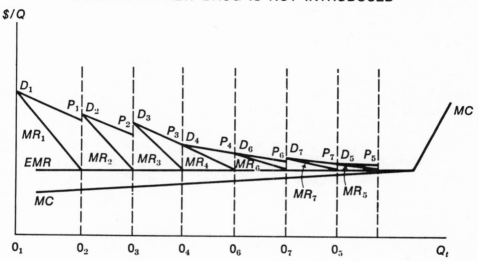

**Figure 3**

MULTI-PRODUCT PRODUCTION IN PERIOD WHEN
SIGNIFICANT NEW DRUG IS NOT INTRODUCED

231

of resource movement within the individual firm. Furthermore, a product that demonstrates some therapeutic superiority over existing products (as in demand curve $D_6$ in Figure 2) should be an important signal for resources to flow to the firm introducing that product. This is very similar to the stochastic model recently described by Mancke.[19] The essence of Mancke's model is contained in the following:

> If, for simplicity, we assume firms to be risk-neutral, then each firm's profit-maximizing strategy would be to invest all of its assets in that bundle of investment projects having the highest net present value. Suppose that all firms do adopt this strategy and, at the time they choose the bundle of projects in which they want to invest, the outcomes of these investments are uncertain. Then, if the magnitude of the successes actually realized on different investment bundles is distributed randomly, we infer that future values of measures of different firms' profit rates, size, market share, and past growth will differ solely because of "chance." Moreover, these differences will be systematic. Specifically, the firms whose investments prove to be most "successful" are those that ought to report the fastest growing profits and ultimately the highest profits and highest profit rates. Also, assuming that there is no systematic tendency for such successful firms to reinvest a smaller (than the average for all companies) fraction of their total profits, these firms will tend to grow faster (because reinvested profits will be larger) and therefore become relatively larger and have a larger market share. Conversely, the firms whose investments prove least successful ought ultimately to report lower profit rates; they will also tend to grow more slowly and therefore become relatively smaller and have a smaller market share.[20]

The result of this stochastic process is exemplified by a demand curve such as $D_6$ in Figure 2 and is desirable from a resource allocation point of view. When new drug therapies are introduced, resources should be attracted to their production, and a firm's market share should be increased. This is the role of profit in a competitive system. When a firm demonstrates that it has been successful in introducing significant new products, its *ex post* profit can be expected to be relatively higher than that of firms which are less successful with their R&D investments. If resources do flow to firms that are "lucky" in this chance situation and if this resource movement is reflected in an expanding market share, then resources are being allocated in a desirable manner.

In addition to illustrating how resources might be allocated in the firm under stochastic conditions, the Clemens model also depicts how drug firms can make product decisions when they have the resource flexibility to engage in multi-product production. This kind of resource mobility can be significant in fostering price-competitive results.

---

[19] Richard A. Mancke, "Causes of Interfirm Profitability Differences: A New Interpretation of the Evidence," *Quarterly Journal of Economics*, vol. 88 (May 1974), pp. 181–93.
[20] Ibid., pp. 182–83.

These price-competitive effects are shown in Figure 3. In this case the firm in the subsequent period is not successful in introducing a significant new drug product. Its competitors have been entering its profitable product areas. At the same time, the firm itself is introducing products into the therapeutic areas of its competitors: $D_6$ and $D_7$. In both of these instances there is an increase in the elasticities of all the demand curves concerned.

Thus, the result of substantial research and development effort in a number of drug firms is a kind of entropy that makes a comparative static interpretation of Clemens's model very realistic in the case of the ethical drug industry. The entropy is one in which new competitive products are a by-product of the R&D process of drug firms, resulting in a systematic impact on the demand curves faced by firms already in the market. The initial market power of significant new drugs sows the seeds of its own destruction. First, as we have seen, it alerts competitors to the profitability of a new or improved method of therapy. Second, the existing drug institutional framework allows competing firms to act upon this profit signal. This comes about because drug research and development which employs the scientific method, is a step-by-step procedure. The introduction of a new product can become an important piece of information to competitive firms by allowing them to fill in an important step of their own research efforts. Furthermore, even though the drug patent temporarily enhances the market power of the originating firm, it also provides a vehicle for the transference of information that, in a sense, is publicized by the issuance of the drug patent.

In essence, this is the "molecule manipulation" which critics of the pharmaceutical industry have castigated as a form of mere product differentiation.[21] Instead of being the sole R&D goal of the firm, this product differentiation is very likely a by-product of the drug research and development process; it makes the demand schedules facing other firms more elastic and the market more competitive (that is, it decreases the ratio of price minus marginal cost to price). This spin-off or by-product phenomenon can also be observed in product areas outside of human pharmaceuticals. There have been spin-offs from human pharmaceutical R&D resulting in veterinary products and in agricultural chemicals. Indeed, many pharmaceutical firms have units that produce and sell these kinds of products.

In the context of Clemens's model, this by-product effect can have important competitive implications. Competitors of a firm that has introduced a new drug are willing to build on their own research and can thus offset some of the advantages that accrue to a competitor who has been successful in the stochastic R&D process. In addition, as long as there is a profitable market for an existing drug therapy, firms have incentives to introduce similar products. This entry can then lessen the steepness of the demand curve faced by the firm that originally introduced the new drug therapy. The model again highlights the idea that the firm can consider several demand curves relative to its rather flexible R&D and pro-

---

[21] Schifrin, "The Ethical Drug Industry," pp. 897–98.

duction processes. This appears to be a nearly unique characteristic of drug firms that may also apply to other R&D-intensive firms. It must be reiterated that the competitive goal of drug firms is not merely to act upon research previously done by others and maximize profits on this activity, but rather to "maximize their profit maximization." To do this they must develop new drugs of their own that have preferred market positions.

In earlier studies of the industry it was assumed that drug promotion expenditures are primarily an entry barrier and that much of this activity is wasteful. This is an area that needs more extensive research, but for the purposes of the present study it is assumed that promotion is neither wasteful nor intended primarily as an entry barrier by a significant number of drug firms. The chief reason for making this assumption is the perception that drug promotion disseminates information that is a joint product of the R&D process. This joint product is demanded by physicians in their use of ethical pharmaceuticals; the level of expenditures on drug promotion may reflect the market value of this demand.

Underlying this assumption concerning drug promotion is the idea that the physician as purchasing agent must be sophisticated. Drug therapeutics is complicated and selection requires more technical knowledge than most purchases. This assumption also considers that physicians apply the scientific method when they make their choice among drug products. Finally, there is the general acceptance by the physician of risk when he prescribes drugs. This should have the tendency to reduce any irrationality in prescribing that could be caused by drug promotion. All of these factors may help explain why physicians even take the time to see drug detail men. This time is a real opportunity cost to the physician and thus may be indicative of the information value of promotion.[22]

The application and adaptation of Clemens's model to the drug industry does not predict that at some time we can expect a competitive equilibrium. The desire of drug firms to develop significant new drugs and their success in doing so prevent this. The model does show that, given enough R&D-oriented firms not specializing their R&D effort, an institutional framework is provided that insures results tending toward competition. Unless there are some exogenous constraints, resources should flow as the competitive model predicts. A primary impediment to this resource flow would be a reduction in the introduction of new drugs.

The essence of the model used in this paper is summarized in this statement by Clemens:

> To assume conditions of competitive equilibrium where all profit margins are equal would be completely unrealistic. Normal profits, necessary to a

---

[22] For articles that relate to the importance of the informational aspects of drug promotion see Raymond A. Bauer and Lawrence H. Wortzel, "Doctors Choice: The Physician and His Sources of Information about Drugs," in Donald F. Cox, ed., *Risk Taking and Information Handling in Consumer Behavior* (Cambridge, Mass.: Harvard University Press, 1967), pp. 152–71; Robert Ferber, "Consumer Economics, A Survey," *Journal of Economic Literature*, vol. 11 (December 1973), pp. 1329–30; Peltzman, *Regulation of Pharmaceutical Innovation.*

firm's long-run existence, are obtained only insofar as average revenues under multiple-product production are equal to average costs. This condition can only be attained by the continuous process of invasion and cross-invasion of markets, by the shuffling and reshuffling of prices and markets which are so characteristic of economic activity.[23]

The analysis that has been outlined implies that in considering the competitiveness of drug firms, it is necessary to look across all of the demand-side markets that these firms face. The demand curves shown in Figure 1 would generally represent quite different demand-side products, but the R&D and manufacturing resource mobility that is assumed means that competitive effects occur as new products are introduced. Thus, it is necessary to consider all of these demand-side markets as a whole.

## Empirical Results

This section presents some preliminary empirical evidence as to the predictive power of the model outlined in the previous section. Specifically, this evidence attempts to measure important aspects of the competitive behavior and performance of a number of leading firms in the drug industry. To do this, data relative to the largest twenty-one drug firms in the United States, as measured by their hospital and drugstore sales, will be presented. These data cover the time from 1962 to 1972.[24] This period was chosen because the use of data for years prior to 1962 may have a tendency to distort the results because of the structural impact of the 1962 drug amendments.

One of the key assumptions of the model of the drug firm presented in the preceding section is that research and development must be institutionalized in a significant number of firms. This is necessary so that these firms can have sufficient R&D capital to strive for innovative new products. In addition, it gives them the technological capability of adding products similar to the existing drug therapy of competitors, thus affecting the price elasticities of existing products. Consequently, drug firms should be able to demonstrate this R&D and manufacturing resource flexibility.

Data are not available allowing direct measurements of how individual drug firms allocate their R&D and manufacturing resources. As a result, it is not possible to measure directly the extent of the R&D effort being devoted to individual classes of drug therapy. Likewise it is not possible to measure directly the amount of R&D diversification across therapeutic classes. However, there are data available indicative of this kind of diversification and thus of the mobility of these resources. Tables 1 and 2 present several of these indicators.

---

[23] Clemens, "Price Discrimination," p. 273.

[24] IMS America, Ltd., *Pharmaceutical Market: Drug Stores and Hospitals* (Ambler, Pa., 1962–73), annual issues.

Column 1 of Table 1 shows the level of research and development expenditures in 1972 for fourteen of the leading twenty-one drug firms. These expenditures were obtained from annual reports, which listed total R&D expenditures for the entire corporate entity. Since the figures do not specifically apply to drug R&D expenditures, they may produce varying degrees of distortion. This distortion could be especially significant for a firm such as Bristol-Myers, which has both pharmaceutical and unrelated subsidiary units. In addition, these expenditure data cover only one year rather than the entire period under consideration. Notwithstanding these qualifications, these R&D expenditures do give some idea of the importance of R&D for most of the twenty-one drug firms. The average R&D expenditure per firm in 1972 for the fourteen firms was $44.9 million (S.D. = $18.8 million).

The pharmaceutical industry and the marketing research firms that serve it have generally classified individual products according to product groups known as therapeutic categories. These categories are viewed as a set of products that have similarities in the diseases treated and in the character of treatment.[25] For the most part, the chemical and biochemical characteristics of the products in a particular category are similar. It has been previously assumed that these categories represent relevant demand-side markets, but recent evidence suggests that this may not be true in every case.[26] Since the chemical characteristics of the products in one therapeutic category may differ from those of products in another category, the number of therapeutic categories in which a firm has product activity can indicate the diversity of its research effort. Such data could include the number of therapeutic categories in which the firm is selling at least one product as well as the number of categories in which the firm is introducing new products.

Columns 2 and 3 of Table 1 show the number of therapeutic categories in which each of the leading drug firms had at least one product for sale. In 1962 there were forty-seven therapeutic categories; in 1972 there were forty-nine. Most of these firms had products in a substantial number of categories in both 1962 and 1972.

To elaborate on this diversification among categories, columns 1 and 2 in Table 2 show the ratio of the number of therapeutic categories in which each of these twenty-one firms had sales to the total number of such classes listed for the years 1962 and 1972. The average firm had products for sale in approximately 60 percent of the available therapeutic categories.

This diversification is indicative of both the manufacturing and the R&D mobility possible within these firms. The fact that these firms have products in

---

[25] Comanor, "Research and Competitive Product Differentiation," p. 382.
[26] A recent study by Douglas L. Cocks and John R. Virts, "Market Definition and Concentration in the Ethical Pharmaceutical Industry," suggests that these demand-side markets may include a single therapeutic category, a combination of categories, or a subcategory within a single therapeutic category. The determination of these markets depends upon possible substitution across therapeutic categories.

## Table 1
## R&D AND MANUFACTURING RESOURCE MOBILITY OF
## TWENTY-ONE LEADING ETHICAL DRUG FIRMS, 1962–72

| Firm | R&D Expenditures ($ millions) (1) | Number of Therapeutic Categories in Which the Firm Had Sales 1962 (2) | 1972 (3) | Number of New Single Chemical Entities (NCEs) 1962–72 (4) | Number of Therapeutic Categories Represented by the NCEs,[a] 1962–72 (5) |
|---|---|---|---|---|---|
| Lilly | 74.3 | 43 | 43 | 12 | 9 |
| Hoffmann-LaRoche | n.a. | 24 | 21 | 9 | 5 |
| American Home Products | n.a. | 38 | 39 | 8 | 6 |
| Merck | 79.7 | 37 | 38 | 12 | 11 |
| Bristol-Myers | 45.0 | 19 | 21 | 10 | 6 |
| Abbott | 31.2 | 36 | 36 | 5 | 5 |
| Pfizer | 44.1 | 26 | 27 | 11 | 6 |
| Ciba-Geigy | n.a. | 26 | 27 | 4 | 4 |
| Upjohn | 50.3 | 34 | 33 | 8 | 4 |
| Squibb | 35.5 | 27 | 29 | 7 | 5 |
| SmithKline | 38.4 | 20 | 25 | 3 | 3 |
| Johnson & Johnson | 56.4 | 27 | 29 | 4 | 3 |
| Schering-Plough | 28.6 | 26 | 24 | 6 | 4 |
| Parke-Davis[b] | n.a. | 39 | 41 | 4 | 4 |
| Searle | 35.9 | 20 | 15 | 3 | 2 |
| Lederle[c] | 44.2 | 25 | 26 | 7 | 7 |
| Sandoz-Wander | n.a. | 25 | 27 | 4 | 4 |
| Robins | 6.2 | 21 | 25 | 4 | 4 |
| Sterling | n.a. | 37 | 35 | 5 | 3 |
| Burroughs Wellcome | n.a. | 28 | 27 | 5 | 4 |
| Warner-Lambert | 59.3 | 27 | 25 | 4 | 4 |

**Source:** Column 1 taken from available 1972 annual reports. These data reflect total R&D expenditures by the corporate entity, including activity not devoted to pharmaceutical R&D. Columns 2 and 3 taken from IMS America, Ltd., *Pharmaceutical Market: Drug Stores and Hospitals* (Ambler, Pa., 1962 and 1972). Column 4 from Paul de Haen, Inc., *de Haen New Product Survey,* vols. 9–19 (New York: Paul de Haen, Inc., 1962–72).

[a] In 1962 there were forty-seven therapeutic categories and in 1972 there were forty-nine categories.

[b] In late 1970 Parke-Davis merged with Warner-Lambert. The data for each have been maintained separately and are shown here separately.

[c] Total R&D expenditures for American Cyanamid.

many therapeutic classes implies some basic knowledge in the manufacturing of a given class of products. This may allow the firm to readily transfer or add to similar manufacturing resources in a different product area. As far as R&D is concerned, this therapeutic category diversity suggests that these firms have at least some basic knowledge in several areas of chemotherapy and can build on this knowledge as scientific opportunities become evident. The diversity shown by these firms may also indicate a degree of marketing resource mobility.

### Table 2
### R&D DIVERSIFICATION RATIOS OF
### TWENTY-ONE LEADING DRUG FIRMS, 1962–72

| Firm | Ratio of the Number of Therapeutic Categories in Which Firm Had Sales to Total Number of Categories[a] | | Ratio of the Number of Therapeutic Categories Represented by the NCEs to the Total Number of NCEs, 1962–72 |
|---|---|---|---|
| | 1962 (1) | 1972 (2) | (3) |
| Lilly | .915 | .876 | .750 |
| Hoffmann-LaRoche | .511 | .429 | .556 |
| American Home Products | .809 | .796 | .750 |
| Merck | .787 | .776 | .786 |
| Bristol-Myers | .404 | .429 | .545 |
| Abbott | .766 | .735 | 1.000 |
| Pfizer | .553 | .551 | .500 |
| Ciba-Geigy | .553 | .551 | 1.000 |
| Upjohn | .723 | .673 | .500 |
| Squibb | .574 | .592 | .714 |
| SmithKline | .426 | .510 | .600 |
| Johnson & Johnson | .574 | .592 | .750 |
| Schering-Plough | .553 | .490 | .667 |
| Parke-Davis | .830 | .837 | 1.000 |
| Searle | .426 | .306 | .667 |
| Lederle | .532 | .531 | 1.000 |
| Sandoz-Wander | .532 | .551 | 1.000 |
| Robins | .447 | .510 | 1.000 |
| Sterling | .787 | .714 | .600 |
| Burroughs Wellcome | .596 | .551 | .800 |
| Warner-Lambert | .574 | .510 | 1.000 |
| Average firm ratio | .613 | .596 | .771 |
| S.D. | .151 | .147 | .187 |

[a] In 1962 the IMS audits delineated forty-seven therapeutic categories and in 1972, forty-nine.

238

Economists concerned with the R&D activity of the drug industry have generally agreed that new single chemical entities (NCEs) represent the most innovative of the new products coming out of the R&D process.[27] An NCE is a new drug (with one active ingredient) that has never been marketed in the United States. In the present analysis, NCEs will be used as the variable that provides the major impetus to the resource movement depicted stochastically by Clemens. In addition, the diversity of therapeutic classes that are represented by the NCEs are an additional indicator of the R&D resource mobility of these leading drug firms.

Column 4 of Table 1 shows the number of NCEs introduced between 1962 and 1972 by the twenty-one firms included in this study. Column 5 shows the number of different therapeutic categories represented by these NCEs. Column 3 of Table 2 shows the ratio of the number of therapeutic categories represented by each firm's NCEs to the total number of NCEs introduced. The average of these twenty-one firms indicates that approximately seventy-five percent of the NCEs a firm introduces represent distinct therapeutic categories.

It is recognized that the above data do not directly measure the diversity or intensity of R&D or the manufacturing resource mobility of these firms. It is also recognized that the basic relationship between R&D effort and new product introduction is lagged, and since the data presented here is *ex post*, this lagged relationship is not totally taken into account. However, these data do give some measure of the diversity of the R&D and manufacturing effort and thus are a reasonable indicator of the resource mobility of these twenty-one firms for the 1962–72 period. The diversification that these data show might also have been expected from a profit maximization standpoint. By diversifying its R&D and manufacturing processes, the drug firm can spread its risk.[28]

The Clemens model is significant in describing the behavior of R&D intensive drug firms for three primary reasons:

(1) The model highlights the idea that a firm in a technological environment can adapt its R&D and manufacturing processes to develop and produce products in several areas of drug therapy. This context emphasizes that the

[27] See Henry G. Grabowski, "The Determinants of Industrial Research and Development: A Study of the Chemical, Drug, and Petroleum Industries," *Journal of Political Economy*, vol. 74 (March–April 1968), p. 294; and Peltzman, *Regulation of Pharmaceutical Innovation*, p. 92. There has been a great deal of debate as to the usefulness or value of the new products coming out of the R&D process of the drug industry. This debate has occurred on both the social and scientific fronts. From an economic standpoint Peltzman, *Regulation of Pharmaceutical Innovation*, pp. 39–46, has demonstrated that new drugs generally do provide economic value.

[28] For a discussion of the importance of this aspect see Thomas R. Stauffer, "Discovery Risk, Profitability Performance and Survival Risk in a Pharmaceutical Firm" (Paper presented at the Second Seminar on the Dynamics of Pharmaceutical Innovation and Economics, American University, Washington, D. C., 14–16 October 1973). This paper will be published in the proceedings of the conference edited by Joseph D. Cooper.

behavior of these firms is determined by profit maximizing decisions that consider several different kinds of drug products.

(2) When an individual firm is successful in developing innovative new products whose demand curves presumably are favorable relative to costs, resources should flow to that firm as the profit incentive dictates. This implies that the firm that is relatively more successful in the stochastic process of finding new drugs should receive an increased market share and an increased *ex post* rate of return.

(3) As firms attempt to develop singular new products, they develop, as a by-product of R&D, products that compete with existing ones. From an empirical standpoint this can be expected to result in a substantial amount of entry into drug markets, market shares should be affected, and price pressures should be evident.

Reasons (2) and (3) imply that there are two, possibly simultaneous kinds of competition taking place in the drug industry. This permits two major hypotheses about drug firm behavior that follow from the Clemens model and its corollary, the Mancke stochastic model. First it is hypothesized that, when a drug firm is successful in developing significant new products, a relatively greater amount of resources will be attracted to that firm, and its *ex post* rate of return will be higher. This implies that there are competitive forces operating and that it would be very difficult in this environment to establish oligopolistic coordination. It is also hypothesized that in seeking unique new products, drug firms also develop products that put competitive pressure on the products of other firms. The remainder of this empirical section will present evidence that addresses these hypotheses.

A preliminary way to test the first hypothesis is to observe the rate of firm turnover occurring among the leading R&D intensive firms in the industry. This will give some indication as to whether these firms have established some kind of oligopolistic coordination. Although industrial organization economists are not in complete agreement on the usefulness of the turnover concept in measuring competition, the concept has been recognized by some as a measure of the competitiveness of a given industry.[29] This turnover concept is felt to have even greater significance in relation to industries with differentiated products.[30] For this purpose, changes in rank by market share of the twenty-one leading firms is an indicator of whether oligopolistic behavior prevails.

Table 3 shows the market share of hospital and drugstore sales and the ranking for the twenty-one leading firms for the years 1962 and 1972. The last column of the table shows the extent and direction of change in rank for each

---

[29] Stephen Hymer and Peter Pashigian, "Turnover of Firms as a Measure of Market Behavior," *Review of Economics and Statistics*, February 1962, pp. 82–87.

[30] Norman Schneider, "Product Differentiation, Oligopoly, and the Stability of Market Shares," *Western Economic Journal*, December 1966, pp. 19–24.

## Table 3

### FIRM TURNOVER FOR THE LEADING TWENTY-ONE FIRMS IN THE ETHICAL PHARMACEUTICAL INDUSTRY, 1962–72

| Company | Market Share of Hospital and Drugstore Sales (percent of industry total) | | Rank in Terms of Market Share | | Change in Rank between 1962 and 1972 |
|---|---|---|---|---|---|
| | 1962 | 1972 | 1962 | 1972 | |
| Lilly | 7.2 | 7.9 | 1 | 1 | 0 |
| Hoffmann-LaRoche | 4.0 | 7.5 | 10 | 2 | +8 |
| American Home Products | 6.1 | 6.6 | 3 | 3 | 0 |
| Merck | 4.9 | 6.0 | 6 | 4 | +2 |
| Bristol-Myers | 3.4 | 4.2 | 13 | 5 | +8 |
| Abbott | 3.9 | 3.7 | 11 | 6 | +5 |
| Pfizer | 3.8 | 3.6 | 12 | 7 | +5 |
| Ciba-Geigy | 4.2 | 3.6 | 8 | 8 | 0 |
| Upjohn | 5.8 | 3.5 | 4 | 9 | −5 |
| Squibb | 4.1 | 3.4 | 9 | 10 | −1 |
| SmithKline | 6.3 | 3.3 | 2 | 11 | −9 |
| Johnson & Johnson | 1.3 | 2.7 | 22 | 12 | +10 |
| Schering-Plough | 2.4 | 2.7 | 15 | 13 | +2 |
| Parke-Davis[a] | 4.6 | 2.7 | 7 | 14 | −7 |
| Searle | 2.2 | 2.5 | 17 | 15 | +2 |
| Lederle | 5.3 | 2.3 | 5 | 16 | −11 |
| Sandoz-Wander | 1.6 | 2.0 | 19 | 17 | +2 |
| Robins | 1.9 | 2.0 | 18 | 18 | 0 |
| Sterling | 2.4 | 1.9 | 16 | 19 | −3 |
| Burroughs Wellcome | 1.4 | 1.8 | 20 | 20 | 0 |
| Warner-Lambert[a] | 2.6 | 1.7 | 14 | 21 | −7 |
| Average absolute change in rank between 1962 and 1972 | | | | | 4.1[b] |

[a] Parke-Davis was merged with Warner-Lambert in late 1970; rank and market shares computed as if firms had not merged. Market share of the combined firm in 1972 was 4.4 percent, or fifth in rank.

[b] Computed with Parke-Davis and Warner-Lambert changes based on their ranks as if they had not merged.

**Source:** IMS America, Ltd., *Pharmaceutical Market: Drug Stores and Hospitals* (Ambler, Pa., 1962 and 1972).

firm: a minus sign indicates decline in rank, a plus sign shows a rise. The average absolute change in rank during this period is 4.1 places. This indicates a relatively volatile industry. Such turnover would be anathema to a group of firms trying to maintain tacit oligopolistic discipline. Also, since this turnover is observed over a relatively short period of time, the likelihood or possibility of tacit oligopoly coordination is small.[31]

This turnover data was, in a sense, "normalized" so that mergers would not significantly affect the results. All mergers, with the exception of the Parke-Davis, Warner-Lambert merger of late 1970, were treated as if the firm existed as a single entity throughout the 1962–72 period. If two drug firms merged earlier in the period, the market shares of both firms in 1962 were combined.

Hymer and Pashigian suggest that an analysis of firm turnover should not include all firms in an industry. A rough measure of the competitive effects of turnover can be obtained by concentrating on leading firms.[32] They also point out that the Spearman rank correlation coefficient is an unreliable indicator of firm turnover, because it is very sensitive to the size distribution of the firms in the sample. To offset this size sensitivity Hymer and Pashigian developed an instability index directly measuring changes in market shares. The nature of the index is such that the higher the index the more unstable are market shares.[33]

From the data in Table 3 an instability index similar to Hymer's and Pashigian's has been calculated for the twenty-one firms in this study. The index is calculated according to the following formulation:

$$I = \sum_{i=1}^{n} \left( \frac{s_{t,i}}{S_t} - \frac{s_{t-1,i}}{S_{t-1}} \right) \tag{1}$$

where

$I$ = index of instability,
$s_{t,i}$ = sales of the $i$th firm at time $t$,
$S_t$ = total industry, hospital, and drugstore sales at time $t$.

Table 4 presents instability indices calculated by Hymer and Pashigian for nineteen two-digit standard industrial classification (SIC) industries. These cover the changes in shares of assets for these industries between 1946 and 1955. As a means of comparison the drug industry instability index is also presented. Note that there is only one industry's instability index higher than the index for the drug industry. This comparison becomes more significant when it is realized that the two-digit industry classes are probably too broadly defined to represent realistic industries. Thus, the instability indices for these industries will have a tendency to be higher than those for more properly defined industries.[34]

The application of Clemens's model to the pharmaceutical industry suggests that a primary cause of this kind of turnover is the innovativeness of individual firms. This turnover can also indicate the direction of resource movement within an industry; when turnover is compared to the stochastic process of discovering

[31] Hymer and Pashigian, "Turnover of Firms."
[32] Ibid., p. 83.
[33] Ibid., pp. 83–85.
[34] Ibid., p. 87.

242

## Table 4
### INDICES OF MARKET SHARE INSTABILITY

| Industry | Instability Index[a] | Number of Firms |
|---|---|---|
| Food | 10.83 | 119 |
| Tobacco | 9.06 | 12 |
| Textile mill products | 9.30 | 61 |
| Apparel | 1.48 | 7 |
| Lumber and wood products | 4.45 | 16 |
| Furniture and fixtures | 3.86 | 8 |
| Paper | 9.63 | 49 |
| Printing | 14.82 | 25 |
| Chemicals | 17.42 | 74 |
| Petroleum | 24.38 | 35 |
| Rubber | 9.16 | 14 |
| Leather | 5.69 | 8 |
| Stone, clay, and glass | 13.25 | 31 |
| Primary metals | 14.25 | 76 |
| Fabricated metals | 8.70 | 51 |
| Machinery (except electrical) | 12.71 | n.a. |
| Electrical machinery | 17.24 | 46 |
| Transportation | 19.92 | 70 |
| Professional and scientific | 17.19 | 19 |
| Drug industry | 22.8[b] | 21 |

[a] All indices are computed with mergers excluded. Hymer and Pashigian calculated their indices on the basis of shares of assets; the calculation for the drug industry is based on shares of hospital and drugstore sales.

[b] Calculated by the author from the data in Table 3.

**Source:** Stephen Hymer and Peter Pashigian, "Turnover of Firms as a Measure of Market Behavior," *Review of Economics and Statistics,* February 1962, pp. 82–87.

new drugs, the firms that are successful innovators should be those that are successful in gaining or maintaining leading positions in the industry. The same firms that are successful innovators, as indicated by the number of NCEs they introduce, should be those that gain or maintain prominent positions in the industry.

Table 5 presents data that support this view. This table groups the twenty-one firms according to whether they gained in market rank, had no change, or declined. The table also indicates the number of NCEs for each of the firms. Of those firms gaining in rank there is at least partial evidence that this was accomplished by their introduction of more NCEs (an average of 7.1 per firm) than those who declined in market rank (averaged 5.1 per firm). In addition, the group of firms that experienced no change in rank between 1962 and 1972 divides into two distinct categories. One category is made up of two firms that maintained ranks one and three and had NCE introductions of the magnitude of those firms which gained market position. In the second category are three firms of a relatively

## Table 5

### TWENTY-ONE LEADING FIRMS' TURNOVER AND INNOVATION IN THE ETHICAL PHARMACEUTICAL INDUSTRY, 1962–72

| Firm | Change in Position | Total Number of NCEs, 1962–72 |
|---|---|---|
| Firms gaining market position between 1962 and 1972 | | |
| Johnson & Johnson | +10 | 4 |
| Hoffmann-LaRoche | +8 | 9 |
| Bristol-Myers | +8 | 10 |
| Abbott | +5 | 5 |
| Pfizer | +5 | 11 |
| Merck | +2 | 12 |
| Schering-Plough | +2 | 6 |
| Searle | +2 | 3 |
| Sandoz-Wander | +2 | 4 |
| Average number of NCEs per firm | | 7.1 |
| S.D. | | 3.4 |
| Firms with no change in market position between 1962 and 1972 | | |
| Lilly | 0 | 12 |
| American Home Products | 0 | 8 |
| Ciba-Geigy | 0 | 4 |
| Robins | 0 | 4 |
| Burroughs Wellcome | 0 | 5 |
| Average number of NCEs per firm | | 6.6 |
| S.D. | | 3.4 |
| Firms losing market position between 1962 and 1972 | | |
| Lederle | −11 | 7 |
| SmithKline | −9 | 3 |
| Parke-Davis | −7 | 2 |
| Warner-Lambert | −7 | 6 |
| Upjohn | −5 | 8 |
| Sterling | −3 | 3 |
| Squibb | −1 | 7 |
| Average number of NCEs per firm | | 5.1 |
| S.D. | | 2.4 |

lower rank which had new product introductions of a magnitude similar to those which lost market position.

These data on firm turnover are the first indication of the kind of competitive structure that may prevail in the ethical pharmaceutical industry. The fact that there is a fair amount of leading-firm turnover in the industry, and that the primary cause of this turnover is innovation, seems to preclude a finding of oligopolistic coordination.

Knowing the rate of innovation of the leading drug firms, which can serve as a very visible measure of how successful they are in the stochastic R&D process, allows a more direct test of the first hypothesis of this paper. This can be done by relating the change in market share of each firm to the number of NCEs it introduced during the period of change and to its rate of return at the end of the period.

To do this a multiple regression of the following form was performed:

$$\Delta MS_i = a + b(\ln RR_i) + c(\ln NCE_i) + e_i \tag{2}$$

where

$$e_i \sim N(O, \sigma^2 I),$$

$\Delta MS_i =$ change in market share between 1962 and 1972 for firm $i$,

$\ln RR_i =$ natural logarithm of the average rate of return for firm $i$ for the three-year period 1970–72,

$\ln NCE_i =$ natural logarithm of the number of new single chemical entities introduced by the $i$th firm between 1962 and 1972,[35] and

$a,b,c, =$ parameters to be estimated.

The expected signs of the regression coefficients are $b > 0$ and $c > 0$. Equation (3) presents the results of this regression analysis:

$$\Delta MS = -10.566 + .450 \ln RR + .323 \ln NCE$$
$$(2.292) \qquad (1.645) \tag{3}$$
$$(R^2 = .307)$$

---

[35] The data used for this regression analysis comes from the data in the preceding tables except for the rates of return. The average rate of return was computed as the average accounting return on stockholders equity for the three-year period 1970–72 as reported in the *Fortune Directory*. There are four foreign firms included, and the *Fortune* data did not adequately report their return on equity. For these firms then, return was computed as the average return of the four firms closest to them in market rank in 1972. There were three U.S. firms whose returns were not reported, or were incomplete. Their returns were calculated in the same manner as the foreign firms. These data include the return on all the activities in which these firms were engaged. Since most of these firms sell products in areas other than ethical pharmaceuticals, these profit rates are distorted. In addition, these rates of return can, at the most, reflect only relative profitability. Several economists have recognized the need for adjusting accounting rates of return to reflect economic reality. For example, see Jesse J. Friedman and Murray N. Friedman, "Relative Profitability and Monopoly Power," *Conference Board Record*, vol. 9 (December 1972), pp. 49–58; and Thomas R. Stauffer, "The Measurement of Corporate Rates of Return: A Generalized Formulation," *Bell Journal of Economics and Management Science*, vol. 2 (Autumn 1971), pp. 467–68.

The t-values are in parentheses under the regression coefficients and the $R^2$ is significant at the 0.05 level. This is offered as support for the first hypothesis.

This analysis of the initial hypothesis of this paper deals with the impact of the R&D process, as reflected in innovation, and how this affects the performance of the individual firm. It suggests that resources are allocated to the firm as the profit incentive predicts. Thus this process represents competitive results. According to the second hypothesis, this process should also show up as price competitive pressure on the individual firm. Data are not available that will allow a direct measurement of this price pressure. However, there are data relative to individual drug markets that are indicative of the kind of price competition that is predicted in the application of Clemens's model to the pharmaceutical industry.

In order to test the second hypothesis, data will be observed on the pricing, entry, and market share characteristics of the leading products in ten markets that account for approximately 80 percent of all retail prescriptions written in the United States. The market definitions employed were recently developed from market research data on how physicians actually use alternative drugs in a given diagnosis.[36] This market definition was seen as a substitute for measuring cross elasticity of demand.

Previous analyses of the pharmaceutical industry have used the therapeutic class to denote relevant demand-side markets, but it appears that in some cases the products in one therapeutic class may actually be substitutes for products in another therapeutic class. In addition, there are cases in which the products in a given subclass are not substitutes for products in the overall therapeutic class. By measuring how physicians use various kinds of drugs, it is possible to group products into relatively meaningful markets. The method is to align therapeutic classes or subclasses according to their use as alternatives. If there are three therapeutic classes A, B, and C, and it appears that physicians use the products in classes A and B for treating a particular diagnosis and products B and C as alternatives for another diagnosis, then all three therapeutic classes are grouped as a set. In other words, a group of products of one therapeutic class that intersects with a group of another class can be combined to form an overall set of products. Intersection is based on the way physicians use various drugs, and it is the intersection of these groups in use that establishes the boundaries of the particular market.[37]

Table 6 presents recent data on the number of firms entering ten markets.[38] An important aspect of the Clemens model is that the institutionalization of R&D

---

[36] Cocks and Virts, "Market Definition and Concentration."

[37] Cocks and Virts, "Pricing Behavior of the Ethical Pharmaceutical Industry," pp. 349–62.

[38] Entry was measured by determining the number of separate corporate entities that had products for sale in that market in 1964 and 1973. The difference in the number of firms between these two years indicates the number of entries that occurred. Care was taken that corporate entities with more than one subsidiary did not inflate the total number of entries into the market. Data source for these calculations is IMS America, Ltd., *Pharmaceutical Market: Drug Stores and Hospitals* (Ambler, Pa., 1964–73), annual issues.

246

in a significant number of firms provides the mechanism for the entry of new firms. From the standpoint of the pure competitive model, ease of entry is a necessary condition for price competition. As can be seen from the table, firm entry not only has been fairly robust in several of these markets, but this robustness appears to be ongoing.

An alternative way of observing whether competitive price forces are operating within a market is to view how volatile individual product prices and market shares are over a period of time. This is done for each of the leading products in these ten markets for the period 1962–71 and the results summarized in Tables 7 and 8.[39] Table 7 shows the market share changes that occurred and Table 8 the changes in prices. The products in each table are listed in the same order so that data on a given line refer to the same product. Figures 4 and 5 give a detailed picture of rank changes over a period of ten years for the leading products in two markets.[40]

The Clemens model is only designed to depict firm behavior, but it also indicates how systematic price competition can occur when several firms are engaged in R&D. The price and market share volatility that occurs among many of the products in these markets gives a strong indication that price competitive forces are operating.

This evidence on the entry, pricing, and market share characteristics of ten important drug markets is offered as support that there are elements of price competition occurring in the drug industry as is predicted by the Clemens model. In addition, a recent study by Peltzman indicates that a primary cause of declining drug prices is the ability of drug firms to develop new drugs.[41]

We have seen one by-product of the institutionalization of R&D in a significant number of firms, namely, the development of new drugs that compete with the existing products of rival firms. It is on this phenomenon that the price competitive performance and behavior outlined above is based. There is good reason to believe that, when there is a strong R&D environment within an individual firm, an additional by-product results: This R&D atmosphere permeates all of the activities of the firm and works toward greater productive efficiency. Assumption (5) of the theoretical model alludes to the idea that research and development can affect the costs of producing drugs in such a way that price competitive pressures result for existing drug products. There are some preliminary data contained in two productivity studies of the industry that indicate that these cost pressures are operating. The rate of increase in the labor productivity of the industry for 1963–72 has been calculated to be significantly greater than the rate

---

39 The data for these are based on Cocks and Virts, "Market Definition and Concentration," and "Pricing Behavior in the Ethical Pharmaceutical Industry."

40 A complete set of data on price changes and market shares for the intervening years not shown is available from the author upon request.

41 Peltzman, in *Regulation of Pharmaceutical Innovation,* pp. 46–48, found that innovation plays an important role in reducing drug prices.

# Figure 4
## MARKET SHARES OF THIRTEEN DRUGS IN THE ANTIHYPERTENSIVE AND DIURETIC MARKET

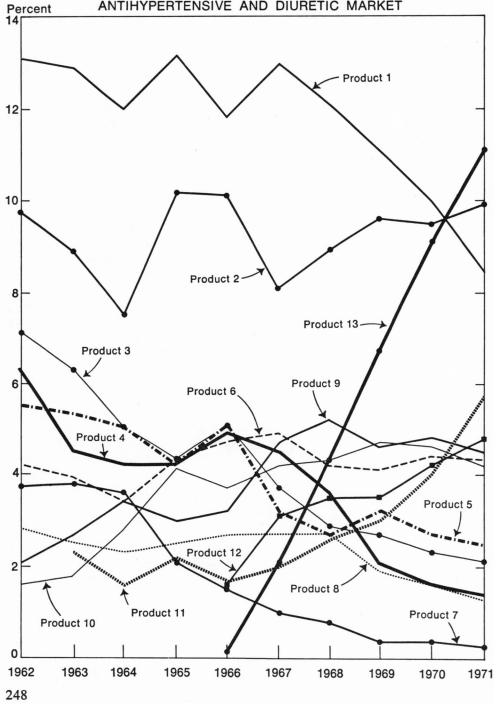

**Figure 5**

MARKET SHARES OF TEN DRUGS IN THE
PSYCHOPHARMACEUTICAL MARKET

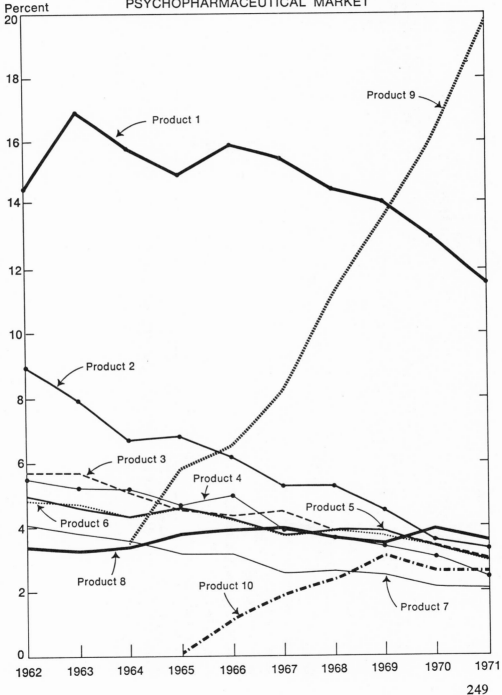

## Table 6

## MARKET ENTRY IN TEN MAJOR PHARMACEUTICAL MARKETS

| Economic Market | Size of Market Sales, 1973 ($ thousands) | Number of Firms in Market 1964 | Number of Firms in Market 1973 | Number of Entrants into Market, 1964–73 | New Manufacturers' Sales as Percentage of Total Sales, 1973 |
|---|---|---|---|---|---|
| Anti-infectives | 793,155 | 211 | 293 | 82 | 0.93 |
| Analgesic and anti-inflammatory | 497,169 | 218 | 272 | 54 | 0.78 |
| Psychopharmaceuticals | 704,557 | 169 | 193 | 24 | 1.97 |
| Cough and cold | 288,084 | 184 | 243 | 59 | 1.45 |
| Antihypertensive and diuretic | 382,986 | 92 | 116 | 24 | 18.04 |
| Vitamin and hematinic | 278,376 | 311 | 394 | 83 | 2.56 |
| Oral contraceptive | 150,923 | 5 | 9 | 4 | 28.21 |
| Anticholinergic and antispasmodic | 97,659 | 101 | 132 | 31 | 2.67 |
| Antiobesity | 72,958 | 127 | 144 | 17 | 9.37 |
| Diabetic therapy | 134,084 | 7 | 7 [a] | 1 | 17.02 |

[a] One firm dropped out of the market.

Source: IMS America, Ltd., *Pharmaceutical Market: Drug Stores and Hospitals* (Ambler, Pa., 1964–73).

# Table 7

## CHANGE IN MARKET-SHARE RANK OF LEADING PRODUCTS IN TEN PHARMACEUTICAL MARKETS, 1962–71 [a]

### Absolute Point-Change in Rank, 1962–71 [a]

| Rank of Product, 1962 | Anti-Infective | Analgesic and anti-Inflammatory | Psycho-pharma-ceutical | Cough and cold | Anti-hypertensive and diuretic | Vitamin and hematinic | Oral contra-ceptive | Antichol-Inergic/antispas-modic | Anti-obesity | Diabetic therapy |
|---|---|---|---|---|---|---|---|---|---|---|
| 1 | −8 | 0 | −1 | −4 | −2 | 0 | −9 | 0 | −1 | 0 |
| 2 | −5 | 0 | −2 | +1 | 0 | −1 | −1[c] | −1 | −2 | 0 |
| 3 | −1 | −1 | −2 | 0 | −7 | −4 | −6[d] | −1 | −2 | −4 |
| 4 | −4 | −8 | −5 | −3 | −7 | +2 | −7[b] | +2 | +1 | +1 |
| 5 | −5 | −5 | −2 | −6 | −4 | +3 | −3[b] | −1 | −5 | −3 |
| 6 | +4 | +1 | 0 | −3 | −1 | −3 | +4[f] | +1 | +5 | −3 |
| 7 | −4 | −2 | −3 | −3 | −6 | −3 | +6[g] | 0 | −2 | −3 |
| 8 | −4 | −3 | +5 | +6 | −4 | −3 | +1[g] | −1 | 0 | 0[d] |
| 9 | +8 | +1 | +8[c] | +1 | +3 | +5 | +4[g] | −1 | +2 | +5[e] |
| 10 | +7 | +4 | +2[b] | +6 | +2 | +4 | +5[h] | +2 | +4 | —[i] |
| 11 | +6 | +6[b] | — | +5[d] | +6[c] | +6 | +5[h] | — | — | — |
| 12 | +6 | +5 | — | — | +7[b] | — | — | — | — | — |
| 13 | — | — | — | — | +12[e] | — | — | — | — | — |

## Table 7 (continued)

### Cumulative Percent Market Shares, 1971

| | Anti-infective | Analgesic and anti-inflammatory | Psycho-pharma-ceutical | Cough and cold | Anti-hypertensive and diuretic | Vitamin and hematinic | Oral contra-ceptive | Anticholinergic/antispasmodic | Anti-obesity | Diabetic therapy |
|---|---|---|---|---|---|---|---|---|---|---|
| Leading four products | 16.8 | 29.2 | 38.3 | 22.5 | 35.2 | 11.5 | 50.8 | 56.3 | 45.7 | 75.4 |
| All above products | 34.0 | 47.8 | 54.7 | 43.2 | 60.6 | 21.7 | 83.5 | 72.4 | 74.2 | 91.8 |
| All others | 66.0 | 52.2 | 45.3 | 56.8 | 39.4 | 78.3 | 16.5 | 27.6 | 25.8 | 8.2 |

**Note:** Interim data 1962–71 available from author.

a + indicates increase in market share; − indicates decrease; 0 indicates no net change.
b Change from 1965, when product entered market.
c Change from 1963, when product entered market.
d Change from 1964, when product entered market.
e Change from 1966, when product entered market.
f Change from 1967, when product entered market.
g Change from 1968, when product entered market.
h Change from 1970, when product entered market.
i Attained sixth rank in year of introduction, 1971.

# Table 8

## PRICE CHANGE OF LEADING PRODUCTS IN TEN PHARMACEUTICAL MARKETS, 1962–71

| Rank of Product in Terms of Market Share | Percentage Change in Price Index[a] | | | | | | | | | |
|---|---|---|---|---|---|---|---|---|---|---|
| | Anti-infective | Analgesic and anti-inflammatory | Psycho-pharmaceutical | Cough and cold | Anti-hypertensive and diuretic | Vitamin and hematinic | Oral contraceptive | Anticholinergic/antispasmodic | Anti-obesity | Diabetic therapy |
| 1 | −29.7 | −11.6 | −15.6 | +10.2 | −8.2 | −3.0 | −19.6 | +11.9 | −1.3 | −22.0 |
| 2 | −6.2 | +5.1 | −6.8 | +28.2 | −11.0 | +12.7 | −9.1 | −6.5 | +4.1 | −10.0 |
| 3 | −66.9 | +4.5 | +6.1 | −6.5 | −1.8 | −4.3 | −8.0 | −1.1 | +0.5 | +14.7 |
| 4 | −34.4 | −5.0 | +5.4 | +37.1 | −0.3 | +14.7[b] | −0.7 | −1.4 | +2.5 | +1.6 |
| 5 | −27.4 | +9.0 | +4.2 | +4.3 | −14.2 | −9.3 | −6.2 | +6.5 | +36.8 | +2.0 |
| 6 | −17.9 | +0.8 | +5.5 | −3.5 | −11.2 | −8.7 | +4.3 | +17.5 | +5.0 | +1.3 |
| 7 | −32.2 | −10.4 | +13.2 | +4.4 | −6.2 | +11.1 | +10.7 | −1.9 | +6.1 | 0 |
| 8 | −7.5 | +8.3 | −35.7 | −0.7 | +0.8 | +6.7 | +14.8 | −0.4 | +19.4 | −43.5 |
| 9 | −52.3 | +6.5 | −6.0 | +26.2 | +1.6 | −13.3 | +6.2 | +7.7 | +2.3 | −23.6 |
| 10 | −19.7 | +8.3 | −10.9 | −4.7 | +12.5 | −24.0 | +3.2 | +17.8 | +28.5 | +1.0 |
| 11 | −59.5 | −11.1 | — | +12.6 | −11.4 | −5.3 | +0.9 | — | — | — |
| 12 | −20.1 | −7.5 | — | — | −8.5 | — | — | — | — | — |
| 13 | — | — | — | — | −11.5 | — | — | — | — | — |
| Aggregate price index of leading products | 68.2 | 98.0 | 91.7 | 102.9 | 92.8 | 99.3 | 78.0 | 100.1 | 105.1 | 86.3 |
| BLS consumer price index for prescriptions | 94.6 | 94.6 | 94.6 | 94.6 | 94.6 | 94.6 | 94.6 | 94.6 | 94.6 | 94.6 |

Note: Interim data 1962–71 available from author.

[a] Base 1962 or year of introduction if later.

[b] Percentage change for 1962–69 only.

253

of increase in the manufacturing sector of the economy as a whole.[42] A study of the total factor productivity of a major ethical drug firm shows that its rate of growth in productivity for the period 1963–72 is approximately three times that of all U.S. nonfinancial corporations.[43]

## Summary and Conclusions

It has been the purpose of this paper to outline a more dynamic analysis of the ethical pharmaceutical industry. The key element in this analysis is the role of research and development in determining competitive behavior among drug firms. Drug firms have a significant incentive to develop new drugs. The results are manifested in the uniqueness of their new drugs and in patents. The model that was applied to the industry indicates that the R&D that establishes the potential market power of new drugs also sets in motion forces that may result in price competitive behavior.

Empirical evidence was presented indicating that competition may be workable in the ethical drug industry. This workable competition was evident in a period in which it has been maintained that the 1962 drug amendments represented a kind of "externality" that had the effect of lessening competition. A significant number of drug firms were shown to exhibit aspects of competitive behavior and performance that would preclude the existence of conscious parallelism.

This paper also suggests that public policy toward the drug industry must carefully weigh the benefits and costs of the existing R&D institutional framework. There is a fundamental relationship between the incentives for innovation that yield new drug products, as well as between the institutionalization of R&D that is the basis for price competition and the temporary firm advantages that may be experienced through the market power of important new drugs. This paper suggests that resource misallocation may be relatively short-lived and may not be as severe as it was previously thought to be. The market power of new products provides the incentives for their own development as well as the means of diminishing the market power of existing drug products. At a minimum, further research on the role of R&D in the drug industry is necessary before clear public policy conclusions can be drawn.

---

[42] Horst Brand, "Productivity in the Pharmaceutical Industry," *Monthly Labor Review,* March 1974, pp. 9–14.

[43] Douglas L. Cocks, "The Measurement of Total Factor Productivity for a Large U.S. Manufacturing Corporation," *Business Economics,* vol. 9 (September 1974), pp. 7–20.

# THE FOLLOW-ON DEVELOPMENT PROCESS AND THE MARKET FOR DIURETICS

*Bernard A. Kemp*

## Introduction

The conventional view of patent protection is that a product patent leads to a one-product one-firm market. Occasionally the market may have a different structure at the sufferance of the patent holder, or as a resolution of an interference or infringement action, or because the patented product happens to be a reasonably close substitute for one already on the market. In the pharmaceutical industry, however, firms have developed and institutionalized a practice whereby, after a breakthrough is marketed, they deliberately attempt to research, develop, and market a new product with similar therapeutic properties. Of course the firm hopes that its product will be an improvement. Even if the follow-on is somewhat differentiated from the breakthrough, it must be suitable for the treatment of the same disease or condition if the firm that developed it is to take advantage of the potential profits available in that market. If one or more firms are successful in developing patented follow-on products, then a number of changes occur in the structure, conduct and performance of the markets involved.[1]

It has been generally recognized by the members of the industry, its critics, and economists, that firms in the pharmaceutical industry frequently develop and market more than one product in the same therapeutic class. At worst, this practice has been viewed with disdain by physicians and even by members of the industry, on the assumption that it leads to duplicative products. At best, it has been considered one of the following: (1) a diversion of resources from one of the primary objectives of the industry, namely, the development of dramatic new products for the treatment of disease,[2] (2) a sort of booby prize for lack of success

---

[1] A companion article, "The Follow-on Development Process vs. the Conventional Patent Protection Concept," in *IDEA: The PTC Journal of Research and Education*, vol. 16, no. 1 (Fall 1974), pp. 31–59, provides a detailed comparison of both approaches and is based on an earlier, more extensive study: Bernard A. Kemp, *The RDTEM Process: The Pharmaceutical Industry's Way around Patent Barriers (As Applied to Diuretics)*, Philadelphia, 1971. Copies of the latter, a privately published monograph, are available from the author.

[2] William S. Comanor, "The Drug Industry and Medical Research: The Economics of the Kefauver Committee Investigation," *The Journal of Business of the University of Chicago*, vol. 39, pt. 1 (January 1966), p. 18; reprinted in U.S., Congress, Senate, Select Committee on Small Business, Subcommittee on Monopoly, *Hearings on Present Status of Competition in the Pharmaceutical Industry*, 90th Cong., 1st and 2d sess. (1967–68), pts. 1–5, pp. 2087,

in meeting that objective,[3] (3) part of vigorous product competition,[4] or (4) an attempt by a firm to differentiate its product in order to mitigate or insulate itself from rivalry and prevent a recurrence of the penicillin or streptomycin experience in which a large number of sellers led to marked price declines.[5]

The practice of developing follow-ons is intimately related to the patent law. Whether the critics of patent policy like it or not, the industry is currently operating under a law by which, as a matter of national policy, the government grants the inventor the exclusive right "to make . . . and sell" the patented product for seventeen years. What has not been appreciated is that the development of additional products of the same subclass makes entry possible when it would otherwise be barred by the patent on the breakthrough drug. The successful implementation of the practice makes that entry possible during the period of patent protection, and the practice itself is an integral part of the resource allocation process.

A discussion of the process by which follow-on products are developed and marketed is of theoretical interest for two reasons. First, it examines the nature and effect of entry where the extreme condition typically assumed does not exist. That condition is that the potential entrant cannot replicate the patented product and consequently is barred just because the product is patented.[6] Second, the process is an elaboration, extension, and specific application of the Schumpeterian hypothesis, which makes it possible to integrate product innovation into the resource allocation process.[7]

The practice also has important policy implications if it can be used to explain and predict the pharmaceutical industry's activities better than the conventional view. If the follow-on development process is the better predictor, then

---

2091; Henry Steele, "Monopoly and Competition in the Ethical Drugs Market," *Journal of Law and Economics,* vol. 5 (October 1962), pp. 133–63; idem, "Patent Restrictions and Price Competition in the Ethical Drug Industry," *Journal of Law and Economics,* vol. 12 (July 1964), pp. 198–223, reprinted in U.S., Congress, Senate, Subcommittee on Monopoly, *Hearings on Present Status,* pp. 1950, 1961, 1965–66, 1972.

[3] Antonie T. Knoppers, in Joseph D. Cooper, ed., *The Economics of Drug Innovation* (Proceedings of the First Seminar on Economics of Pharmaceutical Innovation, 27–29 April 1969) (Washington, D. C.: The American University Center for the Study of Private Enterprise, School of Business Administration, 1970), p. 252.

[4] Comanor, "Research and Competitive Product Differentiation," p. 2073, and Jesse W. Markham, "Economic Incentives and Progress in the Drug Industry," in Paul Talalay, ed., *Drugs in Our Society* (Baltimore: Johns Hopkins University Press, 1964), pp. 172–73.

[5] Comanor, "Research and Competitive Product Differentiation," pp. 2070, 2076.

[6] While the theory of entry in oligopoly examines some of the effects of market imperfections on entry, for example, absolute cost differences, it does not take into explicit consideration the effect on entry of situations where replication of the product is not possible. Joe S. Bain, *Barriers to New Competition* (Cambridge, Mass.: Harvard University Press, 1956); Paulo Sylos-Labini, *Oligopoly and Technical Progress,* translated from the Italian by Elizabeth Henderson (Cambridge, Mass.: Harvard University Press, 1962); Franco Modigliani, "New Developments on the Oligopoly Front," *Journal of Political Economy,* vol. 66 (June 1958), pp. 215–32; Comments and Reply, *Journal of Political Economy,* vol. 67 (August 1959), pp. 410–19.

[7] Joseph A. Schumpeter, *Capitalism, Socialism and Democracy,* 3d ed. (New York: Harper & Brothers, 1950), pp. 72–106.

current corporate and government policies, practices, and procedures will have markedly different effects on profits and socioeconomic welfare than are presently envisioned.

## The Follow-on Development Process

The hypothesis developed here asserts the existence of a process for developing follow-on products. It also asserts that, when the first drug in a subclass is profitable, this process serves—better than the conventional view of patent protection— to explain and predict the actions of firms in introducing additional new drugs and the effect that these additional drugs have on market and socioeconomic performance.

In understanding the process, it is important to recognize that the differentiated products in a class of therapeutic agents usually fall into subdivisions or market segments that we shall call subclasses. For example, broad-spectrum antibiotics are a class, tetracyclines are a subclass, and chlortetracycline is one member of the subclass. The basis for classifying tetracyclines as a subclass is their similar therapeutic properties, not similar chemical structures, even though products of the same subclass frequently are chemically similar.[8] Recognizing this distinction, we may describe three kinds of new drugs:

(1) the breakthrough drug, which defines the class;

(2) those drugs suitable for the treatment of the same disease or condition and consequently fall within the same class but which are different enough from the breakthrough drug or any others on the market to be the first of a subclass; and

(3) new drugs of the same subclass as one previously on the market, which we call follow-ons.

The only other new pharmaceutical products are not new drugs. They are the additional products of previously marketed chemical entities. This paper is only interested in the factors that directly influence the development and marketing of drugs of the third type and the effect of these follow-ons.[9]

**The Process.** The process is one of continual feedback in the development and introduction of follow-on drugs. If the breakthrough product is profitable, other firms will want to enter the market. However, because the breakthrough drug is patented, it is necessary for the firm to research, develop, test, and evaluate a

---

[8] Bernard A. Kemp and Paul R. Moyer, "Equivalent Therapy at Lower Cost," *Journal of the American Medical Association,* vol. 228, no. 8 (20 May 1974), pp. 1009–14.

[9] While this distinction was recognized by some of the other authors, it was not incorporated into their analyses. It should be recognized, furthermore, that an increase in research activity designed to develop follow-ons may serendipitously lead to the development of additional group 1 and 2 types of drugs.

substitute or follow-on product through the approved new drug application (NDA) stage in order to enter the market. In order to understand the implications of the process for development of follow-ons, it is necessary to examine the premarketing and postmarketing phases separately.

In the premarketing phase potential profits lead firms who are not presently marketing a product in the subclass to direct resources into the research and development of follow-ons. The increase in inputs, if successful, will lead to an increase in the output at each of the premarketing stages. These premarketing stages include the development and screening of analogs, three phases of clinical testing, and the FDA approval procedures.[10] Increased activity in these stages will be evidenced by a rise in the number of analogs developed and in the number of drugs with potentially similar therapeutic properties for which patents are applied and awarded. There will also be an increase in investigational new drug (IND) applications submitted to the FDA for drugs of this subclass, in drugs subjected to clinical and other trials, and in the NDAs that are submitted and approved. The successful completion of all steps in the premarketing phase leads to an approved product, one that is ready for marketing.

When the follow-on drug is marketed, there is an additional chemical entity of the same subclass marketed by another company under a different brand name. The new product provides physicians with an additional therapeutic option. If prescribed, the new product will lead to a shift in market shares. The change in market structure will lead to a change in the patterns of rivalry and in the firms' mutually interdependent responses to it. The introduction of the follow-on may also lead to an improved understanding of the modes of action, therapeutic properties, and side effects of the drugs involved. That understanding leads to a shift in demand within the subclass to a pattern more accurately reflecting the value of the products. There may or may not be an increase in output or a reduction in price, but even if there is neither, there will be a redistribution of profits among the firms and a reduction in potential profits available to other outsiders. These changes are brought about by either a decline in their average revenue function or a progressive increase in the cost of developing additional follow-ons for human use as more and more are precluded, or both.

The reduction in profit potential and the changing profits picture are the signals that lead firms to reduce or redirect the resources they commit to the research and development of additional therapeutic agents of the same subclass.[11] The firms' response to the reduction in profits closes the gap in the continual feedback process.

---

[10] Harold A. Clymer, "The Changing Cost and Risks of Pharmaceutical Innovation," in J. Cooper, ed., *The Economics of Drug Innovation,* pp. 111–12.

[11] The development of additional products may reveal gaps in therapy, and firms may attempt to develop breakthroughs to fill those gaps. If they are successful they will market a product that will be in a new and different subclass.

Even though extra profits, and not the development of differentiated products, is the objective of producing follow-ons, there are additional ramifications in the market effect because the products are likely to be differentiated. The different chemical entities frequently have slight differences in therapeutic properties and side effects. The variation can provide a valuable adjunct to therapy. For example, if the patient has an idiosyncratic reaction or the disease becomes refractory to one chemical entity, one of the others may be suitable. Moreover if problems develop with the breakthrough product, others with similar therapeutic properties are still available. At the same time, however, multiple differentiated chemical entities in the same subclass make the physician less certain about the patient's therapeutic response. They tend to discourage the physician from shifting among chemical entities, especially when he knows what to expect from the one he has been using and is satisfied with it. Moreover, in promoting their products, the firms are also likely to emphasize differences, rather than similarities, in order to mitigate rivalry or insulate themselves from it. If the emphasis is successful, the differentiated products provide additional insulation for their market and profits position.

**Distinguishing Features of the Process.** One of the two principal distinguishing features of the follow-on development process is the assertion that this economic activity is a function of potential profits; the higher the profits the greater the amount of resources that outside firms, individually and collectively, are likely to commit to the development of follow-ons. Thus the profits arising from the patent system simultaneously provide the incentives and rewards for attempts to bypass the patents and the signals for continual readjustment in the level of R&D activity. Furthermore, it is important to recognize that the actual profits that any firm can obtain from developing and marketing follow-ons are likely to vary from one outside firm to another; the profit estimates are likely to vary as well. Consequently the R&D activity in the development of follow-ons intended to circumvent patent barriers is responsive to profit potentials and probably will vary among firms.

This is in marked contrast to the conventional, and somewhat simplistic, view of patent protection. A patent gives the inventor the right to exclude others from "making . . . or selling" the new, novel, unobvious product for seventeen years.[12] Frequently that right has been assumed to imply a single-firm monopoly for the patent protection period with product replication and entry occurring after the patent expires. The contemporary academic literature recognizes that the single-firm market structure is not necessarily appropriate. In spite of this conceptual realization, however, the nature and prevalence of other structures for markets for patented products remain unexamined. Even less is known about the price-output and other socioeconomic performance characteristics of the alternative structures that are recognized. Moreover, policy makers, both in government and in industry, typically use the simplistic image as a basis for their recommendations.

---

[12] 35 U.S.C. § 154 (1964).

The conventional view of patent protection is, in fact, one extreme of the follow-on development process. If no resources are devoted to the development of follow-ons, or if the resources used do not result in more products of the same subclass, then—from the viewpoint of market structure, at least—the conventional view of patents is likely to apply. When either of these situations does not apply, the follow-on development process provides the explanation of what occurs. Moreover, the larger the number of follow-ons that are developed and marketed, the more likely it is that the market structure will differ from that predicted by the conventional patent protection concept.

The other basic difference of the follow-on development process is that, to the extent that firms are successful in developing follow-ons, some of the competitive response is transferred from the postpatent period to the time when the patent is in force. This shift reduces the effective control of the patent holder during the life of the patent and distributes the rewards for product innovation among a number of different firms. After the patent expires, firms can enter the market by replicating the product. Consequently, in the end, cost-demand conditions for a particular type of therapeutic agent dictate the number of firms the market will support. This number is likely to be similar in either case. However, the product options presented by those firms are likely to be more varied when follow-on product activity is successful because, after the patent expires, the entrants can replicate the patented product.

## The Follow-on Development Process and Diuretics, 1953–69

Let us evaluate the nature and effect of the follow-on development process in one class of therapeutic agents: diuretics. Diuretics are drugs used to treat edema, a condition where excessive body fluid is retained in the spaces between the cells. This condition is associated with a number of different diseases including congestive heart failure and hypertension. It is usually manifested by swelling, especially in the extremities and sometimes in the abdominal cavity. There are seven major subclasses of single-entity diuretics: theophylline derivatives (principally aminophylline), organomercurials, carbonic anhydrase inhibitors, amisometradines, thiazides and related compounds, potassium-conserving diuretic compounds, and fast-acting diuretics. The last five subclasses involve patented products; except for amisometradines, each subclass has been quite profitable. The four profitable subclasses will be used in the comparison. From a medical, physiological, pharmacological, economic and marketing viewpoint the basic unit is the subclass. Since the economic and market factors that influence profitability are likely to vary from one subclass to another, the factors influencing the success of the process for developing follow-ons vary also. Without a specific examination of these factors, the relevance of comparisons across classes is open to question. Moreover, since there have been only four profitable, patented subclasses of diuretics introduced since 1953, the generality of these results cannot be determined. However, the conditions surrounding their development and success has varied widely (see Tables 1 and 2). Consequently, even if diuretics are not typical of all classes of pharmaceuticals, the wide differences among the subclasses should provide important insights into the nature and effect of the follow-on development process and the conditions under which it or the conventional patent protection concept is the more relevant hypothesis.

None of the four subclasses existed before 1953. By 1969 diuretics was a large market.[13] The estimated value of shipments in 1968 was about $103 million.[14] The value of new prescriptions for diuretics increased nine-fold in fourteen years from 1955 to 1969.[15] In 1969, the four subclasses involved in this analysis amounted to 99 percent of the diuretics market.[16]

**Premarketing Experience.** In the conventional view of patent protection outside firms will not commit any resources to the development of follow-ons during the period of patent protection and none will be developed. Even the sparse data available show a very different pattern of behavior (Table 3). Fifteen additional chemical entities were developed and marketed in the United States, and at least 160—and perhaps many more—were developed and not marketed. One company alone, the one which provided detailed information, developed 156 thiazide analogs. Two of them were marketed. The amount of resources committed to the development of diuretic follow-ons was apparently sizeable. Even if we consider only the eighteen brands of the fifteen single-entity follow-ons that reached the market, the estimated cost of the resources involved is $22.9 million.[17] More resources, perhaps many more, were involved in the development of the twenty-nine combination products marketed by outsiders and an unknown number

---

[13] For a more complete discussion and documentation, see Bernard A. Kemp, *The RDTEM Process*, pp. 51–99.

[14] U.S., Department of Commerce, Bureau of the Census, Industry Division, *Current Industrial Reports: Pharmaceutical Preparations except Biologicals* (MA-28G[68]-1) (Washington, D. C.: Government Printing Office, 1970).

[15] No other comparable data are available for as long a period. See Category 2700 (diuretics) data in R. A. Gosselin, *National Prescription Audit (NPA), Therapeutic Category Report, Ten-Year Trend* (Dedham, Mass.: R. A. Gosselin, 1958), p. 1; *NPA*, 1967, pp. 455–60; and *NPA*, 1969, pp. 371–75. I wish to thank Lea, Inc., and the individual companies involved for their permission to use the Gosselin data.

[16] All market share data is based on the dollar value of new prescriptions as reported in R. A. Gosselin, *National Prescription Audit.* It is based on a sample of retail pharmacies and therefore does not cover all methods of distribution and administration to patients. Consequently results using more complete data could vary somewhat.

[17] The post–1962 cost is based on Clymer's minimum estimate of the allocated cost incurred before a product can reach the market, $2.5 million. See Cooper, *Economics of Drugs Innovation*, p. 117. The pre–1962 cost estimate is assumed to be $1.0 million. According to Clymer, clearance now takes three to four times as long (ibid., p. 110).

## Table 1
## DIURETICS INTRODUCED SINCE 1953

| Subclass and Brand Name | Chemical Entity | Producer | Year of Introduction |
|---|---|---|---|
| Carbonic anhydrase inhibitors | | | |
| Diamox | Acetazolamide | Lederle | 1953 |
| Cardrase | Ethoxzolamide | Upjohn | 1957 |
| Daranide | Dichlorphenamide | MSD | 1958 |
| Neptazane | Methazolamide | Lederle | 1960 |
| Amisometradines | | | |
| Mincard | 1-allyl-3-ethyl-6-amino-tetrahydropyrimidinedione | Searle | 1954 |
| Mictine | 1-allyl-3-ethyl-6-amino-tetrahydropyrimidinedione | Searle | 1956 |
| Rolicton | 1-methallyl-3-methyl-6-amino-tetrahydropyrimidinedione | Searle | 1956 |
| Thiazides and related compounds [a] | | | |
| Diuril | Chlorothiazide | MSD | 1957 |
| Esidrix | Hydrochlorothiazide | CIBA | 1959 |
| Hydrodiuril | Hydrochlorothiazide | MSD | 1959 |
| Oretic | Hydrochlorothiazide | Abbott | 1959 |
| Bristuron | Bendroflumethiazide | Bristol | 1959 |
| Naturetin | Bendroflumethiazide | Squibb | 1959 |

| Potassium-conserving compounds | | |
|---|---|---|
| Aldactone | Searle | 1960 |
| Aldactazide[b] | Searle | 1962 |
| Dyrenium | SK&F | 1964 |
| Dyazide[b] | SK&F | 1965 |
| Fast-acting compounds | | |
| Lasix | Hoechst | 1966 |
| Edecrin | MSD | 1967 |

[a] The other thiazide compounds which were introduced after 1959 are presented in Table 2.
[b] These are combination products.
**Source:** Bernard A. Kemp, *The RDTEM Process: The Pharmaceutical Industry's Way around Patent Barriers (As Applied to Diuretics)* (Philadelphia, 1971), p. 56.

## Table 2

### INTRODUCTION OF THIAZIDES AND RELATED COMPOUNDS, SINGLE ENTITIES AND COMBINATIONS, 1957–69

| Chemo-Therapeutic Agents | Brand Name | Producer | Year of Intro- duction |
|---|---|---|---|
| Chlorothiazide | Diuril | MSD | 1957 |
|   With reserpine | Diupres | MSD | 1967 |
|   As sodium salt | Lyovac Diuril | MSD | 1958 |
| Hydrochlorothiazide | Esidrix | CIBA | 1959 |
| | Hydrodiuril | MSD | 1959 |
| | Oretic | Abbott | 1959 |
|   With reserpine | Hydropres | MSD | 1961 |
| | Serpasil-Esidrix | CIBA | 1960 |
| | Singoserp-Esidrix | CIBA | 1961 |
|   With hydralazine hydrochloride | Ser-Ap-Es | CIBA | 1961 |
|   With potassium chloride | Esidrix K | CIBA | 1961 |
| | Hydrodiuril-Ka | MSD | 1960 |
|   With reserpine | Hydropres-Ka | MSD | 1961 |
|   With meprobamate | Cyclex | MSD | 1960 |
| | Miluretic | Wallace | 1961[a] |
|   With apresoline hydrochloride | Apresoline-Esidrix | CIBA | 1961 |
|   With butabarbital | Butizide | McNeil | 1963 |
|     With reserpine | Butiserpazide | McNeil | 1963 |
|   With mebutamine | Caplaril | Wallace | 1964 |
|   With guarenthidine monosulfate | Esimil | CIBA | 1966 |
|   With deserpidine | Oreticyl | Abbott | 1961 |
|   With pentaerythritol tetranitrate | Perithiazide SA | Warner | 1963 |
| Methyclothiazide | Enduron | Abbott | 1960 |
|   With cryptenamine | Diutensen | Mallinckrodt[b] | 1963 |
|     With reserpine | Diutensen-R | Mallinckrodt[b] | 1963 |
|   With deserpidine | Enduronyl | Abbott | 1962 |
| Trichloromethiazide | Metahydrin | Lakeside | 1961 |
| | Naqua | Schering | 1960 |
|   With reserpine | Matatensin | Lakeside | 1963 |
| | Naquival | Schering | 1964 |
| Flumethiazide | Ademol | Squibb | 1960[a] |
|   With potassium chloride and rauwolfia | Rautrax | Squibb | 1961 |
| Bendroflumethiazide | Bristuron | Bristol | 1959[a] |
| | Naturetin | Squibb | 1959 |
|   With potassium chloride | Naturetin cK | Squibb | 1960 |
| | Rauzide | Squibb | 1968 |
|   With rauwolfia | Rautrax-N (and Modified) | Squibb | 1961 |

Table 2 (Continued)

| Chemo-Therapeutic Agents | Brand Name | Producer | Year of Intro- duction |
|---|---|---|---|
| Hydroflumethiazide | Saluron | Bristol | 1960 |
| With reserpine and porto- veratrine A | Salutensin | Bristol | 1961 |
| Benzthiazide | Aquatag | Tutag | 1960 |
| | Exna | Robins | 1960 |
| With reserpine | Exna-R | Robins | 1966 |
| Cyclothiazide | Anhydron | Lilly | 1963 |
| With potassium chloride | Anhydron K | Lilly | 1963 |
| With reserpine | Anhydron KR | Lilly | 1965 |
| Polythiazide | Renese | Pfizer | 1961 |
| With reserpine | Renese-R | Pfizer | 1965 |
| Chlorthalidone | Hygroton | Geigy | 1960 |
| With reserpine | Regroton | Geigy | 1967 |
| Quinethazone | Hydromox | Lederle | 1962 |
| With reserpine | Hydromox R | Lederle | 1962 |
| Spironolactone[d] With hydrochlorothiazide | Aldactazide (-A)[e] | Searle | 1962 |
| Triamterene[d] With hydrochlorothiazide | Dyazide | SK&F | 1965 |

[a] No longer on market. See Kemp, *The RDTEM Process*, appendix table C–1 for the date of discontinuance.

[b] Originally marketed by R. I. Neisler.

[c] Rautrax-N and Rautrax-N Modified, which contain the same ingredients in different amounts, are treated as one combination.

[d] Both the single entity and combination products drugs are treated in the discussion as potassium-conserving diuretics rather than thiazide combinations.

[e] Aldactazide-A and Aldactazide are the same.

**Source:** Kemp, *The RDTEM Process*, pp. 88–89.

of additional products, the development of which was terminated before they reached the market.

**Postmarketing Experience.** The primary result and the preliminary indication of success of the follow-on development process is its effects on the competitive structure—on the number of chemical entities, of brands, and of companies (Table 4). In each subclass, at least one additional single-entity brand was introduced by outsiders. In thiazides there were fifteen. The follow-ons that were marketed had only a minimal effect on market shares in two of the types, namely, carbonic anhydrase inhibitors and fast-acting diuretics. But they had a marked effect on physicians' prescribing patterns and on market shares for the other two types. The follow-ons came on the market one to four years after the breakthrough

## Table 3

PREMARKETING EXPERIENCE IN DIURETICS: KNOWN ANALOGS
DEVELOPED AND MARKETED BY COMPANIES THAT DID NOT
MARKET THE BREAKTHROUGH, 1953–69

| Subclass | Minimum Number of Analogs Developed | Single Entity Follow-ons | | Cost of Resources ($ millions) |
| | | Number of chemical entities | Number of brands | |
| --- | --- | --- | --- | --- |
| Carbonic anhydrase inhibitors | 5 | 2 | 2 | n.a. |
| Thiazides and related compounds | 165ᵃ | 11 | 15ᵇ | n.a. |
| Potassium-conserving compounds | 12ᶜ | 1 | 1ᵈ | 3.4 |
| Fast-acting diuretics | 2 | 1 | 1 | n.a. |
| Total | 175 | 15 | 18 | 3.4 |

**Note:** These data are incomplete. The numbers shown are only the amount that can be currently documented. N.a. indicates information not currently available.

[a] One hundred fifty-six were developed by one firm alone. The number of additional thiazide analogs that were developed by the 12 other successful companies and by those who were unsuccessful is unknown.

[b] In addition there are 28 additional thiazide combinations not produced by Merck which use these single entities.

[c] SmithKline & French developed eleven of them.

[d] Two other important potassium-conserving follow-ons are combination products; one produced by Searle, who marketed the breakthrough, and one by SK&F, who marketed the follow-on single entity.

**Source:** Kemp, *The RDTEM Process,* pp. 62–76.

(Table 5). The number of brands remained relatively constant. Eventually, however, there were marked changes in the relative importance of the breakthroughs and the follow-ons.

Within each subclass the follow-ons present the physician and patient with differentiated therapeutic options. In some cases they are slightly differentiated; in others, the differentiation is more pronounced. For example, hydrochlorothiazide is produced by three companies under three brand names, presumably by the same process of production resulting in equivalent potency, absorption, and attained blood levels. On the other hand, in the cases of the potassium-conserving compounds and the fast-acting diuretics, the somewhat different therapeutic properties of the follow-ons has been documented in careful pharmacological studies. Yet in each case the follow-on is sufficiently similar to the breakthrough to be included in the same subclass.[18]

---

[18] Practically speaking, it is at this point in the research, development, marketing, and promotion process that Comanor's emphasis on product differentiation comes into play, because typically the pharmacological activity of different chemical entities cannot be predicted beforehand.

## Table 4

### POSTMARKETING EXPERIENCE IN DIURETICS: NUMBER OF SINGLE ENTITY FOLLOW-ON BRANDS MARKETED AND THEIR MARKET SHARE IN 1969

| Subclass | Number of Follow-on Brands Marketed | | Share of Market of Break-through, 1969 (percent) | Share of Market of Single Entity Follow-on Products Marketed, 1969 (percent) | |
|---|---|---|---|---|---|
| | Breakthrough company | Out-siders | | Breakthrough company | Out-siders |
| Carbonic anhydrase inhibitors | 1 | 2 | 97.9 | 0.0 | 2.1 |
| Fast-acting diuretics | 0 | 1 | 90.9 | — | 9.1 |
| Thiazides and related compounds | 1 | 15 | 27.2 | 25.2 | 40.9[b] |
| Potassium-conserving compounds | 1[a] | 2[a] | 11.6 | 40.3 | 48.1 |

[a] Two of the follow-ons were potassium-conserving thiazide combinations. They are treated here as single entity products.
[b] The combination products make up the remaining 6.7 percent.
**Source:** Kemp, *The RDTEM Process*, pp. 72, 75.

## Table 5

### SPEED OF INTRODUCTION OF FOLLOW-ON DIURETICS MARKETED BY OUTSIDERS

| Subclass | Year Break-through Introduced | Number of Years to First Follow-on | Number of Follow-ons 5 Years after Introduction of the Breakthroughs | |
|---|---|---|---|---|
| | | | Brands | Compounds |
| Carbonic anhydrase inhibitors | 1953 | 4 | 2 | 2 |
| Thiazides and related compounds | | | | |
| Single entities | 1957 | 2 | 15 | 11 |
| Fixed combinations[a] | 1960 | 1 | 25 | 19 |
| Potassium-conserving compounds | | | | |
| Single entities | 1960 | 4 | 1 | 1 |
| Combinations with thiazide | 1962 | 3 | 1 | 1[b] |
| Fast-acting diuretics | 1966 | 1 | 1 | 1 |

[a] Three others dropped out of the market, one before the first five years were over.
[b] The same companies produce combinations as well as single entities.
**Source:** Kemp, *The RDTEM Process*, p. 75, Table IV–6.

These changes in market structure led to, or were associated with, secondary changes in the pattern of rivalry, in the firms' market conduct, and in market performance. These patterns were quite different from those which would have characterized a single-firm patent monopoly. The oligopolistic rivalry within each subclass takes the form of elaborate and expensive techniques for discovering the nature of other firms' research activity, market research activity about rival brands, surveillance of their advertising campaigns, especially in the medical journals, monitoring changes in sales, and promoting a company's own brand over a rival's. In part the failure of follow-ons to take a larger share of the market away from the breakthrough company may be due to the promotional activity of the breakthrough company and the difficulty of overcoming the first-of-a-type syndrome. In one case, that of fast-acting diuretics, the company that introduced the breakthrough, Hoechst, was new and small in the U.S. market, although not small internationally. Its successful promotional campaign enabled it to obtain and maintain its market position. Some of the resources required for this activity were used to discover and counteract the effect of promotional strategies of rivals; but in other cases, like the potassium-conserving compounds, the competitive rivalry led to an improved understanding by physicians and pharmaceutical manufacturers too, of the modes of action, therapeutic properties, and side effects of drugs that were on the market previously.

The results for two performance variables, output and prices, and, by implication, for profits were also markedly different from the conventional view. If the factors affecting demand and market price are constant, the expected sales pattern, under the conventional view, for the breakthrough product and consequently for the subclass is as follows: a peak in sales shortly after the introduction of the breakthrough as physicians become aware of and try the new drug, a slight decline to a constant sales level as they integrate it into their patterns of treatment, and a more marked decline when and if new subclasses are introduced.[19] This pattern was reasonably approximated only in the case of the carbonic anhydrase inhibitors. In each of the other cases the sales of each subclass of diuretic increased markedly and continued to rise. The average annual rate of increase ranged from 146 percent for the potassium-conserving diuretics to 2,150 percent for the thiazides. These increases occurred in spite of the fact that two new and important subclasses of diuretics, the potassium-conserving and fast-acting compounds, were introduced after the thiazides and one new one after the potassium-conserving diuretics were marketed.

The predominant expectation in these markets, either as single-firm monopolies or as oligopolies, is price stability, especially for published prices. That is

---

[19] James W. McKie, "An Economic Analysis of the Position of American Home Products Corporation in the Ethical Drug Industry," in U.S., Congress, Senate, Committee on the Judiciary, Subcommittee on Antitrust and Monopoly, *Report on the Study on Administered Prices in the Drug Industry*, 86th Congress, 2d Sess., 1960, pt. 17, p. 9944.

just what occurred. For nineteen of the twenty-five single entity brands—seventeen thiazides or related compounds, four carbonic anhydrase inhibitors, two potassium-conserving compounds and two fast-acting diuretics—*Red Book* prices did not change from the date they were introduced through 1969. In all, 207 product-years were involved, and there were only nine price changes affecting six brands. This is an average of one change every 23 product-years—remarkable price stability.

Admittedly these conclusions about price stability are based on list prices at the manufacturer-retailer level. It is well-known that they do not necessarily reflect the level or variation of actual prices, but it is the only publicly available price information.

The list prices were not the same, however. Consequently, the physician and patient are provided with therapeutic and price options that would not be available in one-product markets. These options made it possible for the physician to prescribe and the patient to receive equivalent therapy at marked price reductions. Price comparisons could be made only for the thiazides and the potassium-conserving diuretics because they are the only types for which potency equivalents could be determined.[20] *Red Book* prices in 1969 for the fifteen brands of thiazides or related compounds based on equivalent potency were the following:

| Price to the Pharmacy ($/bottle of 100s) | Number of Brands |
|---|---|
| 8.75 to 8.25 | 1 |
| — | — |
| — | — |
| — | — |
| 6.25 to 5.75 | 7 |
| 5.75 to 5.25 | 2 |
| 5.25 to 4.75 | 4 |
| 4.75 to 4.25 | 1 |

The most typical price to the pharmacy was $6.00. However, it was possible to get 100 tablets of equivalent potency for 26 percent less by prescribing and buying Lakeside's Metahydrin at $4.44 per bottle of 100.

Metahydrin is one of the two brands of trichlormethiazide; Schering's Naqua is the other. Interestingly, prescribing trichlormethiazide generically would probably result in a higher price to the consumer, since Naqua sells for $5.70 and part of the time the pharmacist would fill the prescription with the higher priced brand.

Market price differences for equivalent therapy exist among the potassium-conserving compounds, as well. For example, on the basis of equivalent daily dose SmithKline & French's Dyrenium is one-third the price of Searle's Aldactone.

---

[20] *Red Book* prices do not fully reflect differences in the channels of distribution or corporate discount policies. Consequently even these published prices may not be directly or appropriately comparable.

Even leaving patient-to-patient differences aside, authorities differ on the potency equivalent of the products in a subclass. There is more agreement among thiazides than among any of the others, and even here the estimates of potency equivalents have a marked effect on the price comparisons. Differences in estimates of relative potency exist for bendroflumethiazide, methychothiazide, polythiazide and cyclothiazide. The spread in potency estimate for polythiazide makes Pfizer's Renese either the least expensive or the most expensive thiazide.

It is difficult to determine potency equivalents even for products like the thiazides, which are considered basically the same. Consequently, even though prices are stable, the development of follow-ons provides physicians with therapeutic options and significant price differences that they would not have in a one-product market. If the published price results reflect actual prices, and if the lower prices are known and taken advantage of by physicians, patients could get lower prices and cost savings for equivalent therapy. For whatever the reason, the market share data indicate that, in practice, physicians have not typically taken advantage of the lower-priced options.

There is no direct evidence of the effect of the introduction of follow-ons on the profits within each subclass. However, the increase in sales and market share for the fast-acting and potassium-conserving diuretics is evidence of increased, rather than decreased, profitability as a result of, or concomitant with, the introduction of the follow-ons. The decrease in market share for the other two subclasses does not necessarily indicate declining profitability in markets expanding as rapidly as these are.

In part the expanding sales for the subclass, especially if prices are in fact stable, is due to the market response that led to an increase in demand. That increase may be due to the dissemination of information, to an improved understanding of the nature of the drug once it is on the market (as with the potassium-conserving diuretics), or to new, previously unrecognized uses and indications like the antihypertensive properties of the thiazides and subsequent diuretics. In fact, there is some evidence that the introduction of additional chemical entities in the same subclass leads not only to expanded sales for the subclass but for the previously marketed products as well. The socioeconomically desirable function of the discovery of new uses, more widespread information, and more rapid expansion of appropriate existing uses may not be independent of the rivalry of multiple firms attempting to get a market niche.

There is also some independent evidence that firms have shifted their research resources in response to this changing profit picture. The marketing of a new potassium-conserving diuretic overseas and the rumors about research activity indicate that firms are actively trying to find analogs for Lasix and for the potassium-conserving compounds. Apparently they are no longer trying to develop additional thiazides or carbonic anhydrase inhibitors.

**Summary.** Between 1953 and 1969 in each of the four subclasses of profitable patented diuretics, follow-on development process describes and predicts the behavior of firms better than the conventional patent protection concept. In each one, firms committed resources during the period of patent protection in an attempt to develop follow-ons. In each type, one or more firms were successful in developing and marketing follow-ons, and this led to a decline in the share of the breakthrough product. In two cases that decline was moderate or marked. Within each subclass the follow-ons provided physicians and patients with additional, more or less differentiated therapeutic options that would not be available in one-product markets. These changes in market structure led to or were associated with an increase in output in three of the four subclasses. And while they do not appear to have led to published price reductions (published prices were remarkably stable), they did make it possible for the physician to provide the patient with equivalent therapy at a lower cost if the doctor was aware of and prescribed the least expensive, therapeutically equivalent option. Apparently firms have responded to the changing potential profit picture in these patented diuretics by adjusting the amount of resources they commit to the development of additional patented follow-ons.

## The Follow-on Development Process and Diuretics, 1970–73

A number of important changes occurred in the diuretics market between the time the base study was conducted and early 1974. The lack of change in some other areas in which change might be expected is also noteworthy. There were no new subclasses. Neither was there a redefinition of them because of changes in the indications for these chemical entities.[21] The only chemical entity that had lost patent protection was acetazolamide, and its product patent expired in 1968. Consequently, the patent structure in each subclass remained basically unchanged.

In spite of the apparently continued high profitability of the fast-acting and potassium-conserving diuretics, no new chemical entities were introduced in those subclasses in the United States.[22] Even though the product patent expired for acetazolamide in 1968, a number of firms, including some large ones, only recently obtained approved new drug applications, and none of those products is on the market yet.

---

[21] See chapter on diuretics in AMA Department of Drugs, *AMA Drug Evaluations*, 2d ed. (Acton, Mass.: Publishing Sciences Group, 1973), pp. 65–77.

[22] It is important to recognize that there are other diuretics, that is, other chemical entities, that are already being marketed in other countries. They include thiazides and related compounds and potassium-conserving diuretics. Some of them are marketed by firms having U.S. operations. For these products, at least, it would not be necessary to go through the entire research and development process and to incur those costs. See William M. Wardell, "Introduction of New Therapeutic Drugs in the United States and Great Britain: A Comparison," *Clinical Pharmacology and Therapeutics*, vol. 14, no. 5 (September–October 1973), pp. 778–79; and pages 165–81, this volume.

## Table 6
## NEW DIURETIC PRODUCTS, 1969–74

| Chemical Entity | Brand[a] | Producer/ Marketer | Year of Introduction[b] |
|---|---|---|---|
| **New chemical entity** | | | |
| Metolazone | Zaroxolyn | Pennwalt | 1974 |
| **Old chemical entities as new products** | | | |
| Hydrochlorothiazide | Thiadril | Vanguard | 1973 |
| | Tenzide | Metro Med | 1974 |
| | Thiuretic | Parke-Davis | 1974 |
| | | American Quinine | 1973 |
| | | Approved Pharmaceuticals | 1973 |
| | | Arcum | 1973 |
| | | Barry-Martin | 1973 |
| | | Cenci Laboratories | 1973 |
| | | Columbia | 1973 |
| | | Pennhurst | 1973 |
| | | Premo Pharmaceuticals | 1973 |
| | | Robinson | 1973 |
| | | Sheraton | 1973 |
| | | Stayner | 1973 |
| | | West-Ward | 1973 |
| | | Zenith | 1973 |
| With reserpine | Hydroserp | Zenith | 1973 |
| | Thiapres | Vanguard | 1973 |
| | | Stayner | 1973 |
| Methyclothiazide | Aquatensen | Mallinckrodt | 1971 |
| Trichlormethiazide | Aquex | Lannett | 1972 |
| | | Robinson | 1973 |
| | | Sherry Pharmaceuticals | 1973 |
| Benzthiazide | Pro-Aqua | Reid-Provident | 1970 |
| | Aquapres | Coastal | 1971 |
| | Diucen | Central | 1971 |
| | Edemex | Savage | 1971 |
| | Lemazide | Lemmon | 1971 |
| | Urazide | Mallard | 1971 |
| | Zide | Luar Pharmaceuticals | 1973 |
| | Hy-Drine | Zemmer | 1974 |

[a] When no brand name is given the product is marketed only under its generic name.
[b] Based on information available as of March 1974.
**Source:** For a list of the sources used see Kemp, *The RDTEM Process,* pp. 60–61.

In the thiazides, however, the patents were still in force: the first one, chlorothiazide, was protected until October 1974. In spite of that, important structural changes and resulting price changes occurred in the thiazide market. One new chemical entity, metolazone, was introduced in 1974 by Pennwalt. (See Tables 6 and 7.) But that was not and is not likely to be the significant change.

**Table 7**

CHANGES IN THE MARKET STRUCTURE FOR DIURETICS, 1969–73

| | Number of Products, Branded and Unbranded | | | |
|---|---|---|---|---|
| | On market 1969 | Discontinued 1969–73 | Introduced 1969–73 | On market 1973 |
| Breakthrough | 1 | 0 | 0 | 1 |
| Single entity follow-ons | | | | |
| Breakthrough company | 1 | 0 | 0 | 1 |
| Others | 15 | 2 | 25 | 38 |
| Combination follow-ons | | | | |
| Breakthrough company | 7 | 3 | 0 | 4 |
| Others | 29 | 6 | 3 | 26 |
| Total | 53 | 11 | 28 | 70 |

Source: Tables 1, 2, and 6.

No less than fifteen new products have been introduced in four of the thiazide compounds. Probably the most important change is in hydrochlorothiazide, the largest-selling single thiazide compound. In 1973 Zenith Laboratories got an approved NDA and decided to market hydrochlorothiazide without a patent license. Not only is it marketing the product directly, but it is reselling to a large number of other firms who are selling both branded and unbranded hydrochlorothiazide. By the end of 1973 there were at least sixteen additional hydrochlorothiazide products available. One of the large sellers is Parke-Davis, which specializes in the hospital market.

There is at least the potential for substantial price reductions. The unweighted average 1974 *Red Book* price for the twenty-two new thiazide products for which price information is available is $3.94 per bottle, $1.78 less than the comparable average 1969 price of $5.72.[23] A number of the firms are selling for less than $2.00 per bottle of 100.

Whatever its cause, the recent shift in the market has important implications for the follow-on development process. In thiazides, at least, the follow-on development process resulted in additional products, additional resources flowing into this market, and lower prices. In spite of that, however, further resource adjustments were possible through the replication of existing products. These adjustments appear to have led to still lower prices. Their effects on the development of other new diuretics is unknown.

There are strong indications that the experience in diuretics was repeated in other classes of therapeutic agents as well. The preliminary indications are that

---

[23] This is an unweighted average and consequently does not reflect actual sales.

## Table 8
### EFFECTIVE TERM OF DIURETIC PRODUCT PATENTS

| Class/Subclass | Number of Chemical Entities | Apparent Effective Length of Patent Protection[a] (years) | Time Elapsed to Second Product in Subclass (years) |
|---|---|---|---|
| Oral diuretics | | | |
|   Carbonic anhydrase inhibitors | 4 | 16.5 | 4 |
|   Thiazides and related compounds | 13 | 19.9 | 2 |
|   Potassium-conserving compounds | 2 | 17.0 | 4 |
|   Fast-acting diuretics | 2 | 14.5 | 1 |
| Single entity oral diuretics | 21 | 18.5 | |

[a] The apparent effective term of patent protection is measured from the issuance of the first approved NDA for the chemical entity to the patent expiration date.

the follow-on development process was also working in corticosteroids, oral anti-diabetics, tranquilizers, and patented broad spectrum antibiotics,[24] as well as for many other classes of therapeutic agents.[25] Apparently a one-product one-firm market does not exist in any of them, and in many cases the market structure has changed dramatically.

### Patents

The changes that occurred in the diuretics market occurred in the context of the patent system. Consequently this study simply does not answer the question of what would happen, either to the introduction of new chemical entities or to the market structure for existing chemical entities, if the patent system were changed. There have, however, been recommendations for both increasing and decreasing the term of pharmaceutical product patents. On the basis of data compiled in this study it is possible to determine the effective patent term for these chemical entities.

In assessing these results, it is important to recognize that there are two concurrent administrative processes, the patenting process and the NDA approval process. If NDA approvals take longer than patenting, then the effective term

[24] Steele, "Patent Restrictions and Price Competition," pp. 1976–95.
[25] Arthur D. Little, Inc., "A Report on the Aspects of Concentration and Product Obsolescence in the Pharmaceutical Industry in the United States," U.S., Congress, Senate, Committee on the Judiciary, *Hearings on the Drug Industry Antitrust Act*, 87th Congress, 1st sess., 1961, pt. 4, pp. 2519–23.

of the patent is reduced and vice versa. Moreover, the dates of patent award and of NDA approval are *not* independent of factors that are within the administrative discretion of the firms involved. Granting that, however, it is interesting to note that the average effective patent term for the twenty-one diuretics is 18.5 years, very close to the nominal legal term. The effective period of patent protection ranges from a minimum of ten years to a maximum of twenty-six. The length of the single-product, single firm monopoly position in the therapeutic subclass, however, was remarkably less. The longest time it took for another product with very similar therapeutic properties to be introduced was four years.

## Conclusions

There is good evidence, both direct and circumstantial, that the follow-on development process describes the industry's activity in the development and marketing of additional drugs of the same subclass. When the breakthrough is profitable, outside firms do commit resources during the period of patent protection in an attempt to develop follow-ons. The process was successful for diuretics as a therapeutic class, although more so for some subclasses than others. The preliminary measures of success are the large number of analogs that have been developed, the number of follow-ons, and the speed with which they came on the market. In diuretics, however, the follow-on development process must be considered somewhat less successful if its performance is judged by the erosion that the follow-ons caused in the market position of the breakthrough firm. The evaluation of its success in influencing market performance is more speculative and mixed, and it suffers from a lack of information. However, in three of the four subclasses, the output for each type increased markedly; list prices changed little; profits did not decline as much as expected; a number of new, differentiated therapeutic and price options were developed and, in some cases, rapidly adopted. Recent entry by the replication of existing chemical entities establishes that even after follow-ons were developed, profits were still sufficiently high to make this alternative form of entry profitable.

Suspending the question of whether the follow-on development process is desirable from a socioeconomic viewpoint, there is no doubt that it is working in two senses: resources are directed into the development of follow-ons and meaningful therapeutic options within the same subclass of therapeutic agents have been developed, marketed, and sustained by physicians' prescriptions and patients' purchases. Moreover, the follow-on development process describes this phase of the industry's activity better than the conventional patent protection concept, which implies that no resources are committed by outside firms in an attempt to develop new drugs in the same subclass during the period of patent protection and that none are developed. For some subclasses of diuretics the structural or performance effect was more limited and the results more closely approximate those expected under the conventional patent concept. This indicates only that the follow-on development process was less successful in those subclasses, not that it was not operating.

The pattern of market conduct described by the conventional view of patent protection is a behavioral option that is opened to the firms. However, it is one that many have not chosen to adopt. Consequently, from their viewpoint at least, expected benefits from the follow-on development process must be worth the extra cost involved and, since they continue to engage in the practice, actual benefits probably exceed the cost. Moreover, in diuretics the unexpected, sizable, and probably unrecognized spill-over effects led to larger benefits than could reasonably have been expected. This does not necessarily prove that from a socioeconomic viewpoint the follow-on development process is better than the practice implicit in the conventional view or that the follow-on development process leads to net social benefits. All that can be said analytically at this juncture is that the value of the resources committed to the practice involves a social cost, the magnitude of which is presently unknown, and that in diuretics the successful implementation of the practice has led to market and socioeconomic benefits that would not be available under the conventional view of patent protection.

In spite of almost universal criticism, the twin practices of molecular modification and me-too-ism take on a very different light in the context of the follow-on development process. They no longer need to take second place to new product development, nor must the marketing of the resulting follow-ons "lead to problems for the company," certainly not from political or social pressure.[26] The practices are, in fact, an integral part of the firms' technique for entry where entry with undifferentiated products is precluded because of patents, of the industry's competitive response, and of the socioeconomic resource allocation process. Moreover, unlike the conventional patent protection concept, the follow-on development process responds to the market signals of profit differentials. Consequently, corporate and government policies, practices, and procedures that reduce the profitability of follow-ons could well have unrecognized and undesirable anticompetitive side effects.[27]

---

[26] Knoppers, in Cooper, *Economics of Drug Innovation*, p. 252.
[27] For a more detailed examination of the policy effects see Kemp, *The RDTEM Process*, pp. 107–12.

# COMMENTARIES

## Yale Brozen

A standard thesis of much of the theorizing (perhaps more accurately designated as hypothesizing) in the literature of industrial organization is that the behavior and performance of firms in more concentrated markets is different from that of firms in less concentrated markets. Also, economics and industrial organization textbooks put forth conceptions concerning entry and the circumstances that will result in greater or lesser entry, given the attractiveness of entry. Telser has tested these standard conceptions, and his tests challenge these views.

Some of the conceptions concerning behavior and the resulting attractiveness of entry in more and less concentrated markets are rivals. Professor Telser has, with his tests, given us a basis for choosing among them. What may be called the Stigler hypothesis states that oligopolists [1] set prices at supracompetitive levels that are more profitable than competitive levels and therefore attract entry, with a consequent decline in the market shares of leading firms in concentrated industries.[2] Unconcentrated industries setting competitive prices attract relatively less entry. We should, then, find a positive correlation between prior concentration and subsequent entry. Professor Telser finds no such relationship. This would seem to imply that oligopolistic price setting is not different from competitive price setting, a finding that leaves us with a large body of sterile, not to say useless, economic literature, unless the relationships he finds in the markets for drugs do not hold for other markets.[3]

---

[1] The largest firms in industries where four or fewer have more than 45 to 50 percent of the business in a market (George Stigler, "Industrial Organization and Economic Progress," in Leonard White, ed., *State of the Social Sciences* [Chicago: University of Chicago Press, 1956]), or more than 60 percent (George Stigler, *Capital and Rates of Return in Manufacturing Industries* [Princeton, N.J.: Princeton University Press, 1963]), or not less than 80 percent (George Stigler, "A Theory of Oligopoly," *Journal of Political Economy*, vol. 72 [February 1964], p. 57).

[2] George Stigler, "Discussion of Papers on Capitalism and Monopolistic Competition: I. The Theory of Oligopoly," *American Economic Review*, vol. 40 (May 1950), reprinted in Y. Brozen, ed., *The Competitive Economy* (Morristown, N.J.: General Learning Press, 1974). Also, see Dean A. Worcester, "Why 'Dominant Firms' Decline," *Journal of Political Economy*, vol. 65 (August 1957), pp. 338–47.

[3] Some evidence points to the Telser findings as probably true in markets other than drug markets. Y. Brozen, "The Antitrust Task Force Deconcentration Recommendation," *Journal*

A rival hypothesis, the Bain-Modigliano-Sylos approach, holds that oligopolists set limit prices, that is, prices that do not attract entry or which prevent entry.[4] This seems to say no more than that they set competitive prices.[5] In that case it seems hardly necessary to have a special discussion of oligopoly unless they mean by limit prices those that are below the competitive level because, for some reason, oligopolists are eager to hold their market shares. In that case, we should find a negative relationship between concentration and entry. Again, Professor Telser finds no such relationship. The rival theories of oligopoly behavior are both demolished insofar as drug markets are concerned.

However, Bain and others argue that limit prices are higher than competitive prices and will still fail to attract entry because there are barriers to entering oligopoly markets. Therefore, oligopolists may make supracompetitive rates of return and still attract no entry if they set limit prices. If a limit pricer finds his market share declining, that is a signal that he has made a mistake in setting his price and he will reduce it to get down to that level which stops attracting entry. With a zero rate of entry into limit priced oligopoly markets, we still should have an inverse relationship between concentration and entry.[6] It remains clear, then, that Professor Telser has demolished the rivals—both sets.

But Professor Telser is not content to stop here. He specifically examines the relationship between the most often named entry barrier, promotion costs, and entry to see whether a greater height to this barrier reduces entry. Instead of finding a negative relationship between the height of this barrier and entry, as posited by Bain, Comanor, et al., he finds a positive relationship. Advertising and other types of promotion are used as a means of entry, not to stop entry.

Professor Telser's analysis also shows that firm size or economies of scale do not constitute a barrier to entry to drug markets. The larger the size of firms (measured by sales in a given therapeutic category) in a given market, the more entry occurs in that market.

of Law & Economics, vol. 13 (October 1970); "Concentration and Profits: Does Concentration Matter?" Antitrust Bulletin, vol. 19 (Summer 1974); "Barriers Facilitate Entry," Antitrust Bulletin, vol. 14 (Winter 1969).

[4] Joe S. Bain, "A Note on Pricing in Monopoly and Oligopoly," American Economic Review, vol. 39 (March 1949), pp. 448–64; Paulo Sylos-Labini, Oligopoly and Technical Progress (Cambridge, Mass.: Harvard University Press, 1962); F. Modigliani, "New Developments on the Oligopoly Front," Journal of Political Economy, vol. 66 (June 1958), pp. 215–32.

[5] R. F. Harrod, "Theory of Imperfect Competition Revised," Economic Essays (London: Macmillan and Co., 1962); H. R. Edwards, "Price Formation in Manufacturing Industry and Excess Capacity," Oxford Economic Papers, vol. 7 (February 1955), pp. 94–118.

[6] The inverse relationship may hold, but not necessarily, even if oligopolists set higher than limit prices, as suggested by Stigler, but still hold them low relative to short-run profit maximizing price in order to minimize (a constrained minimum) attractiveness of entry without being so low that no entry is attracted. B. P. Pashigian, "Limit Price and the Market Share of the Leading Firm," Journal of Industrial Economics, vol. 16 (July 1968), pp. 165–77.

The only barrier to entry that Professor Telser can find is one that is never mentioned in oligopoly theory. It is not economies of scale or capital requirements or absolute cost advantage or promotion; the barrier he finds is number of firms. The larger the number of firms already active in a market, the less entry.

Does that mean that the antitrust dogs have been going after the wrong quarry? Should they be attacking the atomized industries instead of the concentrated industries? Should they be urging mergers instead of undoing and preventing them?

The antitrust dogs may be attacking the wrong quarry in going after the oligopoly or concentrated industries, but that does not mean that the atomized industries are necessarily the right quarry. Professor Telser's finding that may be interpreted as larger numbers of firms constituting a barrier to entry emerges because of the way in which he measures entry: it consists of the proportion of total sales by firms new to a market. But surely enlargement of sales and new product introductions by firms already active in a market, which are probably more frequent when such firms are numerous, can do just as much to improve the allocation of resources and serve consumers as the sales and product introductions of firms new to a market. Does the introduction of a new lifesaving drug by a firm already resident in a market save fewer lives than if it were introduced by a firm new to a market?

Some would answer *yes* to this question. They would argue that the old firm, to protect its old drugs, would price the new drug higher than would a new firm with no old drugs to protect. But we have no evidence pointing in this direction. What little evidence we have points to new drugs being priced higher than old drugs,[7] but it does not distinguish between the new drugs of new firms and the new drugs of old firms. If the market is competitive, it would not pay for old firms to price new drugs any higher than would new firms. And Professor Telser's evidence points in the direction of the drug market being competitive, patents to the contrary notwithstanding. Inventing one's way around a patent is an old story in many industries, and an industry may be more competitive with patents than without. Professor Kemp relates the experience of one drug market which demonstrates that inventing one's way around a patent is a regular feature of drug firm R&D strategy.

A comment is in order here on the frequently derogatory description of the inventing-around process as consisting of molecule manipulation producing me-too drugs that add little to social welfare. In other industries, social policy is directed toward encouraging entry of new firms producing me-too products to compete with established firms. It seems a little strange that the production of me-too products is viewed so disparagingly in the drug industry.

---

[7] Sam Peltzman, *Regulation of Pharmaceutical Innovation: The 1962 Amendments* (Washington, D. C.: American Enterprise Institute, 1974), pp. 34–37.

Perhaps a part of the reason for the dim view of me-too products is the suspicion that research resources are being diverted to their development from more important alternative uses. There is, however, no evidence showing more important alternative uses for research resources or for the capital invested. There is evidence that of the eighteen most important of the 848 new chemical entities introduced between 1940 and 1967, eight were the result of molecule manipulation. Patent incentives, sometimes condemned as the cause of wasteful research in the pursuit of me-too drugs, "appear to have played a major role in inducing the research in thirteen of the eighteen cases." [8]

The second paper in this group gives a picture of rough-and-tumble competition in various drug markets similar to that shown by the Telser analysis. Dr. Cocks adds supporting detail by telling us such things as the number of new firms entering various drug markets between 1964 and 1973. This turns out to be a very large number even in markets where the amount of entry by the Telser measure is small. In the anti-infectives market, where the Telser measure shows new entry to be 0.93 percent, Dr. Cocks's data show a 40 percent increase in the number of firms competing. In the analgesic market, where the Telser measure shows new entry to be 0.78 percent, the Cocks data show a 25 percent increase in the number of firms. And in the diabetic market, where there was no entry measured by net change in number of firms there was very substantial entry by the Telser measure, 17 percent of 1973 sales being those of a manufacturer new to the market after 1964. It appears that there is no static or non-competitive market to be found in the drug industry.

Dr. Cocks's data matched against Professor Telser's may appear to picture a decline in the innovativeness of the industry. While Professor Telser finds that approximately 11 percent of sales in 1972 in the average therapeutic class were made by firms entering after 1963, Dr. Cocks finds that 8.3 percent of sales in 1973 were made by firms entering after 1964. Does this decline from 11 percent to 8 percent when the interval examined is shifted forward by one year lead to this conclusion?

The deduction does not necessarily follow. Dr. Cocks's ten major pharmaceutical markets use a different categorization from Telser's seventeen therapeutic categories. Because many of the Cocks markets are broader than the Telser categories, some of the sales by a new entrant in a Telser category may not show in a broader market definition. A firm introducing a new product could be new to a Telser category but already in a Cocks market, with the consequence that its sales do not show as sales by a new entrant in the latter case. We should expect the Telser measure of entry to produce a lower figure in markets as defined by Dr. Cocks.

---

[8] Larry L. Duetsch, "Research Performance in the Ethical Drug Industry," *Marquette Business Review,* vol. 17 (Fall 1973), p. 136.

The Cocks data also destroy the common fiction of rigid prices for drugs and the fiction of inelastic demands for each of these patented products. Prices are remarkably flexible, thus producing large effects on market position. Leading products in the anti-infective market, for example, suffered price declines from 1962 to 1971 ranging from 7 percent (for product number 8) to 67 percent (for product number 3). The average price decline in this inflationary period for these products was 32 percent, while the consumer price index rose 34 percent. The price of leading anti-infectives fell by 51 percent in constant dollars. That is a remarkable record.

Sales of these products also demonstrate what a complete fiction is the story that the average physician pays no attention to prices in writing prescriptions. Product 11 among the anti-infectives languished at 0.1 percent of the market for five years until it had cut its price by 47 percent. At that point, its market share rose to 0.7 percent, a six-fold increase. Another 14 percent price cut raised its market share another 170 percent. Still further cuts over the next three years amounting to 12 percent raised its market share by still another 68 percent. This would seem to demonstrate a remarkably high price elasticity of demand for a branded patented product, particularly in view of the price cuts of competitive products.

Product number 3 had a fading market position from 1962 through 1969 despite its price cuts, but then a 16 percent price cut in 1970 stopped the decline and added 14 percent to its market share. A further 27 percent cut in 1971 jumped its market share by another 40 percent. The market for ethical drugs responds remarkably vigorously to price changes, the myth of the price-insensitive prescribing physician to the contrary notwithstanding.

There appears to be competition among the products within each class despite whatever unique features each possesses. A product only singular enough to win 0.1 percent of the market over a five-year span won a 310 percent increase in market share when it cut its price relative to most of the other products in its market. A fading product turned itself around and reclaimed a major portion of its market position as it undertook similar price action.

The one quarrel I have with Dr. Cocks's discussion of the R&D strategy of drug firms is his insistence that drug firms seek to develop products with inelastic demands. From what little I know of R&D strategy in this industry, and from what I can infer from the little more I know of R&D strategy in other industries, firms seek to develop profitable products. A product with a very elastic demand can be far more profitable than a product with an inelastic demand. This is simply the old story of a product with a ten cent unit profit being far more profitable than a product with a thousand dollar unit profit if the former has a million unit annual sales while the latter has only one unit annual sales. That leads me to suspect that any drug firm will direct its R&D toward large markets, even though elastic, in preference to inelastic markets if the latter are small. Elasticity of prospective demand is a secondary factor in R&D strategy.

The only important quarrel I have with Professor Kemp is his use of *Red Book* prices for drugs and the inferences he draws from the stability of those prices. The fact that book or list prices are not transactions prices and that the two may diverge widely is an old and well-documented story.[9] A recent study shows little correlation between *Red Book* prices and prescription prices for the obvious reason that there is little correlation between actual wholesale prices and those listed in the *Red Book*.[10] A study of eight major multi-source drugs shows that their actual wholesale prices average 47 percent less than *Red Book* prices.

Professor Kemp's data on the effective patent life of diuretics is no longer representative for more recently introduced drugs. Effective patent life has decreased by more than four years since 1962 as the process of obtaining an approved NDA has lengthened; it may now be as short as ten to twelve years. The return to research on drugs has declined as a consequence of the 1962 amendments, which have both doubled the cost of obtaining an approved NDA [11] and lengthened the process. This lengthening of the time required to obtain FDA approval has both postponed the pay-off on research investment and cut the period of pay-off by reducing effective patent life to considerably less than that shown by Kemp for diuretics. To the extent that this reduces the incentives for introducing new drugs, it dampens the competitiveness of drug markets and increases costs to consumers, a result diametrically opposite that intended by Senator Estes Kefauver with his well-intentioned legislation.

## *Robert B. Stobaugh*

First, I will compare a synthesis of the three papers with studies that are being done for other industries. In chemicals, plastics, and electronics especially, there has been a great deal of work over the last decade or so on the idea of a product life cycle. Those who are familiar with this concept would not find the results of these three papers especially startling.

The product life-cycle work is focused on the growth of individual products in markets over time, with a rapid growth during the earlier part of the product life cycle and slower growth later in the cycle. These changes in growth are accompanied by changes in some of the other variables, such as competition. Initially, there is a monopolist, but gradually competitors come into the market.

---

[9] See, for example, G. Stigler and J. Kindahl, *The Behavior of Industrial Prices* (Princeton, N.J.: Princeton University Press for the National Bureau of Economic Research, 1970).

[10] D. L. Cocks and J. R. Virts, *Prescription Drug Manufacturers' Pricing* (multilith, 1974), p. 10.

[11] Sam Peltzman, *Regulation of Pharmaceutical Innovation*, p. 112, n. 3.

Therefore, one would expect to find, according to the product life-cycle theory, an increase in competition until the market growth slows down later in the cycle.

One finds costs going down because of economies of scale, which are of two types. One is dynamic economies of scale, due to accumulated experience. In many industries, production experience may be the most important type of experience, but one could have other experiences that would lower cost. Static economies of scale are related to the quantity of output in one year, but not related to economies made through greater experience. As cost goes down, even a monopolist would lower prices. As more and more competitors come in, price competition begins. Thus, one would have a lower price as time goes on, due to both a lower manufacturing cost and increased competition. The price can be held up a little longer for a product that can be differentiated than for a nondifferentiated product. All of these elements are discussed in a paper that a colleague and I just completed showing the effects of each of these variables on the price of about eighty chemicals.

Another element to consider in product life cycles is the specialization of different types of firms; some firms are more specialized and bring out original products, or breakthroughs, while others specialize in follow-on products.

Now, I would like to fit the results of the research that we heard today into this general picture of a product life cycle.

The Telser paper is consistent, in that he found that products with rapid market growth attract more competitors than do products with slow market growth. Also, he found that the faster the consumption of a product grows, the lower its price becomes. The Cocks paper shows that the more new entrants there are, the lower the price of a product. The Kemp paper shows that new entries occur, but that the competition confronting any one product is in the form of product differentiation and not lower prices. Of course, the mix of products might change and result in lower average prices for consumers. I will return to this point later. Also, the Kemp paper has a footnote on the strategy of firms, or expertise of firms, suggesting that the breakthroughs were made by the bigger companies and the follow-ons by the smaller companies.

Turning in more detail to the Telser paper, I find that it covered a large number of variables. However, I wonder whether one part of Telser's theory should be expanded. The only factor he mentions that causes supply curves to move to the right, that is, for more merchandise to be supplied at lower cost, is for new entrants to come in. However one firm could expand its facilities and learn to operate them better, and this would result in a lower cost to the firm. Hence, with only one firm, there can be a shift of the supply curve to the right. On the question of whether or not high levels of promotional outlays serve as a barrier to entry, I would feel a little more confident about his results if he had an analysis comparing what the existing firms in the industry were spending for promotional outlays with what the new firms spent when they came in. I realize that such data may be difficult to get, but I think we need more such detailed analyses, especially given the low statistical significance that Telser found concerning the effectiveness of promotional expenditures as a barrier to entry.

Cocks's results on turnover are very important to show the competitive results of R&D. In other words, when new firms come into the market, they do not just assume a minor market share, providing little competition for the firms at the top, but they actually displace the leaders in some of the top positions. In terms of theory, it is not clear to me why he needs the assumption of excess production capacity in order to have his theory operative. Furthermore, he does not confirm this assumption by looking at whether or not the pharmaceutical firms that he studied had excess production capacity. I believe that a better way to look at the idea of excess capacity is not only in terms of production capacity but also organization skills, marketing skills, or technological know-how that the firm can use to produce the other products. I also would like to see an additional test for changes in market share, as these seem to be a function of more competition. One would expect to find that the markets in which there are the greatest changes in market share would have the largest declines in prices.

Professor Kemp's RDTEM, the initials that stand for research, development, testing, evaluation, and marketing, might refer to the development of breakthrough pharmaceuticals as well as to follow-ons. He might rename it RDTEMFOP, with the FOP being follow-on products. But he may want to shorten it.

I think that his paper was useful in combatting what I would consider an obviously outmoded view of patents, although I wonder if it is not striking at a straw person. He refers to Machlup's paper of 1958 describing the theory of what develops out of a patent system. It is hard for me to believe that many people actually think that when a patent comes out there is not innovative activity which often creates new products around that patent. We see such activity in many industries.

A key point in this paper is the need for more work showing that follow-on activity is indeed useful to the nation. As I interpret his paper, Professor Kemp is not quite sure at the end whether it is or not. Of course, he lists some qualitative aspects of costs and benefits, but I think he should explore further whether the mix of products prescribed by physicians is lower in price over time. As I interpret Table 8, a price index of leading antihypertensive and diuretic products would show a drop over time. But I think we should look explicitly at whether the consumer is buying a mix of products at a lower price. If so, then that is an advantage.

Also, we should look more carefully at the level of total service rendered. For example, is the physician getting better service because of marketing expenditures by firms? That is very difficult to determine from aggregate data, but a case-study approach should prove quite useful. It could go into great detail by observing what actually happens rather than by deducing events by observing only aggregate data.

284

I will discuss some of the comments now. As to whether *Red Book* prices are higher than actual market prices, the question should be: Does that difference in price change systematically over time as new competitors come in? I would expect to find that early in a product cycle *Red Book* prices are closer to market prices than they are later in the cycle, when there are more competitors and presumably more price competition. This is an empirical question that certainly needs to be answered.

Nothing has been said in this group of papers about international business, but one possible benefit of an increase in the number of competitors is that they are likely to increase U.S. exports and increase U.S. foreign direct investment which, I believe, improves the U.S. economy. This is a side benefit that we ignore if we just look at the effect on the domestic economy.

To conclude with a speculation, I wonder how people can say that the pharmaceutical industry is not competitive if they look at the kind of data that we saw today.

## Stanley Lebergott

Each of the three papers for this session provides us with novel and important information. To canvass their merits adequately in the time available is, of course, impossible. I shall omit comment on the Kemp paper, assuming there is wide agreement on the importance of what he has effectively labeled "innovating around" a patent.

One of the most interesting contributions by the Cocks paper, and potentially one of the most important, is his rejection of therapeutic categories. He proposes instead groupings of drugs within which physicians substitute. These clinical categories are likely to reflect medical practice more realistically and, therefore, substitution on the demand side. The extent to which this conceptual advance will make an empirical difference in economic studies is a tantalizing question. To this end one would hope that a few studies such as his own and that by Professor Telser might give us two sets of estimates, one based on therapeutic categories and one based on economic markets. We could then see the extent to which this conceptual advance made an empirical difference in economic studies. One would also hope for more discussion by clinicians and biochemists of what to a layman seems an important, and distinctly superior, conceptualization of the drug market.

The first hypothesis tested by Dr. Cocks focuses on the turnover of firms. He computes an instability measure based on shares of sales for the drug firms and then compares this with data for other industries based on shares of assets. But because sales shares are more volatile from year to year than asset shares, his figures for the drug industry are not comparable with those for the other industries. Yet even if the data were comparable, I must admit to doubts about the

Hymer-Pashigian measures. What is the meaning of an instability index that tells us that apparel is a highly stable industry, almost a rock of ages, as compared with petroleum refining or electrical machinery? Does that reflect our normal vision of Seventh Avenue versus the petroleum oligopoly? The H-P measure relates only to a group of leading firms, but leaders in some industries, including drugs, are never secure, and a newcomer can drastically upset market shares.

A second difficulty relates to the theory behind his regression equation (2). Why should that theory stipulate that a firm's profit rate at one point (for example, 1970–72) can cause a rise in its market share during the prior decade (for example, 1962–72)? And if he quite reasonably had assumed (page 240) that introducing NCEs would drive up the rate of return, how can he include both that cause and its result as variables in a single equation to explain a third variable? Including both variables confounds the precision with which the equation measures the contribution of either one per se. Since his economic market share concept seems to me a very important advance, I would hope that he pursues the work somewhat further on the basis of a revised theoretical model.

Professor Telser's admirable study addresses the question of what determines entry into the ethical pharmaceutical industry, clearly a subject of high interest. By focusing on the share of the market achieved by new entrants he provides us with a more penetrating analysis than that offered by studies that merely count new entrants. And by concentrating on the market share several years after first entry he gets rid of the transient ebbs and flows that do not create a durable pattern. The paper offers a variety of theoretical advances, such as its treatment of promotional outlays as a capital investment doomed to depreciate. Furthermore its empirical work marks a notable advance over some prior studies, particularly in its use of invoice data rather than *Red Book* or other list prices. I forbear noting other accomplishments obvious to those who read through it. I should like instead to list some points that I trust will be reconsidered as this important study goes forward.

First, one central finding is that "entry rises with promotional intensity," yet that sentence can be read backwards with equal cogency: promotional intensity rises with entry. For do not firms break into a new market by heavy advertising, by extra work of their detail men? That new entrants spend relatively more than those already in the market is consistent with the nonlinear intensity of promotion that Professor Telser reports in Figure 2. It is not that causation does not run the way Professor Telser states, but that it runs both ways between the measured variables. This means that a different econometric model is required. The use of instrumental variables could bring us closer to the structural model required. I share Professor Telser's doubts about levels of promotional outlays constituting a barrier, particularly if we are dealing with firms that can switch funds between the therapeutic markets being discussed. But a revised model would more closely test that hypothesis.

286

Second, Professor Telser tests his entry hypothesis against the 1967–72 change in market shares, but would the data for 1965–72 change have given much different results? Or those for 1963–70? The choice of a period is, of necessity, an arbitrary one. Some sensitivity analysis would be desirable, for it could tell us the consequence of one arbitrary period versus another. I see this as desirable because the length of the entry period will be too long or too short depending on its ratio to the length of the commercial life of products in the market when entry begins. For categories where the commercial life is short—Dr. Cocks suggested a general average of five years for 1960—you would expect relatively high entry over five years even with low promotion outlays. But for categories with a longer commercial life you would expect relatively low entry rates. Over this period average commercial life was apparently lengthening (Mr. Clymer stipulates for fifteen years near the end). Superimposing this tendency, with its own causes, on the period chosen may bring unclear consequences. I conclude that some sensitivity analysis on the duration for market entry will advance our understanding of the role of both promotion intensity and the other causes.

Third, Professor Telser's analysis deals with the 1964–72 price changes. In his regression to explain such changes he includes all the variables previously used to explain entry. Although he is fairly taciturn on why these variables should be included, I am certain an additional paragraph on his model would warrant them. Why does he include, in addition, the entry variable itself? The correlation of these other variables with entry is very high ($R^2 = .817$). Thus, by including entry he includes them indirectly as well as directly. To clear up the regression coefficients, and thereby the elasticity estimates, it would be desirable to explain price change with merely the entry-determining variables, but not entry—or to create an entry measure not collinear with that set.

Fourth, since his review of his findings in both deft and careful, I do not express doubts about his inferences but merely cavil at his statement that his seventeen observations for drugstore sales and seventeen for hospital sales "constitute thirty-four degrees of freedom." They are statistically independent, but since virtually all hospital prescribing is done by physicians who write the drugstore prescriptions, the underlying behavior choices are by no means independent.

These papers, and others prepared for the session, mark an advance in our knowledge of the interaction between R&D and competitive behavior in the pharmaceutical industry. What is more, they indicate lines of research under way that will continue to expand our understanding in the years ahead.

# HIGHLIGHTS OF
# THE DISCUSSION

The discussion period of the last session served as a lively wrap-up of the topics discussed throughout the conference. Not all of the topics discussed came to an identifiable conclusion, nor were all of the questions answered. Still, some interesting opinions were expressed that will serve to explain some of the implications of the empirical results presented in the three papers. I have tried to summarize the afternoon's discussion in relation to four topics: the physician's response to drug prices, the determination of drug prices, the competitiveness of the industry, and the issue of generic equivalency.

## The Physician's Response to Drug Prices

To summarize briefly, the paper by Dr. Douglas Cocks found that when the price of a drug declined, that drug gained in market share. The obvious implication of this result is that physicians do pay attention to drug prices and prescribe relatively more of those drugs whose prices decline. This result apparently surprised some of the physicians in the audience for, as Dr. Leon Goldberg said, "I am a little surprised that a doctor is going to start prescribing a drug because it is less expensive." Dr. Goldberg asked to what extent Cocks's results might be due to the bulk buying habits of hospitals, and especially the V.A. hospitals. Could it be that hospitals are responding to lower prices while individual physicians do not?

Cocks pointed out that his results could not be attributed to the behavior of hospitals since his data were only for drugs sold at retail drugstores and did not include information on hospital sales.

Having cleared up this point, Dr. Goldberg pointed out the usual argument that consumers have very little to say about the choice of drugs and have to take what the physician prescribes. Dr. Goldberg then asked if a doctor would really change his prescription if he knew another drug was 20 percent cheaper. Several pieces of anecdotal evidence were recounted about certain cases involving particular doctors who would never consider price in their decisions about prescribing. In contrast, Professor Lester Telser, an economist, recounted that he had overheard a detailwoman stressing the lower price of the drug being promoted in her presentation.

Professor Yale Brozen responded that nothing could be proven with only anecdotal evidence and reminded the participants that Cocks had presented "global evidence" that physicians do respond to lower prices in their choices of drugs.

Perhaps the best approach to the question was given by a practicing physician, Dr. Paul Moyer, who explained that his response to knowledge of a lower price of one drug relative to another similar drug would depend on the situation—how important the decision about the drug was in the first place. He pointed out that in the choice of an old [cheap] or new [expensive] sleeping pill for a patient having more or less difficulty sleeping, he would use the cheaper drug. On the other hand, he pointed out that he would not "gamble with someone's septicemic shock on the basis of price." If an economist's generalizations might be allowed, perhaps this is another case (also true of consumers' choices of doctors, dentists, and hospitals) where the greater the length of time the decision maker has and the smaller is the risk of nonprice factors, the greater will be the influence of price considerations. Perhaps this is what Dr. Moyer had in mind when he stated, "Physicians are at least aware in a sort of general way that certain drugs are more expensive than others and, given the therapeutic options [they have, they take] that sort of general knowledge into consideration."

## The Determination of Drug Prices

The discussion of drug prices related to the determination of prices by manufacturers and the pricing practices of retail pharmacies. The discussion of manufacturers' pricing policies was initiated by Dr. Leon Goldberg who wanted to know how a drug company decides what price to charge for a new and unique drug when the company "obviously has a monopoly." Dr. Goldberg mentioned the drugs chlorothiazide and cromolyn.

The reply to Dr. Goldberg was made primarily by Dr. John Virts, economist for Eli Lilly and Company. Dr. Virts's response was that he recognized no cases of outright monopoly and that the "concept of the specific drug" had been dramatically overstated in prior economic literature. He reasoned that individual drugs compete with other drugs in relatively large therapeutic markets and that these larger markets are the relevant ones for economic decision making. Prices for one line of products such as cephalosporin could not be set without considering the larger market for anti-infective drugs (penicillins, cephalosporins, ampicillins). This discussion reminds one of the truism found in the antitrust literature—the more limited one's definition of the relevant market for a seller, the smaller will be the number of sellers in that market. The trick, of course, in any analysis of market performance is to define the market that is relevant to the issue at hand. This, in essence, is what Cocks, Telser, and Kemp have done by discussing how firms compete in therapeutic markets rather than the larger "drug market" or the more narrowly defined markets for a particular brand.

Dr. Virts went on to explain how his company attempts to set prices which maximize gross return. The system essentially is to develop estimates of the volumes that would be sold at various prices. Costs per unit are also estimated for various volumes. The company then attempts to pick the combination of price and volume that maximizes gross return. When asked how well this system had worked for Eli Lilly, Dr. Virts indicated that their record had been less than perfect. However, he stressed that an initial pricing decision was not made for all time and could be changed if the initial price had been set incorrectly. This is an example of the type of price cutting which Cocks found in his study.

Dr. Virts also strongly objected to Professor Kemp's use of *Red Book* prices. He indicated that prices were always fluctuating and were affected by discounts and promotional specials, implying that the *Red Book* prices were not good indicators of actual market prices.

The prices of drugs in the retail market were also discussed at some length. Dr. Louis Lasagna reported that, based on some surveys his department had conducted in the Rochester area, the price of a drug to the consumer was primarily determined by the retail pharmacist rather than by the manufacturer or the physician. He reported that they had found the average price of branded drugs sold in chain drugstores to be less than the average price of generics sold in individual pharmacies. He concluded that the study of the contribution of the pharmacist to the pricing of drugs had been grossly neglected.[1]

Professor Yale Brozen reported on some similar unpublished survey work of retail drug prices in the Chicago area. The method was to have several prescriptions carried around to drugstores by various types of students and then follow this up with a telephone survey of the same drugstores. Professor Brozen reported that the price of one of the drugs surveyed varied from $1.00 to $9.00 with a median price of $3.50. Another varied from $1.16 to $12.50 with a mean price of $4.50. A third varied from $3.81 to $15.45 with a mean price of $7.44. These wide variations in retail drug prices have also been documented in many other cities around the country. Brozen also said that the Chicago study could find no systematic relationship between retail prices charged for drugs and other possible explanatory variables such as ghetto versus non-ghetto locations, buyers who were

---

[1] For recent studies on this topic see John F. Cady, "Structural and Competitive Effects of Retail Trade Regulation: A Study of the Impact of Public Policy in the Retail Market for Prescription Drugs" (Ph.D. diss., State University of New York at Buffalo, September 1974); Allison Masson, "The Changing Legal Status of Prescription Drug Price Posting: Effects and Implications" (Paper presented at American Economic Association meeting, San Francisco, 28 December 1974). For additional studies dealing with the effects of retail restrictions see Alex R. Maurizi and Frederic B. Siskind, "The Impact of Regulations Affecting the Retail Drugstore Industry on the Earnings of Self-Employed Pharmacists" (Unpublished paper, Washington, D. C., December 1974); Lee Benham, "The Effect of Advertising on the Price of Eyeglasses," *Journal of Law and Economics*, vol. 15, no. 2 (October 1972), pp. 337–52.

either black or white, male or female, poorly dressed or well dressed. There was even a large variation in prices at a particular store from one visit to another. Thus, Professor Brozen concluded that there is evidence of very large variation in retail drug prices.

The most obvious point, which was not stated at that time, is that this wide dispersion of retail prices is not consistent with competitive local markets where entry and competition for customers are unrestricted. Of course, there will always be some dispersion of individual drug prices as long as search costs are positive and costs of retailing differ. Some evidence is beginning to appear indicating, however, that the dispersion and level of retail drug prices both tend to be greater in those states which have more restrictions on retail entry and on advertising,[2] a result similar to that found by Benham in studying prices of eyeglasses.[3] Professor Brozen reported that some additional unpublished research at the University of Chicago had found that the most restrictive states had an average prescription price in independent pharmacies of around $4.80 and the less restrictive states had an average of around $3.60 in 1970.

Dr. Crout pointed out that this wide dispersion of retail prices was a major force behind the movement in various states to repeal anti-substitution laws and require drug price posting. He stated that while the FDA is being asked to give testimony on the substitutability of drugs, it had not taken any stand on the issues of anti-substitution laws or price posting, regarding that as a professional problem to be resolved by doctors and pharmacists.

Professor Telser added that because of lack of retail competition in drugs, it was not generally true that substitution of generic prescribing for brand name prescribing would result in lower drug prices. With restrictions on entry and advertising, the pharmacist would sell the drug with the largest markup and thereby increase his monopoly return. Professor Telser was also skeptical of the effects of mandatory price posting, because such a regulation might facilitate collusion among drugstores by making it cheaper for them to detect price cutting. Telser concluded that these two types of laws would probably have little effect on consumer welfare until there are some basic reforms in drug retailing.

**The Competitiveness of the Drug Industry**

While Professor Telser, at the beginning of his paper, very carefully said that his study was not about the competitiveness of the drug industry, Professor Brozen argued that Telser's results point strongly to the conclusion that the drug industry does behave competitively—so competitively, in fact, that only the competitive economic model is consistent with the behavior we observe in the drug industry.

---

[2] John F. Cady, "Effects of Retail Trade Regulation."

[3] Lee Benham, "The Effect of Advertising on the Price of Eyeglasses."

292

The floor discussion of this topic was initiated by Dr. Arthur Carol when he asked Professor Telser if the results of his study actually rejected Stigler's hypothesis of oligopoly behavior, and if so, what variable in Telser's regressions actually rejected Stigler's hypothesis.

Stigler's hypothesis is that oligopolistic industry behavior can be explained by attempts to collude. In his earlier work, Stigler discussed the incentives to collude and reasoned that collusion will occur. In his later work, he outlined the formidable difficulties facing any group of firms attempting to bring about a successful collusion arising from their inability to detect cheating and from enforcement costs.[4] Any persistence of oligopoly must be attributed to economies of scale, differences in productive factors, or legal control of entry (which includes patents).[5] If effective in colluding, these circumstances may, at best, slow the rate of entry into an oligopoly industry charging supracompetitive prices, but the market shares of colluding oligopolists will still decline.

Telser responded to Dr. Carol's question by stating that he really had not had Stigler's hypothesis in mind, but that an implication of the hypothesis that oligopolists collude was that there would be a negative relationship between rates of entry and concentration within the industry; that is, if a small number of firms can collude more easily, then they should be more effective in keeping out new entrants. Since he could find no systematic relationship between concentration and measures of entry in therapeutic drug markets, Telser concluded that the oligopoly hypothesis did not really apply to the pharmaceutical industry. He supported this conclusion by stating that there was too much uncertainty about the discovery, duration, and acceptability of a drug product to make collusion viable in the drug industry. Telser argued that similar conditions existed in other industries such as book publishing, phonograph records, and ladies' dresses so that he would not expect to find any correlation between entry and concentration in these industries where the possibility of collusion would be small.

The Cocks paper can also be used to address the Stigler hypothesis. The Cocks data show that there is a minimum of twenty R&D intensive firms in the drug industry, a number which in and of itself would make tacit collusion very costly. In addition, collusion in the drug industry would require agreement on complex scientific matters which would be very expensive to enforce.

Another discussion relating to the competitiveness of the drug industry concerned the number of drug firms that were involved in the competitive exchange of market shares among the ten markets in the Cocks study. Professor Benjamin Cohen of Yale University pointed out that there is a common allegation that companies introduce new products which take over from their own previously developed product in a particular market so that a company may retain a large

---

[4] George J. Stigler, *The Theory of Price* (New York: Macmillan, 1966), pp. 216–20; see also his "A Theory of Oligopoly," *Journal of Political Economy*, vol. 72, no. 1 (February 1964).
[5] Stigler, *Theory of Price*, pp. 220–27.

share of that market over a relatively long period. Thus it is alleged that market shares and prices of individual drugs can change while a given firm retains a dominant position in that market. Professor Cohen wanted to know if Dr. Cocks could tell him to what extent the changes in market shares in his ten markets involved changes in the firms possessing the leading market share.

Dr. Cocks responded that his study did not address itself to changes in market share of individual firms, but that the number of firms associated with the ten markets were reported in another article.[6] Dr. Cocks added that, while he could not say exactly to what extent the changes in market shares in his ten markets involved changes in firms, in most drug markets there is usually a significant number of firms so that the allegation that control of markets is common was misplaced. Furthermore, he added, his evidence that drug products whose prices declined gained in market share indicated that consumers were benefiting from lower drug prices and that this was the most important aspect of market competition in drug markets.

Mr. Harold Clymer of SmithKline asked Dr. Cocks to what extent the new products in his study were new chemical entities as opposed to multiple-source drugs, combinations, or alternate dosage forms. Dr. Cocks responded that price competition results from the introduction of both kinds of new products. When R&D is carried on by a significant number of firms, Cocks stated that one automatically finds the kind of price competition his study shows even though not all of the new products will be significantly unique. He argued that when this type of research-based competition takes place among firms, entry occurs, prices decline, and consumers benefit.

## The FDA and the Issue of Generic Equivalency

The discussion of drug prices and of generic prescribing led to late-afternoon discussion of the FDA's attempts to maintain quality standards and to assure that multiple-source drugs could be safely substituted. As Dr. Crout pointed out, the issue of generic quality had received a good deal of attention recently because of HEW's announcement of its intention to institute a policy of reimbursing for drugs under Medicare and Medicaid on the basis of the price of the lowest-cost equivalent drug that is "generally available."

Dr. Crout stated that the FDA has a responsibility to assure the quality of drugs on the market, and, therefore, has no authority to allow a low-quality generic to remain on the market just because it is cheaper than other drugs. The FDA's mandate is to set standards of quality and not to permit the marketing of drugs that do not meet these standards.

---

[6] Douglas L. Cocks and John R. Virts, "Pricing Behavior of the Ethical Pharmaceutical Industry," *Journal of Business,* vol. 47, no. 3 (July 1974).

Dr. Lasagna responded that there were "two aspects of the FDA's involvement in standards." The first was that the FDA should see to it that reasonable, defensible standards were being met. The second was to establish standards of quality. Dr. Lasagna argued that more research was needed to "evolve the standards" since he felt that we were a long way from being able to say what the correct standards of drug quality should be. If standards could not be set, Dr. Lasagna reasoned that we could not then identify how many drugs would pose problems of bioavailability.

Dr. Crout responded that he thought bioavailability was a "manageable problem" since it involved only about 40 multiple-source drugs out of the 200 most-used drugs in the country. He recounted that there were only two documented examples of therapeutic inequivalence among brands (digoxin and a thyroid preparation) and three or four other drugs for which there was anecdotal evidence of therapeutic inequivalence. In addition, there were about a dozen or more drugs for which bioavailability problems had been documented.

Dr. Crout also added that it was misleading to say that quality problems with generic drugs were caused by small generic manufacturers since 95 percent of prescription drugs in this country were made by the 100 largest firms. While he thought there were serious differences in quality even among large manufacturers, he felt that this quality control was again a manageable problem for FDA.

Dr. Crout's British counterpart, Dr. J. F. Dunne of the United Kingdom Committee on Safety of Medicines, said that he was surprised by the FDA's decision to attempt to insure generic equivalency. He reported that by British law, his committee was precluded from considering "matters of comparative efficacy." Also, he said, they did not have the data to determine which drugs were "usefully bioavailable" and would therefore be "very loathe" to introduce generic prescribing by any regulation in the United Kingdom.

Dr. Lasagna, responding to Dr. Crout, said that he did not feel comfortable relying on the perceptiveness of doctors and patients to pick up therapeutic inequivalency among drugs when it is said that these same people cannot always tell the difference between a placebo and an active drug. Dr. Lasagna also said that there is wide variation in bioavailability in some drugs which meet current standards and that these poor performances have not been detected clinically. He concluded that a lack of knowledge of problems of clinical bioavailability was not equivalent to saying that there were no problems with generic substitution standards.

Dr. Crout then argued that if the clinician lacked knowledge, there was no rational basis for the doctor or anyone else to choose one brand over another. That was why he concluded that the problem of drug quality was a compliance problem for the federal government and it was the FDA's role to correct the situation.

Mr. Clymer of SmithKline recounted a totally unexpected bioavailability finding his company had encountered in preparing to change a drug from a capsule to a tablet, in that the tablet demonstrated markedly greater bioavailability. He argued that the manufacturer had a strong incentive to study the bioavailability of its own products and most would not put out a product without doing so. If the FDA is to assume bioequivalency, it has one simple standard to evoke, namely, that each manufacturer's product be studied for bioequivalency. Mr. Clymer felt that there had been too many unexpected problems to depend upon extrapolation from *in vitro* testing.

Experts obviously are not in complete agreement about the quality and/or therapeutic equivalency of various manufacturers' products with the same principal ingredient. Part of the problem may be that a regulatory agency can at best guarantee only adherence to some set of minimum standards capable of being tested against a commonly available technology of measurement. These standards may or may not be sufficient to determine some practical level of equivalency among a set of products manufactured by different people from different new materials and using different processes. No such standards could in any practical way guarantee that products would be completely identical. The U.K. regulatory authorities may be less concerned about comparative efficacy of products because of their scheme of economic controls on manufacturers' prices. The U.S. regulatory authorities might be less concerned if there were better understanding of the existence of, and the role of, price competition between drugs. In economic theory, at least, it is clearly possible for a set of products each meeting some minimum set of standards to have different prices. In fact, economic theory of competition forecasts that different prices will result unless the products are absolutely identical in all respects, including the aspects of knowledge about, and certainty about, the nature of those products.

# LIST OF PARTICIPANTS

Alexander, Lois, *Office of Research and Statistics/SSA, Washington, D. C.*

Allen, Robert, *CIBA-GEIGY, Summit, New Jersey*

Altman, Stuart, *Department of Health, Education and Welfare, Washington, D. C.*

Ayanian, Robert, *Department of Economics, University of Southern California*

Bailey, Martin J., *Department of Economics, University of Maryland*

Balter, Mitchell B., *National Institute of Mental Health, Bethesda, Maryland*

Barral, E. Etienne, *Rhone Poulenc Group, Paris, France*

Beck, William T., *Department of Pharmacology, Yale University Medical School*

Binkley, Howard, *Vice President, Pharmaceutical Manufacturers Association*

Blee, Frank, *SmithKline Corporation*

Bloch, Howard, *Department of Economics, George Mason University, Fairfax, Virginia*

Bowes, Kenyon D., *Vice President, Finance, G. D. Searle and Company*

Brown, Richard, *National Science Foundation, Washington, D. C.*

Brownlee, Oswald, *Deputy Assistant Secretary for Tax Policy, Department of the Treasury*

Brozen, Yale, *Graduate School of Business, University of Chicago*

Bunker, John P., M.D., *Department of Preventive and Social Medicine, Harvard Medical School*

Burger, Edward J., Jr., M.D., *Science and Technology Policy Office, National Science Foundation*

Caglarcan, Erol, M.D., *Hoffmann-LaRoche, Inc.*

Campbell, Rita Ricardo, *The Hoover Institution, Stanford, California*

Carol, Arthur, *Economic Adviser, Office of Senator Brock, Washington, D. C.*

Chapman, Carol Ann, *Experimental Technology Incentive Program, National Bureau of Standards*

Clymer, Harold A., *SmithKline Corporation*

Cocks, Douglas L., *Eli Lilly and Company*

Cohen, Benjamin, *Department of Economics, Yale University*

Cooper, Joseph D., *Professor of Government, Howard University, Washington, D. C.*

Crawford, Kent R., *Controller, Lilly Research Laboratories, Eli Lilly and Company*

Crout, J. Richard, M.D., *Bureau of Drugs, Food and Drug Administration*

Curran, John P., *Senior Associate in Public Affairs, Pfizer, Inc.*

Cutler, Jay B., *Minority Counsel, Health Subcommittee, Senate, Washington, D. C.*

DeFelice, Stephen, *President, Bio-Basics International, New York, New York*

de Haen, Paul, *Paul de Haen, Inc., Drug Information Service, New York, New York*

Dickens, Paul, *Office of Research and Statistics, Social Security Administration*

Douglas, Bryce, M.D., *Vice President, Research and Development, SmithKline Corporation*

Dunne, J. R., M.D., *Secretariat of Committee on Safety of Medicines, London, England*

Ebeler, Jack, *Congressional Research Service, Library of Congress*

Einsidler, Jon E., *Senior Associate, Pfizer, Inc.*

Gardner, Vincent R., *Director of Drug Studies, Office of Research and Statistics/ SSA*

Gellman, Aaron, J., *Gellman Research Associates, Jenkintown, Pennsylvania*

Genero, Laura, *American Enterprise Institute*

George, Jim, *Office of Senator Brock, Washington, D. C.*

Goldberg, Delphis C., M.D., *Subcommittee on Intergovernmental Relations, House Committee on Government Operations*

Goldberg, Leon I., M.D., Ph.D., *Committee on Clinical Pharmacology, Department of Pharmacological and Physiological Sciences, University of Chicago*

Goldhammer, Gilbert S., *Subcommittee on Intergovernmental Relations, House Committee on Government Operations*

Grabowski, Henry J., *Department of Economics, Duke University*

Hagan, Charles F., *Assistant General Counsel, Pfizer, Inc.*

Harter, Phillip J., *Experimental Technology Incentive Program, National Bureau of Standards*

Hastings, Richard W., *Director, Government Affairs, CIBA-GEIGY*

Helms, Robert B., *Director, Center for Health Policy Research, American Enterprise Institute*

Henderson, David, *University of California, Los Angeles, California*

Henry, F. W., *Director, Market Planning and Promotion, The Upjohn Company*

Hornbrook, Mark, *Economic Analysis Branch, Bureau of Health Services Research, Department of Health, Education and Welfare*

Hutchinson, Janet, *Director of Consumer Affairs, National Pharmaceutical Council, Washington, D. C.*

Johnson, Thomas F., *Director of Research, American Enterprise Institute*

Kane, Sidney, M.D., *CIBA-GEIGY, Summit, New Jersey*

Kemp, Bernard, *George Washington University Medical Center*

Kitch, Edmund W., *University of Chicago Law School*

Klein, Morton A., *Department of Health, Education and Welfare*

Konopko, Bernard, *Director, Government Marketing, Organon Inc., Rockville, Maryland*

298

Lampert, Herbert, *Montreal, Canada*

Lasagna, Louis, M.D., *Department of Pharmacology and Toxicology, School of Medicine and Dentistry, University of Rochester*

Lehnhard, Mary, *Staff Assistant, House Committee on Ways and Means*

Leventhal, Carl M., M.D., *Deputy Director, Bureau of Drugs, Food and Drug Administration*

Levine, Bertram, *House Interstate and Foreign Commerce Committee, Washington, D. C.*

Lowrance, William W., Jr., *National Academy of Sciences, Washington, D. C.*

Lunsford, Carl D., *A. H. Robins Company, Inc., Richmond, Virginia*

Maurizi, Alex R., *Federal Energy Administration, Washington, D. C.*

Meiselman, David, *Reston Economics Program, Virginia Polytechnic Institute at Reston*

Melmon, Kenneth L., M.D., *San Francisco Medical Center, University of California*

Mitchell, Samuel A., *Research from Washington, Inc., Washington, D. C.*

Mosher, Elissa L., *National Council of the Churches of Christ, Drug Advertising Project, Washington, D. C.*

Moyer, Paul R., M.D., *Doylestown, Pennsylvania*

Muehlhause, Carl O., *Consultant to the Director, Institute for Applied Technology, National Bureau of Standards, Washington, D. C.*

McCabe, Eugene F., *Merck, Sharp and Dohme, West Point, Pennsylvania*

McGhan, William, *American Pharmaceutical Association*

McKitterick, Molly, *F-D-C Reports, Washington, D. C.*

Novitch, A. Mark, M.D., *Deputy Assistant Commissioner for Medical Affairs, Food and Drug Administration*

Oates, John, M.D., *School of Medicine, Vanderbilt University, Nashville, Tennessee*

Page, Irvine H., M.D., *Editor, Modern Medicine, Cleveland, Ohio*

Peltzman, Sam, *Graduate School of Business, University of Chicago*

Peterson, R. B., *Vice President for Domestic Marketing, The Upjohn Company*

Price, Thomas E., *National Council of the Churches of Christ, Drug Advertising Project, Washington, D. C.*

Pullen, Emma, *L. A. Times*

Rawls, Rebecca, *Chemical Engineering News*

Reynolds, James A., *Medical Economics, Springfield, Virginia*

Riley, James W., *Economist, Merck and Company, Inc., Rahway, New Jersey*

Roelofs, Robert, *Organon Pharmaceuticals (Holland)*

Roll, G. F., *Vice President, SmithKline and French Laboratories, Philadelphia, Pennsylvania*

Ross, Walter S., *New York, New York*

Rottenberg, Simon, Ph.D., *Department of Economics, University of Massachusetts*

Russo, James, *Pharmaceutical Manufacturers Association, Washington, D. C.*

Scherer, Frederic M., *Bureau of Economics, Federal Trade Commission*

Schmeck, Harold, *New York Times*

Schuchat, Theodor, *Modern Medicine, Washington, D. C.*

Schwartzman, David, *Department of Economics, New School for Social Research, New York, New York*

Shaw, Daniel L., Jr., M.D., *Vice President, Medical Affairs, Wyeth Laboratories*

Shelton, Lee R., M.D., *Atlanta, Georgia*

Silverman, Stanley N., *Merck, Sharp and Dohme Research Laboratories*

Solomon, E. Barry, *Department of Economics, George Mason University, Fairfax, Virginia*

Somers, Edwin, Jr., *U.S. News and World Report, Washington, D. C.*

Sonnenreich, Michael R., *Medicine in the Public Interest, Inc., Washington, D. C.*

Spavins, Thomas, *Department of Economics, Yale University, New Haven, Connecticut*

Stauffer, Thomas R., *Center for Middle Eastern Studies, Harvard University*

Stetler, C. Joseph, *President, Pharmaceutical Manufacturers Association*

Stobaugh, Robert B., *Graduate School of Business Administration, Harvard University*

Telser, Lester G., *Department of Economics, University of Chicago*

Temple, Robert, *Assistant to the Director, Bureau of Drugs, Food and Drug Administration*

Terselic, Richard A., *Director, Office of Planning and Analysis, Food and Drug Administration*

Tichenor, C. C., *A. H. Robins Company Inc.*

Treichel, Joan, *Science News*

Valliere, Greg, *Washington Forum*

Varley, A. B., *Medical Director, The Upjohn Company*

Vernon, John M., *Department of Economics, Duke University, Durham, North Carolina*

Virts, John R., *Corporate Staff Economist, Eli Lilly and Company*

Wardell, William M., M.D., Ph.D., *Department of Pharmacology and Toxicology, School of Medicine and Dentistry, University of Rochester*

Weidenbaum, Murray L., *Center for the Study of American Business, Washington University, St. Louis, Missouri*

Wells, Benjamin B., M.D., *National Pharmaceutical Council, Washington, D. C.*

Cover and book design: Pat Taylor